*Yakov Abramovich*

# Ya. A. Vinnikov

# Sensory Reception

## Cytology, Molecular Mechanisms and Evolution

With 124 Figures
(173 Separate Illustrations)

Springer-Verlag New York · Heidelberg · Berlin 1974

Professor Dr. Ya. A. Vinnikov
Sechenov Institute of Evolutionary
Physiology and Biochemistry
Academy of Sciences of USSR
194223 Leningrad

Translation from the Russian by W. L. Gray, Cheva Chase/USA,
and Barbara M. Crook, Heidelberg/Fed. Rep. Germany

ISBN 0-387-06674-8 Springer-Verlag New York Heidelberg Berlin
ISBN 3-540-06674-8 Springer-Verlag Berlin Heidelberg New York

# Preface

This book presents a distillation of many years of investigation by the author and his associates on the problem of sensory reception. Both our own data and data from the scientific literature on the electron microscopy, cytochemistry, biochemistry and electrophysiology of the organs of vision, taste, smell, hearing and gravitation, are presented to show that the evolution of the sense organs of all animals on our planet is based on a receptor cell equipped with a motile antenna, a biological recorder of information concerning certain types of energy reaching the animal from the environment. The conversion or encoding of this energy into information is effected with the aid of special protein molecules positioned in the plasma membrane of the antennae. The action of the unit of energy of a stimulus on such a specific protein molecule causes a change of shape, and this is the basis of the trigger mechanism of reception, leading to the stimulation of the receptor cell and the transmission of the information encoded in this cell in the form of nerve impulses to the central nervous system.

The present monograph summarizes over 30 years of working experience by the author and his associates in the field of evolution of sense organs. Material is used here from his earlier monographs: *The Retina of the Eye Vertebrates*, 1947, *The Morphology of the Organ of Smell*, 1957, *The Organ of Corti: Its Histophysiology and Histochemistry*, 1964, written jointly with L. K. TITOVA, and *Receptors of Gravity*, 1971, written with various associates. This material has been updated and includes new bibliographic and experimental data obtained by the author and his associates in recent years. These new data in fact form the basis of the contents of this monograph.

The author dedicates this monograph to all of his associates and students: L. K. TITOVA, A. A. BRONSHTEIN, T. P. LUKASHEVICH-TSIRULIS, R. A. PEVZNER, V. I. GOVARDOVSKII, F. G. GRIBAKIN, M. Z. ARONOVA, V. P. IVANOV, T. A. KHARKEEVICH, G. A. PYATKINA, O. G. GOGNIASHVILI, B. F. ANICHIN, R. A. ABRAMYAN, K. A. KOICHEV, E. G. KOSTANYAN and R. P. TOPOLYANSKAYA. Working with these people has given the author much joy, and it is difficult to overestimate their contribution to this book.

The author is deeply indebted to Professors P. G. SVETLOV, E. M. KREPS, A. I. KARAMYAN, Yu. I. POLYANSKY, O. G. GAZENKO, V. A. GOVIRIN, S. A. NEIFAKH, A. L. POLENOV, E. K. ZHUKOV, N. A. VERZHBINSKAYA, V. S. SHEVELOVA and A. V. VOYNO-YASENETSKII who critically read some sections of the book and made a number of valuable suggestions.

The author expresses his thanks to the authors whose illustrations he has used in his monograph.

It is a great pleasure for the author to thank Prof. G. F. SPRINGER, chief editor of Springer-Verlag's book series, Molecular Biology, Biochemistry and Biophysics, who encouraged me to write this monograph.

The author notes his appreciation of the considerable task undertaken by the translator of this book. He is grateful for Miss B. Billing, Mrs. G. Deus, and Mr. Borsodi for work on the editing of this book.

The author is indebted to his collaborators, Dr. Raisa Pevzner and Dr. Mirra Goldanskaja for the help in editing the English version of the manuscript. The author is also grateful to N. N. Kholodkovskaya, L. F. Bekleshova and M. S. Khabibulina who provided significant assistance in selecting the bibliographic references.

Leningrad, Summer 1974                                    Ya. A. Vinnikov

# Contents

# The Problem of Reception
# and the Evolution of the Cytological
# and Molecular Organization of Sense Organs

Reception is one of the basic problems of biology. It had already been stated fairly clearly, at least for some branches, by the second half of the eighteenth century (LOMONOSOV, 1752—1757, 1756; YOUNG, 1802), but it was definitively formulated only in the first half of the nineteenth century. The question was then expressed as follows: how and where in the various sense organs does the conversion of certain types of physical or chemical energy from the external environment take place, and how adequate are these conversions to the "specific energies" of a given sense organ? (MÜLLER, 1826).

The work of many generations of scientists (morphologists, physiologists and biochemists) was directed toward solving the problem stated above, i.e. finding the point where, in terms of modern information theory (SHANNON, 1963), adequate "coding" or conversion of the energy of an external stimulus takes place. In other words, how is the message translated from the "language of the stimulus" to the "language of the cell" so that it can be transmitted in the form of a nerve impulse to the central nervous system, where it is "decoded".

The accumulation of knowledge on the problem of reception over the past 150 years became possible as a result of accelerating technical progress in morphological, physiological and biochemical research methods, the development of cellular and evolutionary theories, and then of molecular biology. With the aid of the light microscope morphologists could not only see but also understand the purpose of receptor cells; for example, of the rods and cones found in the retina of the eye (MÜLLER, 1886; BABUKHIN, 1863; SCHULTZE, 1866; DOGIEL, 1883, 1888; CAYAL Y RAMON, 1893; ZAVARZIN, 1913, 1941; POLYAK, 1941; DETWILLER, 1943; VINNIKOV, 1947, etc.); of the hair cells of Corti's organ (CORTI, 1851; KÖLLIKER, 1865; CLAUDIUS, 1885; SCHULTZE, 1858; LAVDOVSKII, 1874a, 1874b; HELD, 1902, 1926; KOLMER, 1927; VINNIKOV and TITOVA, 1964, etc.); of the olfactory cells of the organ of smell (TODD and BOWMAN, 1847; LEYDIG, 1851; KOHLRAUSCH, 1853; SCHULTZE, 1856; BABUKHIN, 1872; DOGIEL,

1886; TRETYAKOV, 1916; VINNIKOV and TITOVA, 1957a etc.); of the gustatory cells of the taste buds (LEYDIG, 1851; SCHWALBE, 1867; SCHULTZE, 1862; ARNSHTEIN, 1893; DOGIEL, 1897; HEIDENHEIN, 1914; KOLMER, 1927, etc.). Already in the years between 1840 and 1880 biochemists had detected and separated visual purple in the rods of visual cells of cephalopod molluscs (KROHN, 1839 to 1842; KRÜKENBERG, 1882) and of vertebrates (BOLL, 1877, 1881). It was therefore postulated that the light decomposition products of the purple stimulate the optic nerve endings.

In particular, the achievements of physiologists are significant. They are connected with the investigations carried out by SECHENOV (1863—1865, 1866), HELMHOLTZ (1875, 1896), WEBER (1851), HERING (1931), ANDREEV (1924), GRANIT (1947, 1955), DAVIS (1957, 1958), BÉKÉSY (1960a) and many other scientists, who worked out the basic laws governing the activity of the sense organs at organ level. Only I. P. PAVLOV (1928), however, considered the sense organs as peripheral parts of analyzer systems consisting also of intermediate and central units. PAVLOV's analyzer theory was developed from the standpoint of evolutionary physiology by L. A. ORBELI (1946, 1958) and by his associates and successors: A. V. LEBEDINSKII (1935), A. I. BRONSHTEIN (1950), L. T. ZAGORUL'KO (1948), and is being extended at the present time by G. V. GERSHUNI (1947), V. G. SAMSONOVA (1950), P. O. MAKAROV (1947), P. G. SNYAKIN (1948), A. L. BYZOV (1966), G. A. MAZOKHIN-PORSHNYAKOV (1965) and others. The problem of interoception mechanisms is under development by V. N. CHERNIGOVSKII (1960, 1967) and his associates.

Despite the progress and achievements scored in the physiology of sense organs at the organ and system levels, physiological investigations also continued at the cellular level. They soon led to the establishment of two theories of reception, although these were based exclusively on guesses. According to the first theory, the encoding, i.e. the conversion of the energy of a stimulus in the receptor cells, in achieved by chemical means (BOTEZAT, 1909; LAZAREV, 1916, 1923); according to the second theory, by electrical means (EINTHOVEN, 1908). However, only the research methods of the last two to three decades have made it possible to approach the problem of reception at the level of the molecular and cellular organization of sense organs, and to show that the problem of reception should really be considered as one of the branches of molecular biology.

What is the cellular and molecular organization of sense organs when considered from the standpoint of evolution? A study of the receptor cells in members of practically all phyletic lines of animals made it possible to reach the conclusion that the evolution of the sense organs of animals is based on more or less modified primary or secondary sensory cells, provided with motile flagella or cilia known as kinocilia, and with microvilli or their derivatives known as stereocilia, or "antennae" in our terminology. The motile "antennae" are the first to come into contact with the energy of physical or chemical stimuli from the external environment (VINNIKOV, 1959a, 1959b, 1964, 1965, 1966a, 1966b, 1967a, 1967b, 1969).

The question now arises: How can the antennae of the receptor cells of sense organs, which are so similar from the structural, cytochemical and functional aspects, be capable at the same time of effecting a strictly differentiated reception of the energy of definite stimuli from the external environment? In other words, at what level of organization and by means of what mechanism is a specific differential function of the reception of sense organs achieved? At the present time, more and more data are becoming available, and they indicate that the molecular level of organization of the antennae of receptor cells is involved. It was found that in the plasma membrane of the antennae of receptor cells in practically all sense organs there are located specific protein molecules that assume the role of encoding and converting the energy of a stimulus into adequate, i.e. specific, information for the cell. These molecules thereby perform the function of a primary or trigger mechanism in the process involving stimulation of the receptor cell. The specific information encoded in the molecules and converted in the form of nerve impulses is transmitted through appropriate synapses to the central nervous system, being subjected on the way to a multiple energy increase. In this regard, we must consider as remarkable the contribution made by WALD (1939, 1960, 1961a, 1961b, 1964, 1965, 1968), who was the first to show that photoreception is associated with the molecular organization of the visual pigment, rhodopsin, located in the membranes of antenna disks (rods and cones) of photoreceptors. According to WALD's data, regular conformational shifts and a breakdown of the rhodopsin molecule take place under the action of the energy of one photon. These processes form the basis of the coding of the energy of photons, i.e. of the switching of the trigger mechanism in the stimulation of a visual cell.

Recently, DASTOLI and PRICE (1966) and DASTOLI, LOPIEKES, and DOIG (1968) etc. detected in the taste buds special "sweet-sensitive" and "bitter-sensitive" protein molecules, which can bind sweet and bitter food ingredients. Consequently, the encoding of gustatory molecules, i.e. the switching of the trigger mechanism of taste reception, is also based on a molecular interaction between a gustatory cell molecule and a molecule of the sweet or bitter food substance. Apparently, a similar coding, i.e. trigger mechanism, is the basis of the reception of molecules of odoriferous substances. Evidence of this fact is given by the work of ASH (1968, 1969), ASH and SKOGEN (1970), RIDDIFORD (1970) etc.

Finally, evidence that molecular processes are involved in the perception of a converted auditory stimulus was provided by us (VINNIKOV and TITOVA, 1961, 1963, 1964), since we were able to detect acetylcholinesterase in the antennae (stereocilia) of hair cells of Corti's organ, together with a choline-receptive protein capable of binding acetylcholine present in the endolymph, thus allowing the conversion and encoding of sound and the switching of the trigger mechanism that effects stimulation of the auditory cell. The search for analogous protein receptor molecules in other antennae of sense organs is being vigorously pursued.

Thus, special protein molecules, which are the first molecules to react specifically with the energy of an external stimulus, have been detected in practically all sense organs or exteroceptors, and more precisely in the plasma membrane of the antennae of receptor cells.

The mechanism of reception arising in the course of evolution in various sense organs, is in principle unique. As a rule, this mechanism consists of two interconnected molecular processes: a mechano-chemical process and an encoding process. The first is responsible for the automatic movement of the antennae of receptor cells, and thus contributes to their active interaction with various forms of energy from the external environment. The second process involves an encoding or trigger conversion that occurs under the action of the specific energy of the stimulus, first in special protein molecules located in the receptor membranes of the antennae, from where it is then transmitted in the form of information, i. e. nerve impulses, from the body of the cell through its synapses to the central nervous system.

In this book an attempt is made to examine, from the standpoint described above, the problem of reception and the associated problem of the evolution of the cellular and molecular organization of the organs of vision, taste, smell, hearing and gravity reception, i. e. of the exteroceptors. We present a correlation of the data obtained over many years, mainly in the author's laboratory, on the light and electron microscopy and cytochemistry of the sense organs, also certain literature data on their biochemistry, and a few on their electrophysiology. It is our hope that this will help to reveal the bases for a molecular theory of sensory reception.

Since we consider the special protein molecules in the plasma membrane of the antennae to be the principal sensing structures of receptor cells, we include along with the specific data on each of the sense organs mentioned above a special introductory chapter that briefly presents the information currently available on the structure and development of biological membranes. We consider separately the data on the structure and function of the antennae by means of which contact is achieved, i. e. the "input" and conversion of the energy of a stimulus by the receptor cell. There is a further chapter on synapses through which the "output" of the information converted by the receptor cell is transmitted in the form of nerve impulses to the central nervous system.

Chapter I

# Structure and Development of Biological Membranes

## 1. Introduction

Electron microscopy has shown that what are called biological membranes form the basis of the structural organization of the entire phylogenetic series of living organisms, starting from some viruses and bacteria and ending with the cells of multicellular organisms. As BERNAL (1968, p. 143) points out: "Only after the formation of a membrane around a cell do we really get what can be justly called an organism". Indeed, a membrane is as a rule located at the interface of two media: an external plasma membrane separates the internal medium of the cell from the external medium; membranes of mitochondria separate the mitochondrial matrix from the cytoplasm; nuclear membranes separate the karyoplasm from the cytoplasm; membranes of the endoplasmic reticulum separate the content of cisterns, etc. The functions of membranes, characterized by a great variety, are also in accord with such a fundamental morphological location of membranes.

The first question to arise is: What is the structural organization of membranes which makes it possible for them to perform such a wide variety of functions?

The second question, which is of fundamental importance in understanding the development of cells from the standpoint of evolutionary theory, concerns the origin or biogenesis of membranes. How do membranes develop in present-day cells? Do they develop "*de novo*" in each cell under the effect of the function of ribosomes, i.e. in the final account under the effect of a nucleic code, or does their "assembly" (self-assembly) take place on the basis of an existing "seeding" or matrix from previous membranes, which, of course, does not detract from the role played by a nucleic code? Finally, how are the molecules of receptive proteins built into the membranes? These are the questions we propose to discuss.

## 2. Structure and Chemical Composition of Membranes

In considering the problem of the structure of biological membranes we should keep in mind that, when using the electron microscope, we are in effect dealing with a supramolecular level of organization of biological membranes. Biochemists and biophysicists with the aid of their methods have come close, if we can express ourselves that way, to an investigation of the premolecular level, i.e. to the study of a complex of molecules. On the other hand, the

molecular level of organization of biological membranes is so far only the subject
of hypotheses. Naturally, in investigating the structure of biological membranes
it is sometimes difficult to separate the above-mentioned levels of organization
from each other.

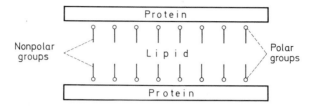

Fig. 1. Membrane model (DAVSON and DANIELLI, 1943)

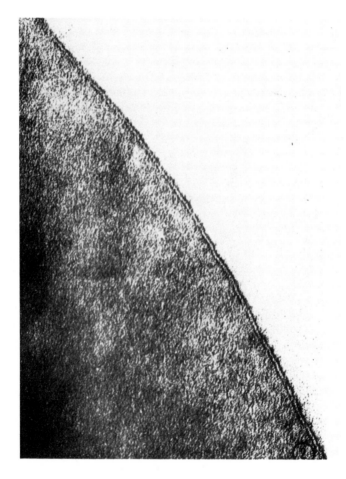

Fig. 2. Structure of unitary membrane. Section across human erythrocyte, fixed with permanganate
($\times$ 280,000) (ROBERTSON, 1964)

A structural model of a membrane (Fig. 1) was proposed for the first time in 1935 by DANIELLI and DAVSON (1935). The investigations of SCHMIDT (1936a, 1936b, 1938), performed about the same time with a polarization microscope, played an important role in forming an idea of the structure of membranes. According to these authors, a membrane consists of a liquid lipid phase of varying thickness and composition with the lipid molecules oriented to the outside by polar groups and to the inside by nonpolar groups; proteins are adsorbed on the exterior lipid layers. It was demonstrated later that the lipids do indeed constitute a bimolecular layer in which the polar ends face outward and the lyophillic nonpolar ends face inward and proteins are adsorbed on both surfaces. It is assumed that the carbohydrates bound to certain membranes face the extracellular medium. At a later date, as a result of electron microscope studies, the well-known ROBERTSON (1959, 1960a, 1960b, 1964, 1967) theory of an ordinary or unit membrane was elaborated. This theory postulates that, as can be seen in electron microscopy patterns, the membrane has a triple layer structure (Fig. 2). The total thickness of the membrane averages 75—90 Å. There are two dense lines each 20 Å thick, while the less dense line separating these two lines measures 38 Å. Such are the data available on the supramolecular structure of biological membranes.

Premolecular data on the organization of biological membranes are based on numerous, but still scattered facts from which it is difficult to build up a system. Under the electron microscope the most stable structure is that of erythrocyte and myelin membranes. These membranes have a very low protein content but contain a high percentage of unique phospholipids, hydroxylic and

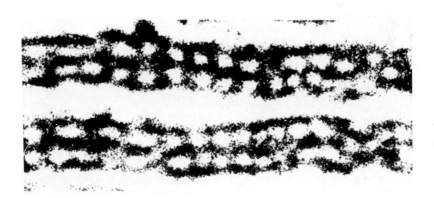

Fig. 3. Globular structure of outer segment membrane in frog photoreceptor (*Rana pipiens*) (× 745,000) (NILSSON, 1964a)

fatty acids. As a rule, these membranes after any kind of fixation exhibit the structure of an unit membrane (KORN, 1966). Other membranes, for example those of photoreceptor disks, mitochondria, endoplasmic reticulum, and the plasma membrane of animal cells, resemble the picture of an unit membrane and exhibit a globular structure, i.e. an organization made up of spherical subunits (Fig. 3). This is seen after certain types of fixation and also after freeze-drying particularly in negative contrast. Hence, SJÖSTRAND (1963, 1967) believes that the lipid phase of a membrane exists in the form of globular micelles which constitute a complex of lipid molecules fitted into a protein matrix. LUCY (1964), however, assumes that the lipid globules are located between two layers of protein (Fig. 4). MÜHLETHALER (1966) on the other hand put forward a concept

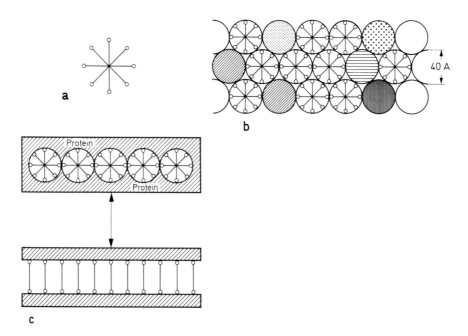

Fig. 4a—c. Diagram showing how phospholipid micelles and protein globules take part in building up the membrane (LUCY, 1964). a Phospholipid micelle; b protein globules and phospholipid micelles in the membrane; c change in the configuration of membranes from a globular to a lamellar configuration

of protein globules immersed in a lipid stroma. Still, most investigators (SJÖSTRAND and ELFIN, 1964; NILSON, 1964a; KAVANAU, 1965, 1966) favor the view that the subunits in biological membranes are formed by lipid globules stabilized by interaction with the surface layer of protein molecules. These subunits have the shape of regular hexahedral or pentahedral prisms of 80—140 Å diameter. The subunits are arranged at intervals of 80—100 Å from center to center and together form the membrane (SJÖSTRAND, 1963; BENEDETTI and EMMELOT, 1967, 1968; KAVANAU, 1965, 1966). ROBERTSON (1966) has also expressed support for these concepts. A globular concept for the structure of membranes was advanced by BENEDETTI and EMMELOT (1968) in their latest study. The isolated membrane of rat liver cells, after being treated with deoxycholate and examined both in sections and by the negative-contrast method, is covered with a thin layer below which the penta- or hexahedral structures are located, and which consists of two rows of globular subunits of 70Å diameter. These subunits are bound by a layer of special firm connective substance some 100—130Å thick. The globular subunits together make up two transparent layers about 50Å thick, separated by an electron-dense line forming lateral coatings around each globule. The coating is resistant to oxycholate, as is the substance known as desmosome with which it appears to be identical (zonula occludens); it consists of a protein which covers and binds the lipid globules (Fig. 5).

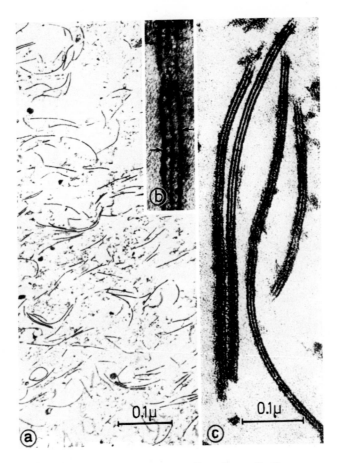

Fig. 5a—c. Structure of isolated plasma membrane of rat liver cells (BENEDETTI and EMMELOT, 1968). a Sectors of isolated membrane at low magnifications (×23,000); b the membrane exhibits a structure consisting of globules (×600,000); c membrane sectors at medium magnifications (×250,000)

Thus, in various membranes not subjected to "rigid" fixation but prepared for electron microscopy by gentler methods, for example, by negative contrast or by freeze-drying, we can observe globular subunits whose shape and size may vary according to the type of membrane. Globular units (mushrooms) are described on the cristae of mitochondria, on the external plasma membrane of liver cells, and on bacterial membranes (PORSONS, 1963; FERNÁNDEZ-MORÁN, 1963; NADAKAVUKAREN, 1964; BIRYUZOVA et al., 1964). Globular subunits have been found in chloroplast membranes of plants and are visible even after fixation with glutaraldehyde (WEIER, BISALPUTRA, and HARRISON, 1966; MÜHLETHALER, 1966). Some researchers assume that the differences observed in the globular organization of microsomes, mitochondrial membranes, and plasma membrane reflect some sort of peculiar molecular differences in their structure (CUNNINGHAM and CRANE, 1966).

Attempts have been made to bind globular structures to the original model of an unit membrane. Thus, STAEHELIN (1968) has carried out a very interesting comparison of the ultrastructure of artificial and biological membranes. Artificial lecithin and cholesterol-lecithin membranes, formed in water and 20% glycerol, after freezing at −150 °C and vacuum-drying exhibited structures which were similar to the structure of an unit membrane. They consisted of two layers each 25—30 Å thick. These two bimolecular layers could be separated by forming cracks between them (ice crystals). In this connection, numerous disks were observed at the site of rupture of nonpolar bonds. Biological membranes, for example the plasma membrane, the endoplasmic reticulum, membranes of the nucleus, of the Golgi apparatus, of vacuoles and myelin (but not membranes of chloroplasts and mitochondria), when treated in the same manner, exhibited a similar structural organization. These membranes were found to consist of a central bimolecular lipid layer coated on both sides with a globular protein. This thin globular protein layer could readily be removed with trypsin. Protein particles form subunits in the form of globules that are held in place on the surface of the bimolecular lipid layer by means of hydrogen bonds and their presence makes the membrane unstable (HAYDON and TAYLER, 1963). A thin layer of a surface-active protein, possibly bound to polysaccharides, is located between these protein globules. Both protein globules and the protein lining are bound to phospholipid molecules. VANDENHEUVEL (1965) believes that only a thin protein monolayer is found on the surface of myelin membranes. The protein molecules can penetrate up to a depth of 10—15 Å into the area occupied by the fatty acids in a bimolecular layer, thus forming lipoprotein complexes.

STAEHELIN (1968) gives an interesting scheme in which he summarizes his observations (Fig. 6). He thinks that during vacuum-freezing the bimolecular lipid layer is split in certain places, in the region of both nonpolar and polar bonds, as a result of which the membrane assumes a globular character. Sometimes this layer can be split lengthwise into two sheets so that only one lipid layer remains, for example, as in the case of myelin (BRANTON, 1967). Since these results, based on the freeze and vacuum-drying method, are not applicable to mitochondria and chloroplasts, Staehelin assumes that these organoids do not possess a bimolecular lipid layer.

Thus, some researchers have reached the conclusion that membranes can have two types of organization, namely a lamellar and a globular organization (O'BRIEN, 1967). We can assume that the lamellar and globular organizations of membranes probably reflect different chemical compositions and therefore

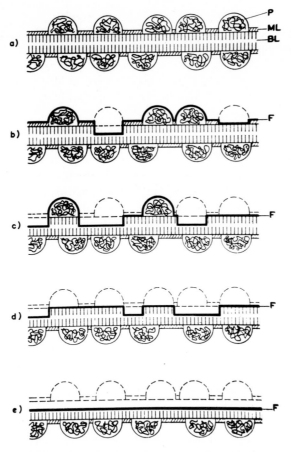

Fig. 6a—e. Membrane model according to STAEHELIN (1968). a The membrane consists of a central bimolecular layer (*BL*), covered on both sides with protein globules (*P*) and a monolayer of nonlipid material (*ML*); b to e possible injuries of the membrane during replica preparation and various methods of treatment (shown by the line *F*)

also different functions. According to WALLACH's data (1969), obtained on replicas of human erythrocyte ghosts the structure of biological membranes depends on the nature of the bonds between proteins and lipids. These bonds determine the conformation of the individual protein molecules.

In this respect, a very interesting theory was elaborated by KAVANAU (1965, 1966). He suggested that biological membranes do not have a static organization but are dynamic and possess a number of systemic properties due to the ability of ATP to convert chemical energy into kinetic energy. Kavanau starts from the classical premise that the molecular organization of membranes is based on a bimolecular lipid layer located between two protein layers. In the bimolecular layer lipids are represented by drop-shaped globules. Such globules would form according to the laws governing surface tension and packing between two protein layers. However, the shape of the globule can change, depending upon the functional state, into a flattened spherical disk or into an elongated rod or small column. Both these shapes are interconvertible. Thus, the lipid globule of the membrane can be defined as a spherical cylinder. Its dimensions can vary: for a disk, thickness 55Å and diameter 150Å; for a small column, length 200Å and diameter 60—80Å. The surface of the spherical cylinders is coated with a layer of protein. Using data on the physics of colloidal lipids as his starting point, KAVANAU postulates that the more dense state of the globule corresponds to a disk and the more liquid state to a column. Conversion of one shape into the other takes place as a result of the conversion of the chemical energy present in membranes ATP into kinetic energy. Depending upon the shape assumed by the spherical cylinders, pores of varying diameter can be formed between them. If the cylinder assumes a disk shape, the pores are naturally closed; if it assumes a rod shape, the pores open and the entire membrane has a sievelike appearance. The presence of such pores permits active transport of substances through the membrane (i.e. water, ions $Na^+K^+$)[1] between the spherical cylinders. KAVANAU thinks this transport is regulated by enzyme proteins. KAVANAU (1965) assumes that the change in the shape of the lipid spherical cylinders and in the conformation of membrane proteins accounts for their ability to undergo contraction and expansion and that a decrease or increase of membrane dimensions does not require the presence of special contractile proteins.

Data published in recent years on conformational shifts of the protein component of membranes (KENNEDY, 1967; SJÖSTRAND and BARAJAS, 1968) indicate that such shifts are responsible for the functional activity of given membranes. Thus, according to KENNEDY (1967) conformational transformations of the membrane structure take place when membranes carry out the functions of electron transfer, oxidative phosphorylation and active transport. The conformation of membrane proteins is determined by their reaction with lipids and polysaccharides, while the membrane as a whole is stabilized mainly by hydrophobic protein–protein bonds and by protein–lipid interactions. Experiments performed by KENNEDY (1967) show that active transport of certain substances (sulfate, amino acids and sugars) is determined by a change in the conformation of specific transfer (messenger) proteins built into the membrane. It was possible to determine differences in the conformation of transfer proteins depending upon whether these proteins are obtained from the membrane in the presence of the substrate being transferred, or in the absence of such a substrate. Thus, the protein and not the substrate undergoes a change during transport through the membrane. The active transport of substances through the membrane is suppressed by energy poisons. However, the energy required for the active transport of substances through the membrane is not used to effect the activation of the substrate, as used to be thought, but rather for the conformational transformation of specific transfer proteins. The concept of a dynamic structural organization of membranes is also supported by PALADE (1967) who found that the exchange of lipids in the membrane is three times as great as that of proteins. Membranes are dynamic. The shape and composition of both lipid and protein subunits

---

[1] The phenomenon of $Na^+$ transport can also be explained by means of an electron-cytochemical method (KOMNIK, 1962).

are constantly undergoing change, and these subunits are capable of "flickering", or "vibrating" or "pulsating" (KAVANAU, 1966).

What, then, is the nature of the chemical compounds which make up the membrane? More and more facts are becoming available to show that, along with the chemical substances common to all membranes, there may also be special chemical compounds. As a result, membranes differ from each other at the molecular organization level in both structure and function (MADDY, 1966). Lipids make up 20 to 30% of the weight of various membranes. The major portion of lipids consists of phospholipids; for example, in mitochondria phospholipids may amount to 90% of the total lipid content (FLEISCHER et al., 1967). Phosphatidylcholine is the major constituent of biological membranes. Mitochondrial membranes, for example, contain a large amount of phosphatidylcholine, but also contain phosphatidylethanolamine, phosphatidylinosite, and diphosphatidylglycerol. In mitochondria from different cells the qualitative composition of the phospholipids is basically the same, but quantitative differences are observed (GREEN and TZAGOLOFF, 1966).

Neutral lipids found in mitochondrial membranes consist of di- and triglycerols, cholesterol and small amounts of carotinoids and ubiquinones (LENINGER, 1966). The amount of these compounds may vary with the type of organism. However, it is important to note that the lipids found in mitochondrial membranes are by no means the same as those found in other cellular membranes, for example in membranes of chloroplasts and bacteria (GEL'MAN, 1967). Thus, cellular membranes may exhibit significant differences in their lipid composition.

Similar relationships are also noted in the case of proteins. Proteins constitute 70—75% of the weight of a membrane (GEL'MAN, 1967), and they are the biologically active components of membranes. The presence of a structural (noncatalytic) protein seems to be an inherent property of all membranes. All membranes contain enzyme systems capable of degrading ATP and converting it into ADP with the liberation of macroergs (GREEN, 1964); modern electron-cytochemical methods make it possible to locate the activity of ATPase in practically all membranes (Fig. 7).

Along with the proteins and enzymes common to all membranes, a different content of enzymes may be found even within the limits of a single organoid, for example, in mitochondria. Thus, by treatment of liver-cell mitochondria with digitonin followed by differential centrifugation, it is possible to isolate three fractions: an inner membrane together with the matrix, an external membrane, and a soluble fraction containing the enzymes located between the membranes. In this case, it was found that monoamine oxidase, kynurenic hydroxydase, and a rotenone-sensitive NADH-cytochrome-C reductase can be detected in the fraction of the external mitochondrial membrane. Succinate cytochrome-C reductase, succinate dehydrogenase, cytochromoxidase, $\beta$-hydroxybutyryl dehydrogenase, $\alpha$-ketoglutarate dehydrogenase, lipoamide dehydrogenase, NAD- and NADH-isocitrate dehydrogenase, glutamate dehydrogenase, aspartate aminotransferase and ornithine transcarboaminase are found in the inner membrane bound to the matrix. Nucleotides and diphosphokinase are found both in the external membrane and in the soluble fraction. Acetylkinase is located between the membranes (SCHNAITMAN and GREENWALT, 1968; SOTTOCASA et al., 1967).

With the aid of electron microscopic methods it is possible to locate the activity of succinate dehydrogenase and cytochrome oxidase in the inner cavity of cristae and in the cavity between the external and inner membranes of mitochondria (LUKASHEVICH, 1964, 1966; SELIGMAN *et al.*, 1968; KARPEL-FRONIUS and

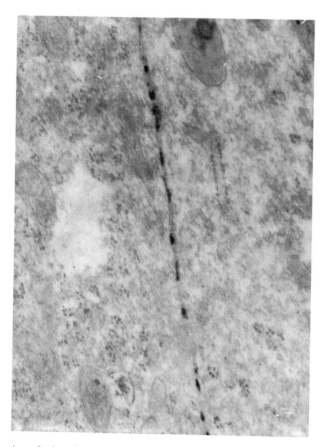

Fig. 7. Localization of adenosine triphosphatase in the plasma membrane of supporting cells of the frog *(Rana temporaria)* olfactory organ. Treatment according to WACHSTEIN and MEISSEL. Preparation of A. A. BRONSHTEIN and G. A. PYATKINA ($\times 84,000$)

HAJOS, 1967; SABATINI *et al.*, 1963). It is important to note that enzymes are apparently located in the external protein layers of the membrane of cristae. At the same time the enzymic sectors are arranged in a discrete manner. As was noted above, ATPase is also characterized by a similar arrangement. We believe that such a discrete distribution of enzymes reflects the manner in which they function. Thus, from biochemical and cytochemical data and the way in which oxidative enzymes are arranged, we can conclude that the two portions of the respiratory chain are located side by side. These results coincide with a review of concepts, according to which the well-known mushroom-shaped subunits on the surface of cristae were considered to be carriers of enzymes effecting the transfer of electrons (GREEN, 1964). Such "mushrooms" are also found in the plasma membrane (BENEDETTI and EMMELOT, 1967) but electron-transfer enzymes are not (WILLIAMS and PARSONS, 1964; GEL'MAN, LUK-OYANOVA, and OSTROVSKII, 1966).

## 3. Development, Differentiation and Growth of Membranes

If biological membranes are characterized by a similar supramolecular and, as a rule, a dissimilar premolecular organization what is the nature of their biogenesis? How are membranes formed from such a large variety of lipids and proteins (catalytic and noncatalytic)? Do cell membranes arise *de novo* in the cytoplasm matrix as a result of the function of ribosomes, or does the development of membranes always require the successive participation of the original premolecular structure, which arose in the early stages of phylogenesis and is transmitted in the form of a "primer" ("prematrix") in the process of ontogenesis from a cell to its daughter cells? Does the construction of a "new" membrane take place by exchange of the lipid and protein components present in an old membrane? If all of these things do occur, then in this case the nucleic code plays only an intermediate role in building the membrane by the synthesis of new proteins, although in some membranes the location of their own RNA has recently been found (ZBARSKII, 1969).

Experiments by a number of researchers indicate that it is possible to reconstruct a membrane from its fragments. For example, it was shown that a cytochromoxidase preparation obtained after treatment with deoxycholate contains up to 30% of phospholipids having the shape of globules 50—100Å in diameter. After removal of deoxycholate, reaggregation of the globules takes place resulting again in membrane formation. Reaggregation of globules occurs only when phospholipids are retained in the preparation or when they are introduced in a micellar form (McCONNEL et al., 1966). In other experiments a pure fraction of 90Å diameter subunits was derived from the inner membranes of mitochondria by treating them with sonic waves. These subunits contained an oligomycin-sensitive ATPase; they could depolymerize at low temperature, whereupon they lost ATPase activity and formed amorphous aggregates. After removal of the subunits the membrane stroma retained an active electron-transfer chain. By fragmentation of mitochondria with salts of inorganic acids under different conditions, it was possible to isolate subunits containing oligomycin-sensitive ATPase, a number of complexes containing certain respiratory-chain enzymes, and also a structural protein. Respiratory enzymes isolated from mitochondria in the presence of stabilizing agents (detergents, deoxycholate), have the appearance of particles of 50 to 120Å diameter. Upon removal of the solubilizing agents, reaggregation of these particles into membrane-like structures is observed (RAZIN, ROTTAN, and RODWELL, 1967). Thus, a membrane can still be restored after artificial fragmentation.

In fact, reaggregation of membranes from solubilized material was achieved from external membranes of mitochondria, chloroplasts, external photoreceptor segments, microsomes and erythrocytes (GREEN et al., 1967). These results are interpreted as indicating spontaneous interaction or self-assembly of subunits liberated from an intact membrane. However, as N. S. GEL'MAN (1969) correctly observed, although reaggregation is indeed a spontaneous process accompanying the removal of detergents or deoxycholate, it can also be effected from fragments of different size as well as from proteins and lipids, and even from proteins alone. Finally, it is impossible to prove the specificity of the reaggregation products. Reaggregation itself is apparently associated with the actuation of the physical and chemical bonds that are responsible for the formation of the supramolecular level of organization of membranes.

Now let us see what happens in a living cell. During cell division in animals and plants the plasma membrane of the mother cell is preserved and is mechanically transferred to the daughter cells. The transfer point of the membrane has been observed under the light microscope and is known as Flemming's corpuscle.

Fusion of sperm with the ovum in Coelenterata, Echinodermata, molluscs, annelids, arthropods and chordates results in the appearance during zygote formation of a mosaic-like plasma membrane, part of which originates from the sperm membrane (COLWIN and COLWIN, 1964).

The membrane surrounding the nucleus consists of two membranes separated by an interval of about 100—300Å. The space between two nuclear membranes is connected with the ducts of the endoplasmic reticulum which apparently open into the intercellular space, i.e. can communicate with external environment. It is known that the cell nucleus rotates at an average speed of between 75 and 280 revolutions/sec. The direction of this motion changes, consequently the entire picture of the nuclear shell and its connections with other membranes is quite dynamic. The nuclear membrane has pores located about 20—40Å apart and 40—100Å in diameter. The inner and external membranes of the nuclear membrane merge along the edges of the pores. These pores no doubt play a very important role in nuclear-plasma relations. During mitosis, while being destroyed at the prophase stage, the nuclear membrane forms a number of fragments, which initially retain a laminated structure but later disintegrate into separate vesicles (BARER et al., 1960; WHALEY et al., 1964). These membrane residues are preserved, together with membrane residues of the endoplasmic reticulum in the cytoplasma around the spindle, while some of these residues can be detected even inside the spindle. During anaphase and telophase, the vesicles of the Golgi apparatus come close to the surface of the karyomeres and then, apparently as a result of their growth or fusion, a new membrane is formed and covers the entire nucleus. With the onset of metaphase, residues of the nuclear membrane begin to move towards the poles of the spindle (ITO, 1960). Some membranes of the endoplasmic reticulum start to proliferate, growing even into the interior of the spindle and into the intervals between chromosomes; this results, already in the telophase stage, in complete enclosure of chromosomes within the nuclear membrane. Nuclear membranes have been the object of a biochemical study by means of differential centrifugation (ZBARSKII, 1969): the nuclear membrane was found to have a high content of ATPase that can be activated by $Mg^{++}$, but to be devoid of ATPase that can be activated by $Na^+$ and $K^+$. The nuclear membrane is thus unable to effect active transport of Na$^+$. According to the same data, this membrane has its own stock of nucleic acids (RNA), which must determine its ability to reproduce (ZBARSKII, 1969).

Membranes of the endoplasmic reticulum have the appearance of vesicles or small ducts of different size and shape, located in the transparent hyaloplasm or matrix. The endoplasmic reticulum bounds a closed space and so forms in the cytoplasm an internal phase separated by a membrane from the external hyaloplasm or matrix. The endoplasmic reticulum is absent in mammalian erythrocytes, but is found in all cells possessing a nucleus. The space enclosed by the membranes can be regarded as an elementary structure of the endoplasmic reticulum.

Membranes of the endoplasmic reticulum that are located on the external surface facing the hyaloplasm with homogeneous granules or ribosomes containing mainly RNA are considered separately as rough membranes of the endoplasmic reticulum. Rough membranes are present in large amounts in growing cells or in cells which synthesize proteins. In histological preparations such cells are characterized by basophilia. At points where glycogen accumulates, for example in the region of what is called the photoreceptor paraboloid, the glycogen granules are located on the exterior surface, thus simulating rough membranes (GOVARDOVSKII and KHARKEEVICH, 1967).

During mitosis membranes of the endoplasmic reticulum undergo fragmentation and only isolated vesicles remain (DALTON, 1961). In other cells outside the spindle region, the membranes retain to a greater extent a structure characteristic for the interphase and are more or less uniformly distributed among the daughter cells. It is believed that after mitosis membranes of the endoplasmic reticulum develop from residues of parent membranes and that these act as a "matrix" or "primer" for the development of a full-grown endoplasmic reticulum of daughter cells.

The Golgi apparatus also consists of membrane-enclosed vesicles and cisternae, but of smaller size, more closely connected with each other, and completely devoid of granules. We shall not dwell here on the various functions of the Golgi apparatus; we shall merely note that it is assumed to play a considerable role in the accumulation and exchange of lipids and proteins (DROZ, 1963; WHALEY et al., 1964; YOUNG and DROZ, 1968; YOUNG, 1968). Separation of the Golgi apparatus into dictyosomes, which are uniformly distributed among daughter cells during cell division, has been observed even under the light microscope.

As a rule, poorly differentiated cells are characterized by a small number of membranes in the endoplasmic reticulum, whereas highly differentiated cells contain a large number of membranes. For example, the endoplasmic reticulum is observed to increase in size three to four times in a hen embryo during differentiation of a nerve cell (KAVANAU, 1965). In the rat ovum it is difficult to detect the elements of the endoplasmic reticulum, but such elements do develop at the two-blastomer stage. Apparently, the endoplasmic reticulum does not exhibit a tendency to multiply during proliferation of a given cell line. It is assumed that after each division, following the build-up of a new nuclear membrane, a new endoplasmic reticulum is formed; this is preserved and functions during the relevant-interphase until the appearance of a final form characteristic of a fully differentiated cell.

The endoplasmic reticulum is labile. Under the action of different experimental effects, such as mechanical action, hypoxia, exposure to a $CO_2$- or CO-containing environment, KCN, high-dose radiation, a sharp increase is observed in the number of endoplasmic reticulum membranes (WALLEY et al., 1964).

In receptor cells of the utricle of the guinea pig labyrinth subjected to radial acceleration at $10\,g$ for 30 minutes, complete disappearance of RNA in the cytoplasm was observed with a simultaneous shift of RNA in the nucleoli towards the nuclear membrane and its exit in the form of nucleolic ribosomes through the pores of the nuclear membrane into the cellular cytoplasma in the direction of its basal pole, that is, in the direction of the gravitational field vector. At the same time, part of the external nuclear membrane was carried along and the escaped ribosomes built, with the aid of membrane "priming", a comple of rough endoplasmic membranes (Fig. 8), which under the light microscope looked like the escaped nucleolus. In this case, we are talking about the process of protein reparation which begins in the receptor hair cell following a sharp increase of its function under the effect of acceleration. However, exit of nucleolic

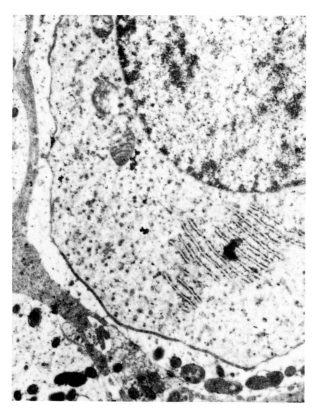

Fig. 8. Formation of spirally shaped sector of rough endoplasmic reticulum in the receptor cell of the utricle of a guinea pig, subjected to radial acceleration at $10\,g$ for 3 min ($\times 10,000$)

RNA and creation of a helical complex of rough membranes take place according to some kind of rhythm also in the normal life activity of the labyrinth receptor cells, since it is observed in individual cells under conditions of relative rest. Experimental effects merely provoke a more rapid appearance of this phenomenon, as indicated by the fact that practically all receptor cells are involved in this process (VINNIKOV et al., 1963a, 1963b).

Biochemical observations by SIEKEVITZ (1967) on the biogenesis of endoplasmic reticulum membranes in newborn rats have shown that formation of the membrane base, namely lipids and structural proteins, takes place in a parallel manner. This base is a finished stroma, which is then encrusted by other enzyme proteins already present in the cell. According to the conception of Siekevitz, biogenesis of membranes is not a single act, but rather a multi-stage process. Membrane components are not formed in the cell in a synchronous manner, but there exists rather a definite process which acts as a signal for the organization of all membrane components.

In concluding this section we can conclude that cellular membranes in one way or another always develop in a successive manner, at the expense of older membranes and as a result of their growth.

At present, the most distinct pictures of the differentiation and growth of cellular membranes can be observed in certain derivatives of the plasma membrane. Of great significance here are the synapses in animal nerve cells; these structures are essentially specialized sectors of the plasma membrane found at the junction of nerve cells with each other, with the receptor cells and with the cells of motor organs. In early embryogenesis there are no synapses, but only the usual membrane contacts between cells. According to the data of TITOVA and GRIBAKIN (1967), at later stages of embryogenesis the plasma membrane of one cell is converted into a presynaptic membrane, whereby the membrane becomes thicker and doubles in size, while additional structures, the so-called synaptic rods, sometimes develop. The presynaptic membrane is separated from the postsynaptic membrane by an intersynaptic gap but the two membranes are at the same time connected with each other by means of a suture (ROBERTSON, 1964). A high acetylcholinesterase activity is observed in synaptic membranes. Cutting of the nerve fiber causes atresia of synaptic membranes (SMITH and RASMUSSEN, 1963). Functional load can apparently be accompanied by a change in the membrane structure (DE ROBERTIS, 1964; ARONOVA, 1967). Synapse membranes contain RNA and DNA, as a result of which nerve endings can synthesize protein independently of the nerve cell body and process (AUSTIN and MORGAN, 1967, 1968). Thus, autoreproduction of specific proteins in synapse membranes is apparently possible.

A considerable number of studies have been devoted to the development of myelin. As we know, myelin membranes of myelinated fibers are essentially sectors of external plasma membranes of Schwann cells; these sectors are enriched with a definite set of lipids and proteins. In embryos, the folds of this membrane enclose the axon, and the latter is densely surrounded by the cytoplasm of the Schwann cell (Fig. 9A). Then, as the axon becomes more and more deeply embedded, the plasma membrane in the gap area draws together and its two layers become joined along their external surface, thus forming a double membrane or mesaxon. During the further development of the myelinated fiber the Schwann cell slowly rotates along its axial cylinder, thus ejecting the whole cytoplasm (GEREN, 1954). Its plasma membrane, winding up in the form of a coil, forms a compact laminated zone, known as myelin. Thus, myelin formation, i.e. differentiation of myelinated fibers, occurs simply by compact packing of a multiple coiled mesaxon, namely an axon-directed sector of the plasma membrane of a Schwann cell. Unfortunately, this concept of the development of the myelin membrane is based so far on a comparison in one field of vision of electron microscope images of myelinated nerve fibers in the process of development. We do not know of any single study concerned with an analysis of the build-up of bulk myelin, of its growth, and of the manner in which phospholipids and proteins are incorporated into its membranes excluding the works of RAWELINS (1973). The work done so far allows us to reach the descriptive conclusion that myelin is a derivative of the growing plasma membrane of a Schwann cell. Thus, the development and differentiation of myelin membranes are associated with an already present primer or matrix, i.e., with an "indifferent" plasma membrane of an embryonic Schwann cell. The new myelin membrane is thus the result of differentiation and growth of a preceding plasma membrane.

A subject which has been more extensively studied in this respect is the growth and differentiation of the surfaces of the plasma membrane in the embryonic photoreceptors, which are converted into the external segments of rods and cones. These processes, which in principle are very similar to the development of myelin membranes, will be examined in detail during the description of the visual cell. Here we shall merely point out that photoreceptor membranes develop as a result of the formation of folds in the plasma membrane of the embryonic cilium of the photoreceptor cell (Fig. 9B). A protein known as opsin is supplied into these folds from the cell cytoplasm; opsin forms a molecule of rhodopsin by binding an oxidized vitamin-A molecule (retinal) supplied by the pigment layer of the retina, as can be verified by appropriate experiments. For example, if the contact between embryonic photoreceptors and the pigment epithelium through which vitamin A is supplied is disrupted, there is underdevelopment of the outer segment and membranes of its disks. Apparently, disjunction of the visual and pigment layers prevents the possible

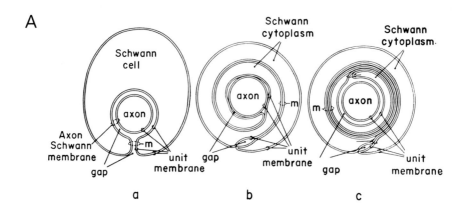

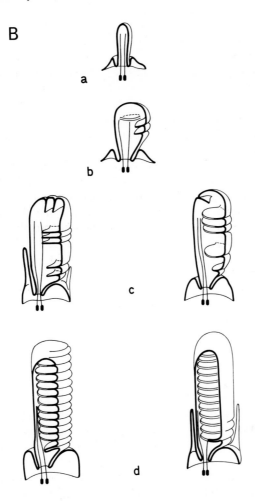

Fig. 9 A and B. Diagram showing the development of myelin and of outer segments in the rods and cones of a chick embryo. A. a Is the earliest stage at which one Schwann cell is associated with one axon with a short mesaxon (*m*); in b the mesaxon is elongated into a spiral; c shows another stage in the formation of compact myelin (ROBERTSON, 1964). B. a cilium of embryonic cell; b first presumption of disks; c and d formation of disks of cones and rods (GOVARDOVSKII, 1967)

establishment of a molecular bond between oxidized vitamin A and opsin, and this is accompanied by disruption of the process involving the growth and differentiation of membranes of photoreceptor disks (GOVARDOVSKII and KHAR-KEEVICH, 1965, 1966a, 1966b). These conclusions can be confirmed in tests with experimentally induced vitamin-A deficiency (DOWLING and GIBBONS, 1961).

In rats and reptiles under conditions of prolonged (4—6 months) vitamin-A deficiency, atresia and destruction of disk membranes and of the entire outer segment is observed. Thus, in these tests it is possible to establish not only the succession of membranes, but also the mode of their development, which takes place by encrustation and intussusception of the preceding membrane primer. Disruption of the supply of encrusting substances results in atresia of the membrane.

*Development of Mitochondria and Plastids.* During the process of evolution mitochondria occur already in Protozoa but not in bacteria, where their function is performed by protoplast. They are well expressed in yeasts and are present in cells of all plants and animals.

There are four theories of the origin of mitochondria. The first theory postulates that mitochondria are synthesized: *de novo* in the cytoplasm from spherical structures having a diameter of 80—340 millimicrons (NILSSON, 1964a). However, an attempt to test this theory, made in our laboratory by GOVARDOVSKII and TSIRULIS (1969) on the same object, the photoreceptor ellipsoid, has shown that this is far from true; mitochondria were found to be concentrated in this region as a result of movement out of the remainder of the cell from which they disappear completely. They then divide by constriction. The second theory starts from the assumption that the cytoplasm contains a premitochondrial matrix of microbodies, 0.1—0.3 micron in diameter, and that these are mitochondrial precursors (BERGER, 1964). However, it is possible that we are dealing here with lysosomes, and this matter is being investigated at the present time. The third theory, which has a great deal of support, starts from the concept of extensive development of mitochondria from plasma and nuclear membranes, and from membranes of the endoplasmic reticulum, including the Golgi apparatus (ROBERTSON, 1964). Supporters of this theory point to a number of electron microscope patterns and present diagrams which at first glance seem to illustrate the theory in a satisfactory way, so long as we do not consider that we are confronted simply with images showing expansion of mitochondria.

The fourth theory, which was formulated back in the era of the light microscope, assumes that mitochondria multiply by division with the aid of constriction. In addition to being supported by direct photographs of mitochondrial division, this theory is also based on data obtained with mitochondria of *Neurospora crassa*, labeled with $\alpha H^3$ and $\alpha C^{14}$-choline and transferred to a nonradioactive medium. It was found that the number of mature mitochondria increases by division and that these mitochondria transmit their radioactive label to daughter mitochondria (TRUMEN and KORNER, 1962). A decisive factor in support of this theory was the detection of RNA in mitochondria (TRUMEN and KORNER, 1962) and the detection of DNA strands in the mitochondrial matrix (NASS and NASS, 1963). Further, it was shown that the DNA content, calculated for a single mitochondria, is sufficient for the synthesis of mitochondrial proteins (SCHATZ et al., 1964). These data force us to assume that mitochondrial DNA effects the reproduction, storage and transmission of information, i.e. that mitochondria are able to reproduce themselves (KAZAKOVA, 1965).

The DNA of mitochondria of *Neurospora crassa* (molecular weight about $13 \times 10^6$) differs sharply from nuclear DNA in the magnitude of its buoyant density and its resistance to the action of DNAase (LUCK, 1967). It was demonstrated that mitochondrial DNA can be replicated independently of nuclear DNA. Mitochondria of *Neurospora crassa* contain DNA, RNA-polymerase, ribosomes and ribosomal RNA. The RNA of mitochondria differs in composition and sedimentation properties from the ribosomal RNA of cytoplasm. RNA and enzyme systems for protein synthesis have also been found in the mitochondria. Consequently, the latter contain all the components necessary for genetic autonomy. The assumption has been made that mitochondrial DNA is associated with the phenomenon of cytoplasmic heredity. By microinjection from one fungus strain into another it was shown that hereditary properties of mitochondrial DNA are transmitted from the donor strain to the recipient strain. It was also shown experimentally (LINNANE, 1967) that proteins of the respiratory chain located in mitochondrial crista are synthesized by a protein-synthesizing mitochondrial system, while enzymes of the external mitochondrial membrane are formed in ribosomes of the cytoplasm. All these facts lead us to believe that mitochondria undergo successive development at the expense of preceding mitochondria, and that this development is a process no less autonomous than the development of the endoplasmic reticulum and the nucleus.

According to Shimper's old theory (SCHIMPER, 1885) the development of plastids is autonomous. However, FREY-WYSSLING and MÜHLETHALER (1965) believe that plastids develop from special initial particles, formed apparently as a result of division and budding of the plastids themselves. In the dark, not only is the formation of chlorophyll suppressed, but that of lamellar chloroplast structures too (MÜHLETHALER and FREY-WYSSLING, 1959; PARKER and SIEGENTHALER, 1966; HASE, 1967). According to some data, plastids contain DNA and RNA (FREY-WYSSLING and MÜHLETHALER, 1965). According to later data obtained by SIEKEWITZ (1967), the biogenesis of chloroplast membranes is intimately connected with the process of chlorophyll synthesis. It is assumed that this membrane is formed from several proteins and lipids, with chlorophyll playing a decisive role in its formation, and that then various enzymes are built into the main stroma.

## 4. Conclusion

Thus, biological membranes constitute one of the oldest and most constant (in regard to structure) forms of supramolecular organization. They always include a bimolecular layer of lipids with protein layers coating both sides of these lipids. The chemical composition of membranes, even though the lipids and proteins are constant, can vary to a great extent depending upon the functional purpose of the membranes. Membranes are made up subunits of pentagonal or hexagonal globular shape. The globules are constantly changing the original state and position of the protein and lipid molecules that make up their composition, and as a result of this the membrane "breathes", "flickers", or "pulsates". Membranes have regulatory properties characteristic of structures with a systemic organization. They contain ATPase and are able to convert the chemical energy of ATP into kinetic energy, which not only enables them to maintain their structure but also makes it possible for them to fulfill their various functions. Membranes of receptor cells of sense organs are capable of reacting directly with specific types of energy from the external environment.

The above-mentioned evidence concerning the development of cellular membranes shows that they apparently never originate *de novo*, but always develop on a pre-existing matrix or "primer", namely a pre-existing membrane ("Omnis membrana e membrana"). Many organoids consisting of membranes (mitochondria, chloroplasts, synapses, etc.) apparently possess their own set of nucleic acids responsible for their reduplication. This is a way of considering the genesis and development of the membranes as a whole as well as the development of organoids consisting of membranes. Consequently, ROBERTSON'S concept (1959) of a broad mutual conversion of membranes into different cellular organoids should be abandoned. In general, the growth and differentiation of cellular membranes, as demonstrated by present-day data, takes place in the following way: the matrix or "primer" is encrusted by already manufactured protein, lipid, or carbohydrate molecules earlier synthesized in the appropriate organoids (proteins in ribosomes, lipids most probably in the Golgi apparatus, etc.). These molecules, moving from their site of production, enter into the composition of membranes and form definite physicochemical bonds (covalent, hydrophilic, electrostatic, polarization, disperse, LONDON, VAN DER WALLS); they then occupy spatial positions, prepared for them in advance, in the architecturally constant supramolecular membrane assembly: lipid globules in the bimolecular layer, and protein and other molecules on the lateral, inner, and external surfaces. Thus the growth and differentiation of membranes are now known to take place by means of a complex process of intussusception or encrustation (KAVANAU, 1965; VINNIKOV, 1966d).

It is important to note that the problem of reception, which is the subject of this book, is most intimately connected with the structure, chemical composition, development and function of biological membranes.

# Chapter II

# Ultrastructural and Molecular Organization of Antennae

## 1. Introduction

The antennae of receptor cells can consist either of microvilli and the stereocilia that result from their differentiation, or of kinocilia, the flagellum, and its derivatives.

Microvilli were detected soon after the introduction of the electron microscope on the surface of cells of the small intestine (PALAY and KARLIN, 1959) and kidney tubules (RHODIN, 1954, 1958). Subsequently it was found that microvilli can be detected on the surface of practically any epithelial cells facing into a free cavity. Thus, in our laboratory they have been described on the surface of the supporting cells of lateral-line organs, the utriculus, the sacculus (ARONOVA, 1967; ABRAMYAN, 1968, 1969; VINNIKOV, GOVARDOVSKII, and OSIPOVA, 1965a, 1965b; VINNIKOV et al., 1965) and of the organ of Corti (KOICHEV, 1969a) in the inner ear of vertebrates, on the surface of supporting cells of the gravity receptor of cephalopod molluscs (VINNIKOV et al., 1967) (Fig. 10) and of the olfactory organ of vertebrates (BRONSHTEIN and PYATKINA, 1968). Microvilli usually accompany cilia and flagella on the surface of ciliated (OKANO and SUGAWA, 1965) and receptor cells (Fig. 74, IV, V) (VINNIKOV et al., 1965a, 1965b, 1965c). However, in some receptor cells only microvilli may be present, for instance, in taste cells of vertebrates (NEMETSCHEK-GANSLER and FERNER, 1964, and others), in the rhabdomes of the visual cells of arthropods and, in particular, of insects (FERNÁNDEZ-MORÁN, 1958; GRIBAKIN, 1967a, 1967b), and molluscs (RÖHLICH and TÖRÖK, 1963; WOLKEN, 1958; MILLER, 1958; EAKIN, 1963; BARBER et al., 1967), and in the receptor cells of the vomeronasal organ (ALTNER et al., 1970).

Kinocilia are very widely distributed in receptor cells. Thus, flagella-kinocilia crown the olfactory knob of olfactory cells of vertebrates (Fig. 74, IV, V), as well as the chemoreceptor cells of insect sensilla (BRONSHTEIN, 1966; BRONSHTEIN and PYATKINA, 1968, 1969b; SLIFER, 1961; IVANOV, 1966, 1968, 1969a, 1969b). The gravity organ of higher crustaceans contains receptor cells equipped with a flagellum of the kinocilium type (SCHÖNE and STEINBRECHT, 1968). Peripheral processes of receptor cells of mechanoreceptors and the hearing organ of insects are crowned by a flagellum-kinocilium (GRAY, 1960; IVANOV, 1966, 1968, 1969a, 1969b). The photoreceptor cells of vertebrates consist of a modified flagellum, surrounded by microvilli (GOVARDOVSKII and KHARKEEVICH, 1965, 1967). Cells with kinocilia are found in the light-sensitive organs of the lancelet *Branchiostoma*

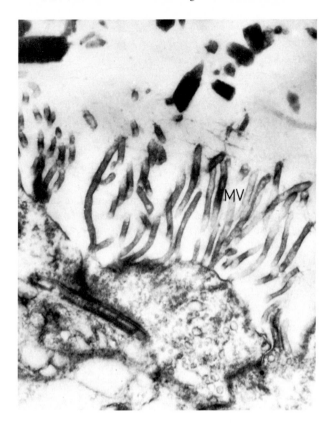

Fig. 10. Microvilli (*MV*) on the apical surface of a supporting cell in the gravitation receptor of the octopus *Ommatostrephes sloanei pacificus* ( × 44,000) (VINNIKOV *et al.*, 1971)

*californiensis* (EAKIN, 1963, 1966). In the eye of echinoderms, e.g. the starfish *Hernica leviuscala*, photoreceptor cells are equipped with mobile flagella-kinocilia (HARNACK, 1963; EAKIN and WESTFALL, 1964). The organization of receptor cells of the aboral organ in ctenophora is associated with kinocilia (HORRIDGE, 1964; VINNIKOV *et al.*, 1971). Kinocilia crown the peripheral processes of the receptor cells of the auricular organ of the planaria *Dugesia tigrina* (MCRAE, 1967). Flagellate structures (-kinocilia) are found in photoreceptor cells of the annelid *( Branchioma vesiculosum )* (LAWRENCE and KRAUSE, 1965) and, according to our data, in receptor cells of the gravity organ of *Arenicola*. Kinocilia are found in receptor cells of the nematode *Xiphenema index* (ROGGEN *et al.*, 1966). Finally, kinocilia are also found in the photoreceptor cells of chaetognatha (EAKIN, 1963).

Along with kinocilia, stereocilia often occur in receptor cells and are as a rule combined with the kinocilia. Hair cells of vertebrates possess, along with clusters of "immobile" hairs, stereocilia that have developed from microvilli (TITOVA and GRIBAKIN, 1967;) a single mobile flagellum-like hair-kinocilium which is clearly apparent in organ of Corti of birds (VINNIKOV *et al.*, 1965) and in young mammals (KIMURA, 1966). Similar kinocilia and stereocilia are found in receptor structures of the labyrinth of vertebrates: in the gravity organ (utricle) (Fig. 11), in the vibration organ (sacculus), in the crests of the ampullae of the semicircular canals, the organ of angular acceleration, and in lateral-line organs (FLOCK and WERSÄLL, 1962a, 1962b; LOWENSTEIN, OSBORNE, and WER-SÄLL, 1964; VINNIKOV, 1964, 1965a, 1965b; ARONOVA, 1967).

In specialized derivatives of lateral-line organs that act as electroreceptors, for instance in Lorenzini's ampullae in the skate *(Raja)* stereocilia disappear in receptor cells and only kinocilia are preserved (WALTMAN, 1966). However, in teleosts *(Ameiurus, Chatonemus)* both stereocilia and kinocilia disappear in electroreceptor organs; there is also a significant simplification in both receptor cells and nerve endings located a long way from these cells (BARETS and SZABO, 1962; MILLINGER, 1964). Organs of gravity, i.e. statocysts in gastropods, bivalves and cephalopod molluscs, according to our findings, contain otoliths and receptor cells crowned with numerous kinocilia and stereocilia-like microvilli (Fig. 114A) (VINNIKOV *et al.*, 1967, 1971).

A

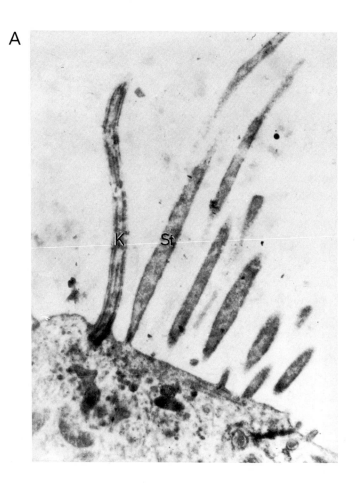

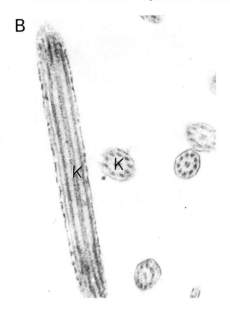

Fig. 11A and B. Stereocilium (*St*) and kinocilium (*K*). A. On the apical surface of a receptor cell in the pigeon utricle ( × 23,000) (VINNIKOV *et al.*, 1965a). B. Kinocilium of the frog olfactory receptor cell, as seen in longitudinal and cross section ( × 31,000) (BRONSHTEIN and PYATKINA, 1969)

Along with vertebrates and molluscs, typical stereocilia are found in Coelenterata: they have at the apex of cnidocilium of the stinging cells or cnidoblasts typical stereocilia surrounding on all sides one giant kinocilium (SLAUTTERBACK, 1967; HORRIDGE, 1969).

Mention should be made of the growing number of studies dealing with the organization of the sense organs in different types of multicellular organisms, in which antennae are described having the form of microvilli, stereocilia and particularly kinocilia crowning the receptor cells.

## 2. Microvilli

Microvilli are most clearly differentiated on the surface of epithelial cells, where they are distributed in the form of more or less regularly alternating columns of long, narrow, cylindrical cytoplasm processes, covered by an extension of the plasma membrane. Each process averages 1.5 micron in length and 80 millimicrons in diameter. Microvilli greatly extend the absorbing surface of the epithelial cell. The microvilli region is characterized by a high activity of alkaline phosphatase, invertases and maltases (MILLER and GRANE, 1961). One finds on the surface of microvilli a PAS-positive substance, identified as α mucopolysaccharide. In the electron microscope this substance is seen to be present in the form of condensates with a diameter of 25—50Å, which are directly connected to the surface of the plasma membrane (Fig. 12) (ITO, 1965; BOYD and PORSONS, 1969). The mucopolysaccharides on the surface of microvilli are

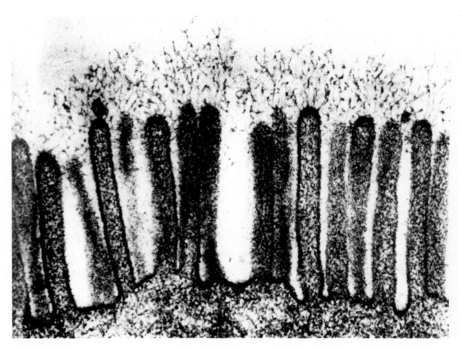

Fig. 12. Microvilli on the surface of intestinal cells of the bat. Mucopolysaccharides are located between the microvilli ( × 85,000) (ITO, 1965)

the first to contact substances being absorbed through the plasma membrane into the villus.

Whereas in the intestine and in some sections of kidney tubules microvilli regularly alternate in palisadelike structures more or less closely adjacent to each other, in ciliated or receptor cells their number is relatively small, and they are as a rule located around the base of the cilium (Fig. 37). At the same time, the regularity of their cylindrical form may be disrupted; moreover, some microvilli can form dichotomous ramifications. On sections through microvilli, a coating plasma membrane and a cytoplasm content in the form of a light matrix can be observed. Inside the microvilli, central fibrillae or tubules of diameter 40—50Å can be seen. Some investigators assume that microvilli effect contraction and retraction with the aid of these fibrillae or tubules (BOYD and PORSONS, 1969). Microvilli always extend into the lumen in the form of straight columns perpendicular to the cell surface and do not usually exhibit any bends or random deviations.

How is the visible elasticity or turgor of microvilli achieved? Either it is the result of their general packing, or else they contain some kind of structure, still unknown, which imparts to them elasticity characteristics. The first assumption does not, of course, exclude the second, but so far concrete data in this respect are lacking. Nevertheless, results obtained in our laboratory and in others show that when the functional state of the cell is modified, for example during prolonged illumination of rhabdomes (RÖHLICH, 1967; GRIBAKIN, 1969a,

1969b), it is possible to observe a drawing out and even some disintegration of microvilli. Motion pictures showing the movement (contraction) of microvilli in intestine and kidney tubules were obtained experimentally by adding to the medium $K^+$, $Na^+$ and certain other substances (THUNEBERG and ROSTGAARD, 1969). It has been suggested that the number of microvilli may vary according to the functional state of the cell (POLIKAR and BO, 1962). What, then, is the function of microvilli? In the first place, they help to create additional, sometimes quite significant cellular surface area, located at a definite point of functional application, for example, in the intestine or in kidney tubules. In the intestine, microvilli apparently, contribute to parietal digestion processes (UGOLEV, 1967), and in the kidney tubules they promote the reabsorption of water and sodium ions (NATOCHIN, 1968; VINNICHENKO, 1967). Thus, microvilli are functionally associated with the permeability processes which take place on the plasma membranes coating them. What is the purpose of the microvilli in ciliated and receptor cells? Here too, some special processes associated with permeability apparently take place in the microvilli. In some cases, a light-sensitive pigment, or rhodopsin is located in the plasma membrane of microvilli, for example in rhabdomes of insect photoreceptor cells. Under conditions of vitamin-A deficiency a change is observed in the plasma membranes of rhabdome microvilli (CARLSON et al., 1968). Thus, microvilli can perform a direct receptor function through the interaction of the rhodopsin molecules located in their coating plasma membrane with the quantum energy of photons, i.e. they can perform the function of antennae.

# 3. Stereocilia

Stereocilia develop from microvilli of embryonic cells (TITOVA and GRIBAKIN, 1967); they are core-shaped tubes located on the surface of a receptor cell; their length can vary from 4 to 5 μm and their diameter from 0.10 to 0.15 μm. They are coated with an extension of the cellular plasma membrane (see Fig. 11). Stereocilia have been found and studied with the aid of the electron microscope in the cnidoblasts of Coelenterata and considered to be receptor-effector cells (SLAUTTERBACK, 1967), (Fig. 106c), and especially on the apical surface of hair cells of lateral-line organs (FLOCK, 1965b, ARONOVA, 1967), of the membraneous labyrinth, and Corti's organ of vertebrates (VINNIKOV, 1969).

Stereocilia contain a large number (75 or more) of densely packed fibrillae which practically fill their entire lumen. Each fibrilla has a diameter of 30—40 Å. In lateral-line organs and in the labyrinth of vertebrates, the fibrillae are consolidated at the base of stereocilia into a compact filament, which then breaks down into separate fibrillae, penetrating the cuticular disk of the cell. Usually about 20 fibrillae enter this disk and form the root of the stereocilium, which runs in the cuticle duct and has a width of 1.5 μm. The root fibrillae enter the conical space of the duct and taper off to terminate at a depth of 0.4 micron from the cell surface (FLOCK and WERSÄLL, 1962a, 1962b; FLOCK, 1965b). In the cnidocilia of cnidoblasts of Coelenterata, the fibrillae of the stereocilia can penetrate deep into the cell cytoplasm (SLAUTTERBACK, 1967).

On the surface of receptor hair cells and cnidoblasts stereocilia are always located together with mobile flagella-kinocilia. Whereas the number of stereocilia ranges from 20 to 80 or more, there is generally only one kinocilium.

However, in the receptor cells of statocysts of cephalopod molluscs the number of kinocilia may amount to 80 or more (VINNIKOV et al., 1967).

A cluster of stereocilia is always arranged in relation to a kinocilium. For instance, in the lateral-line organ and in the inner ear of vertebrates stereocilia are arranged in 6 to 7 parallel rows, and each row consists of 5 to 6 stereocilia. The stereocilia are slightly angled within the row, so that the entire set of stereocilia in cross section form a W shape with the kinocilium located in the center of the W. Thus, the position of the kinocilium in such a cluster is always

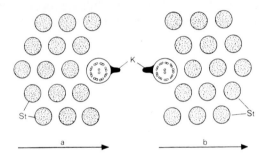

Fig. 13a and b. Diagram showing the position of kinocilia (K) in relation to a stereocilia (St) bundle (LOWENSTEIN et al., 1964). The arrows indicate the direction of shearing force acting on the bundles during cupula displacement: a excitatory displacement; b inhibitory displacement

spatially determined, i. e. polarized (Fig. 13). Electrophysiological tests have shown that stimulation of a receptor cell does not result in its excitation unless the stimulus is directed toward the stereocilia cluster. If it is directed toward a single kinocilium, then the cell is inhibited during stimulation (FLOCK and WERSÄLL, 1962a, 1962b; LOWENSTEIN and WERSÄLL, 1959). However, in the cnidocil of a cnidoblast 12 to 20 pairs of stereocilia in the form of an oval surround the hypertrophied kinocilium; this kinocilium is visible in the light microscope as a giant core (SLAUTTERBACK, 1967). In the receptor cell of statocysts of cephalopod molluscs 4 to 5 stereocilia-like microvilli also surround the centrally located kinocilium; as a result, stimulation in any direction is excitatory. Practically analogous relationships are found in the photoreceptor cells of vertebrates.

What is the function of stereocilia? First, their definition as immobile structures must be rejected. Both their ultrastuctural organization (the presence of a fibrillary apparatus) and their location on the surface of receptor cells provide convincing evidence, despite their great variability, of the ability of stereocilia to deviate from the original axis under the action of a graded stimulus. This deviation, depending on the functional activity, can be single or multiple. In our laboratory, we were able to record such a deviation during functional activity in lateral-line organs (ARONOVA, 1967), in the utricle and sacculus of the inner ear of vertebrates (VINNIKOV et al., 1971; ABRAMYAN, 1969), and in Corti's organ of birds and mammals (GOGNIASHVILI, 1967a, 1967b; KOICHEV, 1969a, 1969b). Evidently, such single or multiple deviations of a core-shaped stereocilium are specifically the result of a stimulus causing excitation. Such mechanical deviation triggers a whole chain of chemical processes connected with the conformation of the molecules (located in stereocilia) of a number of biologically active chemical substances.

It was already established with the light microscope that a whole series of enzymes is located in stereocilia of receptor cells of the mammalian organ of Corti, namely alkaline and acid phosphatases, phosphorylase, and acetylcholinesterase, which is an enzyme present in endolymph and associated with the hydrolysis of acetylcholine (see Fig. 95A) (VINNIKOV and TITOVA, 1961, 1964). The availability of the electron microscope enabled substances to be found in stereocilia which are clearly acetylcholinesterase (KIMURA, 1966) and adenosine-triphosphatase (NAKAI and HILDING, 1967). Finally, with the electron microscope it was possible to trace in the plasma membrane of stereocilia changes in the permeability of sodium ions, depending upon the functional state of the cell (KOICHEV, 1969b). It has been postulated that the deviation of stereocilia in the macula region of the inner ear of vertebrates leads to their depolarization, in view of the deformation of the polysaccharide molecules (hyaluronic complex) located between the stereocilia, which in this case can generate potentials of 10 to 100 mV (DOHLMAN, 1960a, 1960b).

Thus, the stereocilia of receptor cells should be considered as enzymatic antennae, the stimulation of which is a complex mechanochemical process resulting in excitation of the cell (VINNIKOV and TITOVA, 1961, 1964). Mechanochemical processes of stereocilia stimulation will be discussed in greater detail in the appropriate chapter.

## 4. Flagella and Cilia (Kinocilia)

The most widely distributed structure of antennae, with which we associate the perception of a stimulus, is the mobile cilium or flagellum or derivatives of these. As shown above, practically all receptor cells of all sense organs (with rare exceptions) are equipped with such structures (VINNIKOV, 1964, 1965a, 1965b, 1966a, 1966b, 1966c, 1967, 1968, 1969).

Cilia or flagella of receptor cells are very similar in their structural, chemical and functional organization to the cilia and flagella found in all other cells including spermatozoids of both unicellular and multicellular organisms, and in certain plants and animals. Flagella are longer and thicker than cilia. There can be one or several flagella in a cell; cilia, as a rule, are present in lager numbers.

The majority of flagella or cilia have a circular or oval form in cross-section. They are of more or less constant diameter, varying from 0.15 to 0.3 μm.

Flagella are always thicker and more massive than cilia. Both have a cylindrical, rounded or pointed at the top; they are covered by an extension of the cellular plasma membrane. Inside the flagellum is a thin membrane, the so-called axoneme, containing a pair of central fibrillae, surrounded by a ring consisting of 9 pairs of peripheral fibrillae (Fig. 14). Sometimes the plasma membrane can envelop

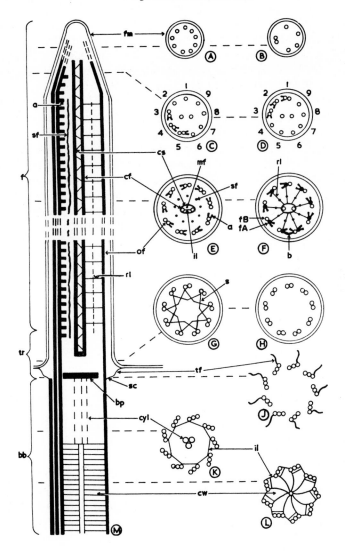

Fig. 14. Structural diagram of a flagellum (HOLWILL, 1966). M. longitudinal section; A. to L. corresponding cross sections. A., B. apex; C., D. levels at which peripheral fibrils terminate; E., F. structural
organization of the main portion of the body of the flagellum; G., H., J. structural organization
of the transition zone; K., L. structure of basal bodies (branching off and uncoiling of peripheral
fibrils). Designation of structural details, based on electron microscopic data: *1—9* numbering
of peripheral fibrils; *a* shoulders; *b* bridges; *bb* basal body; *bp* basal plate; *cf* central fibrils; *cs*
central sheath; *cyl* cylinders; *cw* substance of fibrils; *f* substance of flagellum; *fA* subfibril A; *fB*
subfibril B; *fm* plasma membrane of flagellum; *il* interfibrillar link; *of* outer fibrils; *rl* radial link;
*s* stellate structure; *cs* distal end of subfibril C; *sf* accessory fibril; *tf* transmitting fibrils; *tr* transition
area; *sc* central sheath

10 to 20 groups of fibrillae at the same times. Such fused flagellae can be
called "macroflagellae".

The almost universal presence of a constant formula for the number of fibrillae ($9 \times 2 + 2$) and the similarity of their spatial arrangement in all flagella of protozoa, animals and plants has not yet been explained. The most plausible assumption is that this formula is due to the rationality or geometry of their mode of packing (ASTBURY, BEIGHTON, and WEIBULL, 1955; SERRA, 1960), although some authors believe that such a packing is the result of their structural and phylogenetic characteristics (SATIR, 1962). Sometimes the central pair of fibrillae may be absent, for example, in visual cells of vertebrates or in insect sensilla cells. Although it was assumed earlier that the absence of central fibrillae is a sign of the immobility of a cilium or flagellum, for example in the sense organs (FAWCETT, 1961), it has been found that the central pair of fibrillae may be absent even in obviously mobile flagella (HOLWILL, 1966). As we shall see later, the number of fibrillae can sometimes increase or decrease.

In some cases it is possible to distinguish in addition 9 thin, so-called secondary fibrillae, located between the central and peripheral fibrillae (see Fig. 14). The diameter of the central fibrillae is about 240Å and the distance between their centers 300Å. It is assumed that a line drawn perpendicular to the axis running across the two central fibrillae indicates the direction of the motion of a flagellum (SATIR, 1962).

The peripheral fibrillae form 9 doublets, measuring 250—370Å. The long axis of the doublets is inclined by 5 to 10° to the tangent drawn to the circumference of the flagellum opposite the center of the doublet. Consequently, one of the two subfibrillae (the A fibrilla) is nearer to the center of the flagellum. Two processes having a thickness of 50Å and a length of 150Å (the so-called "shoulders") branch out from this fibrilla, which is slightly thinner in diameter. Both the central and peripheral fibrillae exhibit a helical structure in longitudinal cross-section (GIBBONS and GRIMSTONE, 1960). Negative contrasting has shown that the fibrillae are hollow cylinders, whose walls consist of 10 oriented subfibrillae 35—40Å thick and 88Å apart (PEASE, 1963).

The fibrillae do not extend to the top of the flagellum and usually end at different levels (HOLWILL, 1966). The two central fibrillae originate in the vicinity of what is called the basal plate at the base of the flagellum or cilium, whereas the 9 peripheral fibrillae extend beyond the basal plate into the basal body, from which they originate. The basal body is a hollow cylinder with a diameter of 120—160 millimicrons and a length of 350 millimicrons. The hollow central portion of the body, as seen in the electron microscope, has a low electron density. The cylinder of the basal body is formed by 9 triplets. Frequently, a so-called basal foot extends from the basal body; at present, the start of the cilium's pulsation is associated with this basal foot (Fig. 15) (GIBBONS, 1964). If there are radial connections between neighboring triplets, then in cross-sections structures of the "cart-wheel" or "mill-wheel" type can arise in the region where the flagellum passes into the basal body (MANTON, 1964). It should be noted that DNA and RNA have been found in the composition of the basal body (centrioles) (FAWCETT, 1961; FAURÉ-FREMIÉT, 1961; GALL, 1961); it has consequently been assumed that they are able to reproduce. The division of basal bodies, preceding cell division, was detected in the light microscope.

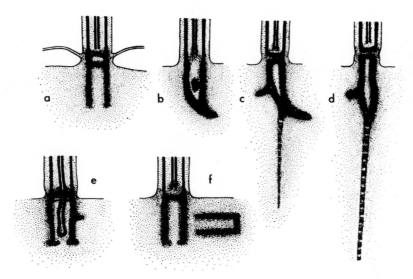

Fig. 15a—f. Diagram showing variations in the shape of basal bodies (FAWCETT, 1961). a Simple basal body; b oblique basal body; c and d basal bodies from which branch out a pedicle and a rootlet cross-striated at the bottom; e the two central fibrils extending deep into the cytoplasm (very rarely observed); f second basal body, or centrosome, located near the basal body of the cilium

With the exception of some animal spermatozoids, fibrous structures, or rootlets, branch off from the base of basal bodies and penetrate deep into the cytoplasm with a striation period of 400—500—700 Å. Such rootlets can branch out and reach the level of the nucleus and in some cases become attached to the inside surface of the cellular plasma membrane by means of a special cementing substance (Fig. 16a, b) (VINNIKOV et al., 1968). It is not yet clear whether these rootlets are contractile or whether they merely constitute the supporting apparatus of the flagellum. Is any kind of information transmitted along the rootlet? If so, in what direction: from the cell to the flagellum, or vice versa? In some cases, the basal bodies are connected by means of a tubular system instead of rootlets (BRONSHTEIN and PYATKINA, 1968).

The motion of flagella is usually considered to take place in the form of space waves, i.e. as plane or oarlike beats (ULEHLA, 1911). The motion of most animal and plant flagella is characterized by plane waves, while the motion of cilia occurs in oarlike beats. It was assumed that all vibrations start at the base of the flagellum and are then propagated to the top (LOWNDES, 1945; BROWN, 1945). However, it was found that in some organisms the motor wave in the flagellum starts from the top and travels towards the base (BAKER, 1961; BOVEE et al., 1963; HOLWILL et al., 1965, 1966). In both unicellular and multicellular organisms the motion of the flagellum is an automatic process, controlled by the cell itself.

In order that the flagellum may perform its beats, it must be able to contract or bend; it must also be able to resist bending or, more correctly, it must be able to unbend; finally, it must maintain phase differences between adjacent parts of the flagellum in such a way as to ensure the propagation of a coordinated wave. This wave is propagated along the stem of the flagellum without a decrement of amplitude (HOLWILL, 1966). In some cases the amplitude of wave propagation increases upon approaching the tip of the flagellum (GRAY, 1955). It is assumed that active retractile units are evenly distributed along the entire length of the flagellum (NACHIN, 1958). At the same time, it is also necessary to assume the presence of compression to guard against the destruction of the structure under the action of forces created by retractile elements. Thus, we must assume the presence in the flagellum of retractile, compressing and conducting systems, which are somehow adapted to certain definite structural elements of the flagellum, in all probability the fibrillary apparatus. Indeed, when flagella of certain protozoa

A

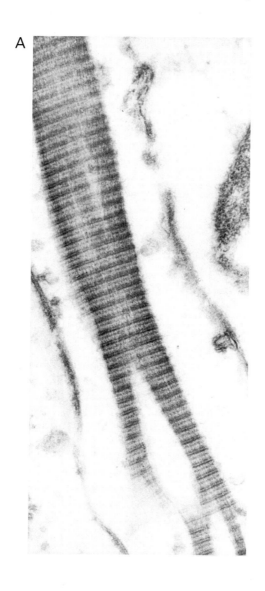

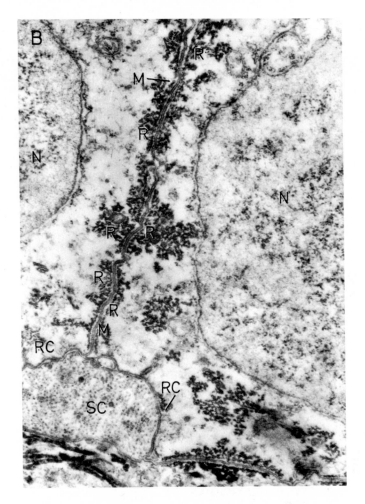

Fig. 16 A and B.  Rootlets branching off from basal bodies (VINNIKOV *et al.*, 1968, 1971). A. Longitudinal section of cross-striated rootlet branching off basal body of a receptor cell in the statocyst of the crab *(Paralithodes camtschatica Tilestos)* (× 40,000). B. Attachment of distal ends of rootlets *(R)* to the inner surface of the plasma membrane *(M)* of receptor cells *(RC)* in the crista of the squid *(Ommatostrephes sloanei pacificus)*; *N* cell nucleus; *SC* supporting cell (× 48,000)

are fractionated, it is possible to isolate a protein fraction with ATPase activity, for instance, dinein (GIBBONS, 1963) or flagellin (BURNASHEVA, EFREMENKO, and LYUBIMOVA, 1963; BURNASHEVA and RASKIDNAYA, 1968). Cytochemical investigations of sperm tails and cilia of rotifers showed that the ATPase activity is located in the peripheral fibrillae (GIBBONS, 1963; LANSING and LAMY, 1961; NELSON, 1958), more precisely, in the shoulders of peripheral fibrillae. A supporting role is generally ascribed to the central fibrillae (SATIR, 1964, 1967, 1968), although contradictory statements have also been made (KINOSITA and MURA-KAMI, 1967).

How is the rhythmic nature of the pulsation achieved? Some investigators, as stated above associate it with impulses coming from the stem of the basal body (GIBBONS, 1964). However, this rhythmic character is, apparently, an intrinsic property of the retractile structure of the flagellum (MANDELKERN, 1967). It was established long ago that formation of rhythmic waves can be induced in isolated flagella, killed with glycerol, by adding physiological concentrations of ATP (HOFFMAN-BERLING, 1955; ALEKSANDROV and ARRONET, 1956). BRONSHTEIN (1964) was able to reproduce this phenomenon on flagella-antennae of mammalian olfactory cells. Isolated dead flagella respond to temperatures and changes in viscosity in the same way as living flagella (HOFFMAN-BERLING, 1955; HOLWILL and SILVESTER, 1965). Thus, as in muscles, the fibrillary system of a flagellum contains a retractile protein similar in its properties to actomyosin, possessing ATPase activity and capable of undergoing a molecular interaction with an energy source, namely ATP, according to the scheme of conversion of chemical energy into mechanical work discovered some time ago by ENGELHARDT and LYUBIMOVA, 1939—1942).

What is the contractile mechanism of the flagellum? If we assume that the 9 pairs of peripheral fibrillae constitute the basic substratum for the contraction of the flagellum, then, taking their structural organization as a starting point, two hypotheses can be made: 1. the concentration of the flagellum is considered as the result of the sliding of fibrillae against each other; 2. contraction is due to conformational changes of the protein molecules in the fibrillae. In other words, the situation is the same as with theories of muscle contraction.

According to the hypothesis of a sliding filament, the two components of a peripheral pair of fibrillae move in relation to each other or in relation to a counter-pair of fibrillae. And, indeed, the fibrillae do terminate at different levels, which means they could slide against each other. The fibrillary structure of the flagellum consisting of thin and thick fibrillae resembles a striated muscle, while the transverse bridges of a muscle are comparable to the radical cross-bars of the flagellum. An original mechanism, based on the interaction of fibrillae, was proposed by SATIR (SATIR, 1964). According to his data, the peripheral fibrillae—and probably the two central fibrillae—contain myosin whereas the matrix contains actin. Motion is the result of interaction between the fibrillae and the matrix, and also the result of rotation of the central pair of fibrillae. The central fibrillae are enclosed in the basal plate and have a fixed position at this level. However, above this point, at the moment when the effective stroke begins, the central fibrillae are twisted relative to each other in such a way that the line connecting two fibrillae forms an angle of about 100° with the line connecting the central fibrillae at the level of the basal plate. As soon as the impulse, which is conducted along the membrane of the flagellum, reaches the level where they are twisted, the central pair of fibrillae begins to straighten out until at the end of the effective stroke the fibrillae are straightened out along the entire flagellum. It is assumed that chemical bonds establish a new configuration of the central fibrillae until the impulse reaches the tip of the flagellum, and then the last bond cleavage stimulates the effective stroke. Rotation of the central fibrillae is accompanied by migration of the bridge connecting two neighboring fibrillae; moreover, the bridge is always located on the axis perpendicular to the line connecting the central fibrillae. Criticisms of the mechanism of sliding filaments were expressed by GIBBONS and GRIMSTON (1960). They believe that if fibrillae did not exhibit any twisting along their entire length, which apparently does take place, then formation of a sinusoid wave would induce motion in opposite directions at different points of the same fibrillae. Therefore, the fibrillae would have to be elastically extensible. A system involving the sliding of elastic filaments against each other is considered by these authors as rather improbable.

The second hypothesis attempts to explain the contraction of flagellar or ciliar fibrillae as due to a change in the configuration or conformation of their protein molecules. This contraction could be the result of twisting or folding of the peptide links in a protein molecule. Fibrillae are thought to consist of globular protein molecules arranged in the form of a helix (ANDRÉ and THIÉREY, 1963; PEASE, 1963). The coils of the helix could change as a result of elongation or contraction of the diameter of the globules by an appropriate · magnitude, thus effecting the change in the length of the fibrilla required to induce the motion of the flagellum. The hypothesis that a globular substance is in fact the retractile unit was confirmed by data obtained by SILVESTER and HOLWILL (1965). In experiments on the reactivation of isolated flagella with the aid of ATP these authors showed that, under definite conditions, the rate at which dephosphorylation of ATP molecules takes place corresponds to the rate necessary for the activation of retractile units, distributed in an identical manner in globular units. However, a molecular interaction between fibrillae and a matrix is not excluded in this hypothesis. If we accept HOLWILL'S (1966) proposal that contraction takes place as a result of conformational changes of retractile units distributed along the flagellum, then the amplitude of its pulsation would be regulated in such a way that the strain developing in that unit would change in time. It is assumed that the retractile unit is associated with a bound ATP molecule during the greater part of its pulsation period (SILVESTER and HOLWILL, 1965). Contraction is induced by mechanical stimulation of units which then dephosphorylate ATP. If each retractile unit is shortened by the same amount, then the amplitude of the wave will depend upon the number of units developing strain in any given interval of time, and that number is determined by the time following stimulation in which the unit develops strain. Relaxation of the system is accompanied by replacement of ADP by ATP.

From cilia of *Tetrachymena piriformis* segments about 1 μm long were isolated; these may possibly be considered as the retractile elements (HOPKINS and WATSON, 1964). Experiments conducted recently by ASAKURA et al. on the self-assembly or biosynthesis of flagellins of salmonella (ASAKURA, EGUCHI, and YINO, 1967) also provide indirect proof for the presence of such retractile elements. Flagella of various *Salmonella* species were subjected to the action of sonic waves and fragments were obtained. At the same time, a flagellin monomer was isolated from flagella. Fragments of both flagella and flagellin are unable to reaggregate at room temperature at neutral pH. When fragments of flagella are added as a "primer" to a flagellin solution a rapid reaggregation of molecular flagellins into filament-like formations, resembling flagella, is observed. On the basis of their experiments, ASAKURA *et al.* (1967) conclude that the self-assembly of flagella takes place as a result of transconformation of flagellin molecules.

Thus, processes determining the pulsation of flagella take place at the molecular level as a result of mechanochemical phenomena occurring in the protein globules that enter into the composition of their 9 pairs of peripheral fibrillae (SCHERAGA, 1967). From an energy standpoint, as shown above, the beating of cilia or flagella takes place as a result of the interaction of a retractile protein containing high-molecular-weight ATPase with low-molecular-weight ATP generated and supplied by the cellular mitochondria. Consequently, the interaction of motile antennae (flagella or cilia) of receptor cells with a specific type of energy from the external environment, i.e. with a stimulus, is achieved by means of the universal mechanochemical phenomenon (ENGELHARDT, 1957), which is the basis of a wide variety of forms of biological motion.

# 5. Conclusion

Thus, the motile antennae of receptor cells are the means by which these cells actively come into contact with a given type of energy from the environment. Antennae can include microvilli and stereocilia, which are the product of their differentiation, but mainly kinocilia, i.e. flagella, cilia and their derivatives. As a rule, all of these structures, which can be found together on the surface of the same cell, are characterized by a motility that can be expressed to a greater or lesser degree. The structural apparatus of the antennae consists of fibrillae; the number of the fibrillae in a flagella can be represented by the formula $9 \times 2 + 2$ or $9 \times 2 + 0$. From the basal body where these fibrillae originate, a system of striated rootlets can branch off, the purpose of which is still not clear. Whereas the central fibrillae apparently play a supporting role and indicate the direction in which the antennae are to move, the 9 pairs of peripheral fibrillae constitute the basic substratum of contraction, which is responsible for the ability of antennae to move. The fibrillae of microvilli and stereocilia have not yet been investigated in this respect.

At present there are two opposed theories concerning the contraction of a flagellum: 1. that contraction is the result of the sliding of fibrillae against each other; 2. that contraction takes place as a result of conformational changes in the protein molecules in fibrillae.

In any case, peripheral fibrillae contain a myosin-like protein, that displays ATPase activity. This protein undergoes a molecular interaction with the ATP generated by adjacent mitochondria. We believe that the contraction of fibrillae in stereocilia or of membranes in microvilli proceeds according to the mechano-chemical rules which form the basis of the interaction between ATP and ATPase. Thus, the energy basis for the motion of the antennae of receptor cells is a particular case of the universal mechanochemical phenomenon. The motion of the antennae is essential to the act of reception.

Chapter III

# Structural and Cytochemical Organization
# of Synapses

## 1. Introduction

The results of structural, cytochemical and pharmacological studies of the synapses of sensory organs were usually examined from the standpoint of their similarity with what we know about the synapses of the central nervous system (DE ROBERTIS, 1958, 1964; DE ROBERTIS et al., 1961; WHITTAKER and GRAY, 1962; GRAY, 1963, 1967, 1969; ROBERTSON, 1964; ECCLES, 1964; WHITTAKER, 1965, 1967; GRAY and GUYLLIERY, 1966; ROBERTS et al., 1967). Among peripheral synapses, nerve–muscle connections in vertebrates have been studied most extensively (COUTEAUX, 1958; BIRKS, HUXLEY, and KATZ, 1960; ROBERTSON et al., 1960b). At the same time, it is quite obvious that the differences in their structural and cytochemical organization must also be clarified. No less important is the clarification of the question whether synapses of receptor cells are mediator-ones (i.e. they transmit a stimulus by liberating a chemical substance) or whether they are ephaptic (i.e. they operate by means of electrical transmission). Finally, what are our present concepts of synaptic transmission in general? This is the range of problems we propose to examine in this chapter.

## 2. Organization of Synapses

The term "synapses" (SHERRINGTON, 1897) is used to designate specialized sectors of the plasma membranes of nerve cells or their extensions, through which are realized the structural and functional contacts of nerve cells with each other, with receptor cells, or with effector elements. The ultrastructural organization of synapses in the central nervous system is fairly uniform (PALAY, 1958; DE ROBERTIS et al., 1961), but it may well be different in the sensory and motor organs. However, in all cases it is always possible to distinguish in synapses a presynaptic membrane, which is usually thickened, an intersynaptic cleft consisting of a narrow homogeneous space having a width of $200-300 \text{Å}$[1] and cross-striated with connecting filaments, and a thickened post-synaptic membrane (Fig. 17). In the central nervous system, synapses are classified as type-1 and type-2 synapses. Type-1 synapses are found only on dendrite stems and on their intumescences or spine. Type-2 synapses are found on the stems of

---

[1] The width of the intersynaptic cleft in the motor end-plate is $600-700 \text{Å}$ (GRAY, 1959).

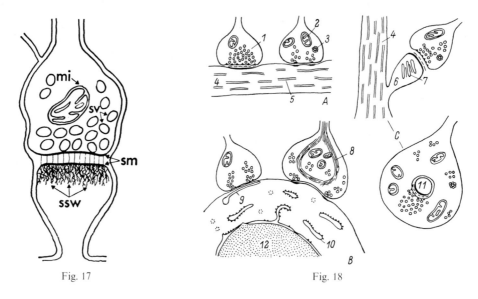

Fig. 17                                        Fig. 18

Fig. 17. Diagram of synapse from the cerebral cortex (DE ROBERTIS, 1967). *mi* mitochondria; *sv* synaptic vesicles; *sm* intersynaptic cleft with cross threads; *ssw* subsynaptic network

Fig. 18 A—C. Diagram of synaptic structures (GRAY, 1967). A. Type-I synapses; B. type-II synapses; C. spine structures. *1* Synaptic vesicles; *2* mitochondria; *3* complex vesicle; *4* dendrite; *5* tubules; *6* spine; *7* spine apparatus; *8* ring of neurofibrils; *9* synaptic sac; *10* endoplasmic reticulum; *11* postsynaptic process (spine); *12* nucleus

dendrites and perikaryons. Both types start from the conversion of an axon, which loses its myelin sheath in this process, into a special expansion, the so-called presynaptic knob (Fig. 18). The latter contains special characteristic vesicles, known as synaptic vesicles, and mitochondria, and its plasma membrane forms a synaptic thickening in the region of contact. In type-1 synapses, the synaptic vesicles and individual mitochondria are concentrated near the thickened sector of the membrane. The synaptic cleft is usually 300 Å wide. The post-synaptic thickening of the membrane is particularly dense. Type-2 synapses also contain mitochondria and synaptic vesicles, but the thickening of the membrane is limited to a small portion of the area of synaptic contact, and the cleft facing the thickened sectors is only 200 Å wide and does not contain a clearly visible layer of extracellular material; in addition, the post-synaptic thickening is denser than the presynaptic one.

According to recent data, synaptic vesicles develop as invaginations of the plasmic membrane of the nerve ending. The vesicles are arranged in a regular pattern being "packed" into a substance lining the inner protein layer of the presynaptic membrane; from this position their contents can be injected into the synaptic cleft (Fig. 19) (AKERT, 1973).

A few words now about the so-called spines. They have nothing in common with the "spines" visible under the light microscope, but in the electron microscope they can be seen as short, blunt extensions of the neuroplasm, located on the peripheral sections of dendrites where synaptic contacts are effected. The tip

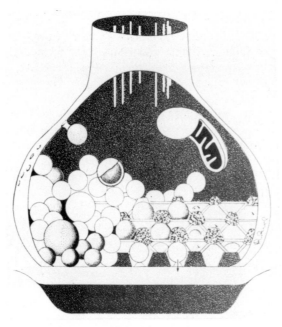

Fig. 19. The presynaptic vesicular grid. Schematic representation of its structure and dynamics (for further comments, see text). (Reprinted from AKERT *et al.* in Structure and Function of Synapses, Eds. G. PAPPAS and D. P. PURPURA, p. 83, New York: Raven Press 1972)

of a spine is shaped like a small isolated, pear-shaped body and is in contact with the presynaptic knob (WHITTAKER and GRAY, 1962). Some spines contain a special organoid, known as the spine apparatus, which consists of several small plates or rods (see Fig. 18). In the central nervous system the spine apparatus is most frequently found in the dendrites of pyramid cells. It used to be believed that the spine apparatus is found only in the central nervous system of mammals, but synaptic rods or plates can be found in synapses of frog lumbar sympathetic ganglion (TAXI, 1962). Similar structures are also observed in lower and higher vertebrates, and by no means only in the central nervous system but also in synapses of sensory organs. Thus, the bases the of central processes of visual cells, from cyclostomes to mammals (DE ROBERTIS and FRANCHI, 1956; SJÖSTRAND, 1958; BOROVYAGIN, 1962a, 1962b, 1966; COHEN, 1963a; DOWLING and BOYCOTT, 1966; EVANS, 1966; GOVARDOVSKII, 1967), are provided with numerous recesses into which enter the interlocking peripheral extensions of bipolar and horizontal cells, which thus effect synaptic contacts. The plasma membrane of a photoreceptor, namely the presynaptic membrane, frequently forms what are called synaptic rods or plates; these are double folds 2—3 µm long and several tenths of a micron wide (see Fig. 38). Although in central neurons spine data are kept separate from plates. The plate as well as the spine apparatus in central neurons is always surrounded by a cluster of synaptic vesicles 300—400Å in diameter. In the photoreceptor body, mitochondria are generally absent in the presynaptic region.

Analogous structures were also detected in the synaptic region of secondary sensory receptor cells in the acoustico-lateral system of lower vertebrates. Thus, two types of nerve endings, "light" and "dark", are located close to the base of the receptor cells of the lateral-line organs of fish. The dark endings contain a considerable number of synaptic vesicles and are considered to be efferent endings. The light endings contain a small number of vesicles and it is assumed that they are afferent endings (HAMA, 1962; FLOCK, 1965; ARONOVA, 1968). Large endings of this type can penetrate deep into the body of the cell or may simply form contacts with its base. In the synaptic region of the receptor cell one or more dense synaptic rods or corpuscles can be seen, located at a distance of 600Å from the cell membrane (Fig. 20). These synaptic rods differ

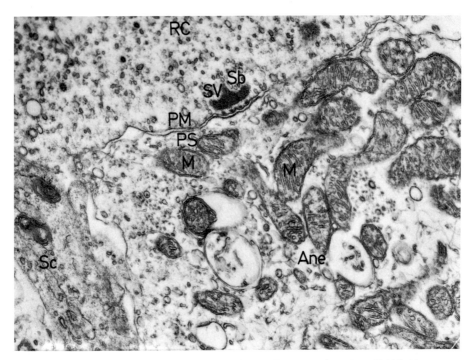

Fig. 20. Synapse in a lateral line receptor cell of the pike *(Esox lucius)* (× 50,000) (ARONOVA, 1968). *Sb* Synaptic body; *RC* receptor cell; *Sc* supporting cell; *SV* synaptic vesicles; *PM* presynaptic membrane; *PS* postsynaptic membrane; *Ane* afferent nerve ending; *M* mitochondria

little from the "spine" rods or synaptic rods of photoreceptors. They are also surrounded by synaptic vesicles of 350Å diameter. The synaptic membranes of the receptor cell and nerve ending form a wavy line. An additional membrane, the accessor, can also be observed inside the receptor cell. Analogous synaptic structures with synaptic rods, provided with synaptic vesicles, have also been described in type-I and -II cells of the utricle of the inner ear in higher vertebrates (WERSÄLL, FLOCK, and LUNDQUIST, 1965; VINNIKOV, 1967a, 1967b; VINNIKOV et al., 1971). However, such structures are apparently absent in synaptic contacts between fila olfactoria endings, which are branched in the form of telodendrons and filled with synaptic vesicles, and dendrites of mitral and other cells in the region of olfactory glomerules of mammals, although the pre- and postsynaptic membranes are developed to a significant extent in these structures.

A few words now about synaptic vesicles. As we know, concentration and liberation of the mediator of synaptic transmission is associated with these vesicles. Among the usual vesicles, with homogeneous contents, there are also vesicles that contain a dense corpuscle in the center. It is assumed that the two types of vesicles contain different mediators: the former acetylcholine, and the latter catecholamines. Sometimes, both types of vesicles are located in the same nerve ending (RODRIGUES-ECHANDIA, 1967, 1968; DE ROBERTIS, 1969). However, their origin is far from clear. Some researchers think that vesicles bud off from small ducts and tubules connected to the endoplasmic reticulum of the perikaryon. Such small ducts and tubules are found in axons but mainly in dendrites (PALAY, 1958). However, other researchers assume that synaptic vesicles develop by pinocytosis from the plasmic membrane of the nerve ending (AKERT et al., 1969, 1973).

On the basis of electron micrographs showing the spatial distribution of presynaptic vesicles and their various shapes after glutaraldehyde fixation of nerve tissue, attempts are being made to carry out a morphological mapping of excitatory and inhibitory synapses (BODIAN, 1966a, 1966b; USHIZONO, 1965, 1967, 1968; PAPPAS et al., 1968). Some researchers assume that synapses that have synaptic vesicles of circular or spherical shape are predominantly excitatory, while synapses whose synaptic vesicles have an ellipsoid shape are inhibitory. For example, the well-known inhibitory synapses of the crayfish contain synaptic vesicles of ellipsoid shape (USHIZONO, 1965).

Synapses with ellipsoid vesicles (and hence assumed to have an inhibitory function) were described in motor neurons of the spinal cord (BODIAN, 1966a, 1966b) and around the soma and processes of Purkinje cells in the cerebellum (LARRAMENDI and VICTOR et al., 1967). However, in certain fish synapses of the motor neurons that control the swim bladder contain neither ellipsoidal nor spherical vesicles (PAPPAS, 1968).

Certain synapses that contain ellipsoidal synaptic vesicles are actually electro-genous and not mediator synapses (PAPPAS and BENNETT, 1966a, 1966b). Conse-quently, the differentiation of excitatory and inhibitory synapses on the basis of the shape of their synaptic vesicles is still far from reliable.

Thus, the ultrastructural organization of synapses whose function is associated with the liberation of a mediator is basically similar in both the central nervous system and the sensory organs. We believe that their function exhibits the same similarity.

## 3. Synapses with Chemical Transmission

It is generally accepted that most synapses perform their function by means of a chemical mediator, usually acetylcholine (ECCLES, 1966). Proof of this fact is provided by the above-mentioned electron microscopic data and primarily by the presence of synaptic vesicles. By the fractional centrifugation of brain homogenates, it was possible to isolate a subfraction consisting of vesicles containing bound acetylcholine (HEBB and WHITTAKER, 1958; DE ROBERTIS et al., 1962). WHITTAKER (1967) has also studied the distribution of enzymes which catalyze the synthesis of acetylcholine (acetylcholine transferase, cholinacetylase and the acetylcholine-hydrolyzing enzyme, cholinesterase). Cholinesterase was found in the soluble cytoplasm of nerve endings, located in scraps of the outer membrane of the nerve terminal. As WHITTAKER correctly points out, this finding is in agreement with histochemical observations under the electron microscope, showing that this enzyme is located on the outer membrane of the cholinergic axon and the nerve terminal (LEWIS, SHUTE, and SILVER, 1967). Calculations show that a synaptic vesicle contains on average 2,000—6,000 molecules of acetylcholine (ECCLES, 1966; WHITTAKER, 1967), i.e. vesicle acetylcholine constitutes a relatively stable reserve of mediator, which is sensitive to osmotic action and survives the isolation procedure. Small amounts of free acetylcholine have also been detected in the original homogenates; this points to the existence of free cytoplasmic acetylcholine, which is found in the entire cholinergic neuron (WHITTAKER, 1969).

Other amines can also be isolated from synaptic vesicles, for example, oxytryptamin (MICHAELSON and WHITTAKER, 1963), noradrenaline (LEVI and MAYNERT, 1964) and histamine, not enclosed in mast cells (MICHAELSON and WHITTAKER, 1963). Results obtained for dopamine (LAVERTI et al., 1963) and for amino acids of stimulants and depressants, on L-glutamate and γ-aminobutyrate, are still contradictory (WHITTAKER, 1967). Apparently, noradrenaline is located in synaptic vesicles in a manner similar to acetylcholine.

With the aid of histochemical methods it has been shown that acetylcholinesterase is located in the cytoplasm of vegetative nerve cells of the central and peripheral nervous systems, as well as on their synaptic surfaces (KOELLE and KOELLE, 1959; FUKUDA and KOELLE, 1959). The location of acetylcholinesterase in nerve–muscle synapses was already well established in the 1950's (COUTEAUX and TAXI, 1952; PORTUGALOV, 1955; COUTEAUX et al., 1958). With the advent of the electron microscope it became possible to establish the exact location of acetylcholinesterase in motor end-plates (LEHRER and ORNSTEIN, 1959). Its location in embryonic and differentiated nervous system was described by GEREBTZOFF (1955). In the retina, the location of acetylcholinesterase has been demonstrated in the inner reticular layer (LEPLAT and GEREBTZOFF, 1956), in the outer segments of photoreceptors and their synapses (EICHNER, 1958), and in the embryonic retina (SHEN, GREENFIELD, and BOELL, 1956). In olfactory cells, acetylcholinesterase was first detected by BARADI and BOURNE (1959a, 1959b), then by BRONSHTEIN (1965) and other investigators. In the synaptic zone of taste buds it was described by BARADI and BOURNE (1959a, 1959b) and PEVZNER (1964b, 1966). Acetylcholinesterase was detected in the stereocilia and synapses of Corti's organ in mammals (VINNIKOV and TITOVA, 1958a, 1958b, 1961, 1963, 1964). Its location was described in detail in embryonic (TITOVA, 1968) and definitive labyrinth structures of vertebrates (TITOVA and VINNIKOV, 1965; VINNIKOV, TITOVA, and ARONOVA, 1965), and in synaptic terminals and receptor structures of the lateral-line organs of fish (TITOVA and ARONOVA, 1964; ARONOVA, 1968).

Thus, in view of the extensive occurrence of acetylcholinesterase in receptor structures of sense organs and the presence of synaptic vesicles, apparently filled with acetylcholine, in their presynaptic region, we can assume that nerve conduction in the receptor cells of sensory organs is effected primarily by means of a so-called cholinergic mediator system.

Careful studies performed by biochemists, using the differential centrifugation method, have shown that acetylcholinesterase is located in the synaptic membranes (pre- and postsynaptic) in what are called synaptosomes. The latter do not contain any $Na^+$- or $K^+$-ATPase, adenylcyclase, p-nitrophenol phosphatase, RNA, DNA, or other substances (GLEBOV, 1968). In sectors of postsynaptic membranes, along with acetylcholinesterase, molecules of a protein are present, called cholinoreceptive protein because it is adapted to interact with acetylcholine molecules (MIKHEL'SON, 1967).

Nerve endings can synthesize protein independently of the perikaryon (AUSTIN and MORGAN, 1967, 1968). It has also been shown that acetylcholinesterase can apparently be synthesized in axons (FUKUDA and KOELLE, 1959). However, convincing data are available, indicating that the synthesis of acetylcholinesterase and acetylkinase is mainly associated with microsomes of the rough endoplasmic reticulum. Acetylcholinesterase ("internal"—KOELLE and STEINER, 1956) can be detected in the region where Nissl's substance is located. Consequently, the organized sectors of the endoplasmic reticulum of a nerve cell, namely Nissl's granules, must be the site of synthesis of the active protein, i.e. acetylcholinesterase. In a similar manner cholinacetylase is synthesized in the endoplasmic reticulum under the action of RNA, and is then transported along the axon in the same way as acetylcholinesterase. The enzymes synthesized in the vicinity of Nissel's substance and the acetylcholine granules formed in the region of the Golgi apparatus are able to move forward because the endoplasmic reticulum extends almost to the nerve terminal[2], i.e. up to the synapse. In regard to the formation of acetylcholine it is also assumed that this compound can be synthesized with the aid of acetylcholinesterase in nerve endings, directly in the synaptic vesicles (HEBB and WAITES, 1956; ECCLES, 1966). It is known that proteins, newly formed with the aid of nucleic acids in the perikaryon region, move along the neurites at a velocity of 240 mm/day. These proteins continuously replace axoplasm components which are consumed during the processes associated with life activity. It is assumed that in the synaptic membrane region acetylcholinesterase is oriented in such a way that its active centers are located outside the bimolecular lipid layer. Thus, functional "external" (NACHMANSON, 1950; BURGEN and SHIPMAN, 1951; FUKUDA and KOELLE, 1959; KOELLE et al., 1959) acetylcholinesterase is located most conveniently to effect the rapid hydrolysis of acetylcholine, which is liberated both during the resting period (miniature potentials) and during the period of synaptic transmission of a nerve impulse.

---

[2] Acetylcholine is synthesized in the nerve cell from choline and acetate (or its precursor), with the enzyme cholinacetylase and coenzyme A(CoA) taking part in the reaction. The synthesis occurs in two steps: 1. formation of an active acetate (acetyl CoA) from acetate or its precursor and CoA with participation of transacetylase, using energy obtained from ATP (SHAPOT, 1954); 2. the actual synthesis of acetylcholine from acetyl CoA and choline in the presence of the enzyme cholinacetylase (NACHMANSON, 1959). For additional details, see VINNIKOV and TITOVA (1964).

How is a synapse made to function by chemical transmission? In other words, what is the nature of the molecular processes upon which the mechanism of this function is based?

Both in the state of relative rest and in the state of stimulation a process is assumed to take place, whereby acetylcholine is liberated from the synaptic vesicles and penetrates into the intersynaptic cleft. A "quantum" of acetylcholine, ejected from a single vesicle under conditions of relative rest, reaches the surface of the synaptic membrane and causes in this membrane a local, nonpropagating subthreshold change in potential, known as a miniature potential (FATT and KATZ, 1951). Under stimulation the release of acetylcholine from synaptic vesicles becomes synchronized, so that acetylcholine is liberated simultaneously from several hundred or thousand synaptic vesicles (DEL CASTILLO and KATZ, 1956). There are indications that, after stimulation, the number of vesicles in the presynaptic region can vary (DE ROBERTIS, 1958). Some authors claim to have observed a migration of presynaptic vesicles through the presynaptic membrane into the intersynaptic cleft in the direction of the postsynaptic membrane, followed by an emptying of the vesicles (DE ROBERTIS, 1964). Other authors, on the contrary refute claims of this sort (BENNETT, 1964).

The released acetylcholine, apparently by simple diffusion, traverses the synaptic cleft in a time of 1 msec (DEL CASTILLO and KATZ, 1956) and reaches the postsynaptic membrane. It was noted a long time ago that the postsynaptic membrane is highly sensitive to acetylcholine, nicotine and other substances causing local stimulation of the membrane and that a decrease in sensitivity to these substances occurs under the effect of curare. Such properties of the postsynaptic membrane were attributed to the presence of a special cholinoreceptor in the membrane. It has now been shown that the cholinoreceptor is a protein molecule adapted to react with a molecule of acetylcholine (NACHMANSON, 1959; CAVALLITO, 1962; TURPAEV, 1962; MIKHEL'SON and KHROMOV-BORISOV, 1964; KOELLE, 1965).

Recently, it has been possible to isolate from subsynaptic membranes and to study under the electron microscope a macromolecule of cholinoreceptor, which was found to be a lipoprotein capable of changing its structure during action and binding, for example, with 5-hydroxytryptamine and other substances that block transmission in synapses (DE ROBERTIS, 1971).

The chemical nature of the cholinoreceptive protein has been studied by MIKHEL'SON (1967). The cholinoreceptor has two active sectors. The anionic sector (designated by a small circle in Fig. 21) establishes an ionic bond with

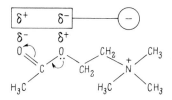

Fig. 21. Diagram of cholinoreceptor (MIKHELSON, 1967). For explanation, see text

the cationic head of acetylcholine. The role of anionic sector can be performed by a carboxylate, i.e. the anion of a dibasic amino acid (aspartic or glutamic acid), or by the anion of a phosphoric acid derivative (CAVALLITO, 1962), i.e. the mercapto group of cysteine (TURPAEV, 1962). The second active sector is some kind of dipole arrangement, which effects a dipole–dipole interaction (BAR-LOW, 1960) with the strongly polarized ester portion of the acetylcholine molecules. This sector is analogous to but not identical with the esterase sector in cholinesterase. In the cholinoreceptor this sector does not carry an esterase function and is not acetylated; it can be called an "esterophilic" sector (KABACHNIK, BRESTKIN, and MIKHEL'SON, 1965).

The cholinoreceptive properties of the postsynaptic membrane are determined not only by the structure and number of cholinoreceptors per unit of membrane surface, but also by their arrangement relative to each other (Fig. 22). Moreover,

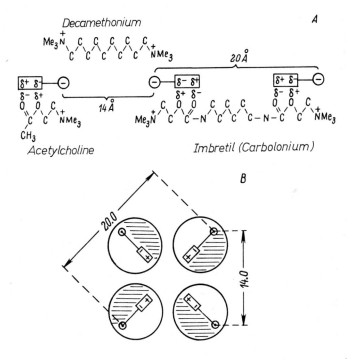

Fig. 22 A and B. Diagram showing arrangements of cholinoreceptors on the postsynaptic membrane of skeletal muscles in higher vertebrates (MIKHELSON, 1967). A. Linear arrangement; B. tetramerous structure

it is possible to trace how the transition occurs during the course of evolution from a disordered, random arrangement of individual cholinoreceptors to their arrangement in a definite order, for example, the transition from a monopolar to an oligomeric structure, etc. The fact of arrangement seems to impart to cholinoreceptors some sort of energy or kinetic advantages (MIKHEL'SON, 1967). As a result of the interaction of acetylcholine with the protein of a cholinoreceptor, which is accompanied by a change in its conformation, there is a change in the properties of the postsynaptic membrane which alters its ionic permeability. This induces a change in the velocities and direction of the ionic currents, primarily of $K^+$ and $Na^+$, across the membrane, and also a redistribution of the electrical charges on both sides of the cellular membrane (i.e. depolarization) and sets off an entire complex of biochemical processes which ultimately lead to stimulation of the cell.

Removal of acetylcholine in the region where the cholinoreceptor is located plays a very important role in this process, since its removal is absolutely indispensable for the restoration of the original state of the postsynaptic membrane. This function is performed by acetylcholinesterase located, as stated above, in the structure of the synapse. As we know, during the action of substances which destroy acetylcholinesterase, the intensity and duration of action of acetylcholine increase. When the enzyme is completely inactive, as a result of a concentration of acetylcholine in the region of the receptor membrane, the transmission of stimulation is blocked (TURPAEV, 1962). It is assumed that cholinesterase hydrolyses only free acetylcholine, thus shifting the equilibrium system to the left: acetylcholine + cholinoreceptor → acetylcholine − receptor complex. This results in the liberation of the receptor from acetylcholine and restores the properties of the postsynaptic membrane. Since, as a result of the high activity of acetylcholinesterase, the rate of hydrolysis of acetylcholine is very high, the process of restoring the properties of the postsynaptic membrane is terminated several milliseconds after stimulation (ECCLES, 1966).

Thus, interaction of the mediator with the receptor protein is the primary reaction which forms the basis of the process involving the transmission of stimulation through the synapses. Along with cholinoreceptive proteins, adrenoreceptive proteins have also been discovered (NICKERSON, 1965; TURPAEV, 1967; MANUKHIN, 1968). This interaction of the acetylcholine mediator with protein constitutes the trigger mechanism for synaptic transmission in its bioelectric expression (NACHMANSON, 1967). Therefore, neuron excitation is preceded by the liberation of a mediator, and it is this liberation that is responsible for the directed flow of ions from depolarized presynaptic terminals of axons to postsynaptic membranes of dendrites or of the perikaryon, or to presynaptic terminals of other axons. The nature of the specific interaction between the mediator and the membrane is determined both by the chemical nature of the mediator and by the structure and condition of the reacting membrane. Stimulation occurs as a consequence of a change that results in the depolarization of the membrane. Inhibition is the result of the liberated substances blocking the action of excitatory influences directed toward the same membrane. It has been demonstrated that $\gamma$-aminobutyric acid, which is present in oval synaptic vesicles, is a mediator of inhibition (ROBERTS, 1967; DE ROBERTIS, 1967; UCHIZONO, 1965). Two enzymes associated with this system, namely glutamic acid decarboxylase and $\gamma$-aminobutyric acid aminotransferase, have a different location. Thus, decarboxylase, which reversibly catalyzes the formation of $\gamma$-aminobutyric acid from L-glutamic acid, is found in nonaminoergic nerve terminals; on the other hand, aminotransferase is located in the mitochondria in the same manner as succinate dehydrogenase (DE ROBERTIS, 1967). It is assumed that in the central nervous system of vertebrates the stimulating mediator is liberated by axodendritic terminals, whereas the inhibiting mediator can be liberated by both axo-axonal and axo-somatic synapses (ECCLES, 1966). It has further been shown that immediately after depolarization the substance which directly induces synaptic inhibition is liberated according to the feedback principle from its compound or bound form, and is released from the postsynaptic zone into the extraneuronal synaptic medium in an amount corresponding to the degree of depolarization (ROBERTS, 1967). Thus, inhibition is effected by the same ionic and electrical mechanisms as stimulation (ECCLES, 1966).

Until recently, researchers have focused all their attention on the energy stimulation of synaptic transmission by means of mediators, in particular, the acetylcholine located in the synaptic vesicles. However, attention should also be directed to the fact that any presynaptic region, whether in the central nervous system or in receptor cells, must necessarily be provided with mitochondria. Their presence has been considered as clear evidence that their energy metabolic activity, as suppliers of ATP, somehow plays a part in the function of nervous conduction (ECCLES, 1966). However, there was no direct cytochemical and morphological proof of this. We have now been able to demonstrate (VINNIKOV et al., 1966; VINNIKOV, 1967a; 1967b) that during transmission of a nervous stimulation there occur definite morphological and cytochemical shifts among the synaptic mitochondria, whose energy resources, together with other substrates and enzymes of the cholinergic system, are also involved in the trans-synaptic switching of the nervous impulse. Such shifts have been observed in the receptor cells of the utricle of the inner ear in various types of vertebrates, from fish to mammals, both in a state of relative rest and when subjected to single and multiple radial acceleration effects.

As was demonstrated in research carried out by ENGSTRÖM, ADES, and HAWKINS (1962), WERSÄLL (1956, 1961), LOWENSTEIN, OSBORNE, and WERSÄLL (1964) and in our laboratory (VINNIKOV and TITOVA, 1962a; VINNIKOV et al., 1965), receptor cells of the utricle in animals have a cylindrical form (type-II cells) or a goblet-shaped form (type-I cells). Goblet-shaped cells are generally surrounded by a giant cup-shaped nerve terminal; this means that a considerable area of their outer plasma membrane is, in fact, a presynaptic membrane. In the utricle of birds and certain mammals from 2 to 5 receptor cells may be embedded in such a nerve bowl, which contains mitochondria. The cylindrical receptor cells carry on their base several small button-shaped nerve terminals.

A study of the receptor cells of the inner ear utricle in animals which were sacrificed either in a state of relative rest or immediately after exposure to radial acceleration, has shown that the mitochondria of receptor cells may be in intimate contact with the presynaptic membrane, i.e. they can abut tightly against this membrane (Fig. 23). This "adjoining" of presynaptic mitochondria can be observed particularly clearly in receptor cells of the utricle of mammals where the presynaptic region contains very large numbers of elongated mitochondria, even when the animals are in a state of relative rest. As a result of the close contact of these mitochondria with the presynaptic membrane, the mitochondria form structures consisting of four membraneous layers, two mitochondrial and two synaptic, separated from each other by very narrow intervals.

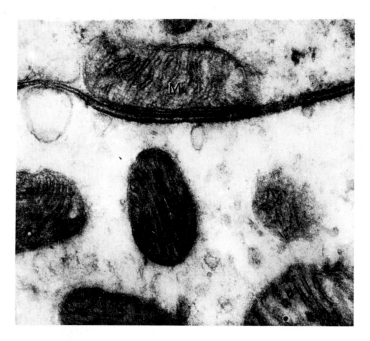

Fig. 23. Presynaptic region of type-I receptor cell in the mouse utricle after centrifugation at $10\,g$ for 3 min ($\times 64{,}000$) (VINNIKOV, 1967a). $M$ mitochondria

In experimental animals, the adjoining of mitochondria in the presynaptic region of both type-I and type-II cells is expressed in an extremely clear manner. Adjoining mitochondria stretch out along the presynaptic membrane and swell slightly. Their membranes become somewhat thinner, and the interval between the external mitochondrial sheaths and the presynaptic membrane becomes barely visible. If, on their way towards the presynaptic membrane, the mitochondria encounter any kind of obstacle, for example a synaptic rod with vesicles, they can bend like an amoeba and go around it, but their peripheral tips still abut tightly against the presynaptic membrane. Some of the mitochondria of cup-shaped nerve endings also swell strongly. At the same time, other mitochondria of the nerve ending remain in their previous state or swell insignificantly. Similar changes are also observed in the mitochondria of button-shaped nerve endings; these changes are particularly clearly expressed in the pike. Since the rod-shaped mitochondria in the receptor cells of the pike are generally quite long, only part of their surface comes in contact with the presynaptic membrane, while the tips of mitochondria some distance away bend over and branch off (Fig. 24). In some cases, it was possible to observe the adjoining of mitochondria to the presynaptic membrane also in dark and apparently efferent, button-shaped nerve endings containing numerous synaptic vesicles.

Thus, the adjoining of mitochondria to the presynaptic membrane in utricular receptor structures of the inner ear in vertebrates can be observed quite clearly, and it can be regularly induced or strengthened by the action of appropriate

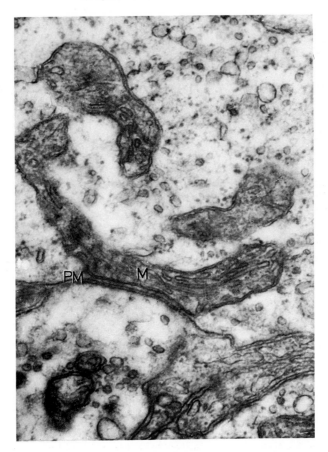

Fig. 24. Receptor cell of the pike utricle after centrifugation at 10 g for 10 min. Presynaptic mitochondria (M), with its middle portion adjoining the presynaptic membrane (PM) ( × 90,000)

experimental effects. This fact, in our opinion, constitutes convincing morphological proof that the mitochondrial apparatus is involved in the conducting function
of a nervous impulse. This phenomenon is also supported by cytochemical
results obtained with the same research objects.

The endogenous dehydrogenase activity, which reflects the total activity of
dehydrogenases and associated endogenous substrates and coenzymes, is clearly
apparent both in mitochondria of receptor cells and in nerve fibers, in button-
shaped nerve endings, and in a particularly striking manner in the nerve calyces
encompassing type-I cells. At the same time, in addition to large mitochondria,
which are readily visible in the light microscope, a weak diffuse activity can
also be detected over the entire cytoplasm and axoplasm. The endogenous dehydrogenase activity is particularly well expressed in the receptor cells and nerve
endings of reptiles and birds. As can be established visually, prolonged and
multiple experimental effects result in a clearcut decline in the endogenous
dehydrogenase activity in swollen mitochondria of receptor cells and nerve end-

ings. As a rule, in nerve endings such effects were seen to produce migration and longitudinal redistribution of mitochondria towards the periphery.

Investigation of succinate dehydrogenase in mitochondria of receptor cells and nerve endings of the utricle revealed an extraordinarily high activity of this enzyme. In animals in a state of relative rest, the enzymic activity of succinate dehydrogenase can be detected in rod-shaped or granular mitochondria of receptor cells and nerve endings (Fig. 25A). When subjected to experimental acceleration, mitochondria form characteristic clusters in the apical portion of the cell body over the nucleus, mainly in the region of the nerve calyx, where it is difficult under the light microscope to distinguish between the cellular cytoplasm and the neuroplasm of the nerve terminal (Fig. 25A). Visually, the enzymic activity in mitochondria of receptor cells and nerve endings of the utricle, especially in reptiles and birds, is exceptionally high. In view of their small size and large number, the mitochondria merge when seen under the light microscope to form a continuous silhouette that reproduces the outlines of nerve fibers and cup-shaped terminals, which are dyed a bright blue by formazan deposited in the mitochondria. However, a noticeable decline in the enzymic activity of succinate dehydrogenase is observed after two or three exposures to an experimental acceleration effect. At the same time, at the cell periphery and in the synapse region, the swollen mitochondria (as observed under the light microscope) change their orientation and line up in rows (Fig. 25B). This behavior apparently corresponds to the adjoining of mitochondria to the presynaptic membrane, as observed under the electron microscope.

A study of the activity of lactico dehydrogenase, malico dehydrogenase and alcohol dehydrogenase has shown that the above enzymes are also located in mitochondria of receptor cells and nerve endings in the inner ear utricle of vertebrates. Experimental effects as a rule somewhat reduced the activity of these enzymes.

From the cytochemical results thus obtained, we can see that the activity of dehydrogenase in mitochondria of receptor cells and nerve endings is quite high, particularly in the synaptic region. In response to experimental effects mitochondria not only change their position in space by moving close to the presynaptic membrane, but also exhibit a change in the activity of dehydrogenases located in the mitochondria. This fact no doubt reflects the special role played by synaptic mitochondria in the conduction of a nervous impulse.

In experimental animals subjected to the effect of radial acceleration changes were observed, not only in mitochondria, but also in synaptic vesicles which, as pointed out earlier, contain acetylcholine. Swollen or depleted synaptic vesicles, or their "shadows" which had apparently already ejected their contents into the intersynaptic cleft, appeared in the synaptic region in the vicinity of the presynaptic membrane and synaptic rods. Isolated swollen or depleted synaptic vesicles of irregular shape were also observed in the cytoplasm of the nerve terminal. In regard to the pictures purporting to show the migration of such vesicles through the synaptic membranes, described for the first time by DE ROBERTIS (1958), the vesicles were apparently observed in isolated cases at places where the synaptic membranes are thinner or form folds, when the cross-section plane underwent a change. Such events were not observed on broad elongated

A

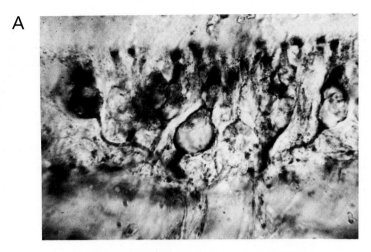

B

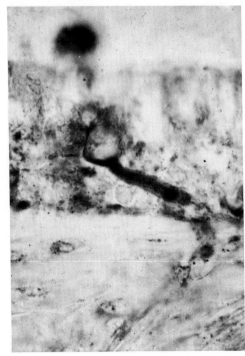

Fig. 25 A and B. Activity of succinic dehydrogenase in mitochondria of type-I receptor cells and in cup-shaped nerve endings of the utricle of the land tortoise (VINNIKOV, 1967a). A. State of relative rest; B. after centrifugation (18 periods of 20 revolutions each, at a velocity of 40 rpm with 10 sec stops between periods) Micrograph, eyepiece 10; immersion, objective 60

synaptic membranes with a clearly apparent intersynaptic cleft. For this reason, the question concerning the passage of synaptic vesicles through synaptic membranes in our objects is left open for the time being.

It is possible that the adjoining of mitochondria to the presynaptic membrane would facilitate the supply of energy for the processes of electrogenesis associated with the transmission of nervous impulses in the synapse region. It is also possible that the fact that mitochondria lie close to cell membranes and that the activity of mitochondrial enzymes varies are both phenomena of a more general character, and that they reflect processes involving autoregulation of energy consumption by the cell in one or another of its territorial portions. Whether this is so or not is a question which other investigations must clarify. At present we can only conclude that, in addition to a cholinergic and adrenergic mechanisms, the participation of an oxidative Krebs cycle, oxidative phosphorylation and electron transfer, associated with mitochondria, is also necessary for the transmission of a nervous impulse in the synapse region, at least in the receptor cells studied here. It is possible that these energy systems interact with each other in the synaptic region.

## 4. Ephaptic (Electrogenous) Synapses

Although there can be no doubt that synaptic transmission operates through mediators in both the nervous system and receptor cells of the sensory organs, data have recently been published, in particular on the lower vertebrates, which force us to admit the validity of previously stated assumptions (ARVANITAKI, 1942; ARVANITAKI and CHALANOZITIS, 1949) concerning the possibility of an electrogenous-ephaptic transmission of excitatory and inhibitory synaptic phenomena. The structural and functional organization of electrogenous synapses is relatively simple, since it naturally lacks any mechanisms associated with mediators. In electrogenous synapses, electron microscopy shows the presence of two closely adjoining membranes, which together form a complex about 140 Å thick, i.e. not exceeding the total thickness of both membranes (BENNET et al., 1967; PAPPAS and BENNET, 1966a, 1966b). Following permanganate fixation, an intermediate line can be observed between these membranes at the point where they are in close contact with each other; when other types of fixation are used, this line is frequently not seen. The electrophysiological and morphological properties of such a close membrane connection demand a special study. In certain species of polychaeta and crustaceans the nerve stems contain giant axons, subdivided into segments by cross partitions. Impulses are propagated along these segments in any direction at a comparatively high velocity (ECCLES, 1966), so that the partitions do not exert any significant effect on longitudinal current movement along the central part of giant fibers (BULLOCK, 1945). In the electron microscope, the membranes of each segment are seen to lie very close to each other, so that the total thickness of the partition is approximately 200 Å (HAMA, 1959, 1962). Electrogenous synapses, formed by bridges between neurons, have a similar structure (PAPPAS, 1968). In these synapses, however, symmetrically distributed small vesicles can be observed, which apparently are formed at the expense of tubules of the endoplasmic reticulum. Electrogenous synapses were studied in special experiments where propionate or acetate was substituted for chlorides in the physiological solution. Under these conditions, an increase was soon observed in the number of junctions between segments, accompanied by a divergence (drawing apart) of the membranes, which allows Schwann's cell processes to penetrate into the spaces (PAPPAS, 1968). When the tissues were immersed in a normal solution of chlorides, the picture became normal and returned to its original state, both in its morphological and electrophysiological expression. This shows that electrogenous synapses are flexible and that their properties can easily change depending upon the conditions present.

In some cases electrogenous and mediator transmission appear to be combined within the same synapse. When an isolated presynaptic fiber forms a very extensive synaptic contact with the mediator synapse, a considerable portion of the electric current generated by the presynaptic impulse can pass through the postsynaptic element and can stimulate it in the same manner as in segmental synapses. Thus, both orthodromic and antidromic electrical transmission are observed in the large cup-shaped synapses of the chick ciliary ganglion (MARTIN and PILAR, 1963a, 1963b). The functional significance of this dual transmission was determined by recording the double junction potential in the postganglionic nerve stem with intervals of about 2 msec between components (MARTIN and PILAR, 1963b).

Cup-shaped synapses are found around type-I receptor cells in the inner ear utricle of higher vertebrates, which, as was stated above, nevertheless possess all the characteristics of mediator transmission and are very similar to the synaptic structures of the ciliary ganglion in birds (DE LORENZO, 1960; SZENTÁGOTHAI, 1963; D'YACHKOVA and HAMORI, 1967; SMIRNOV, 1967). We can assume by analogy that the synaptic cleft in these synapses has a much greater shunting conductivity and that electrical transmission in these synapses must be noneffective (DE LORENZO, 1960; SZENTÁGOTHAI, 1963). HAMILTON in his study (1968) considered cup-shaped synapses of type-I cells to be not only chemical but also electrogenous synapses. However, we can agree with ECCLES (1966) that it is still not known whether electric conduction is a feature of the cup-shaped structure only and whether it is indeed absent in other synapses.

Along with an excitatory function, electrogenous synapses may also perform an inhibitory function. Thus, detailed investigations involving the use of intra- and extracellular recording of the activity of Mauthner cells with the aid of microelectrodes inserted at specific locations have shown that the activation of certain synapses in these cells creates a depolarizing current that acts upon the axon hillock to cause inhibition of the Mauthner cell (FURUKAWA and FURSHPAN, 1963).

According to ECCLES (1966), synapses with electrogenous transmission generally have a high reliability factor in the conduction of impulses and are characterized by rapid action, since electrical synaptic transmission does not differ greatly from transmission along a continuous nerve fiber. Further investigations are necessary to show whether electrogenous synapses are found between the receptor cells of sense organs and their associated neurons.

## 5. Conclusion

The above review shows that there are no basic structural, cytochemical and functional differences whatsoever between synapses connecting receptor cells with neurons and neurons with each other. In regard to synaptic transmission, the receptor cell acts like a neuron. The receptor cells transmit information, encoded in the form of a nervous impulse, basically by means of a cholinergic or adrenergic trans-synaptic mediator mechanism. This mechanism is closely associated with a general cellular oxidative system, concentrated in the mitochondria, which supplies macroergs as a result of ATP cleavage by ATPase. An electrogenous method of synaptic transmission is also possible. However, since the information encoded in each sense organ is different, we are inclined to believe that every synapse will also have its own individual, structural, cytochemical and functional characteristics.

# Chapter IV

# Vision

## 1. Introduction

The evolution of the visual cell in animals is striking in both the parallelism and divergence of its structural, cytochemical and functional organisation. The visual cell (photoreceptor) is always equipped with a flagellum (cilium) or microvilli which, moreover, serve as receptor antennae. EAKIN (1962, 1963, 1966, 1968) distinguishes two lines of evolution of photoreceptors: 1. ciliate or flagellate receptors, in which the photoreceptor plasma membrane develops at the expense of modified cilia or flagella; 2. rhabdome photoreceptors, in which photoreceptor membranes develop at the expense of microvilli independently of cilia. Eakin assigns to the first (flagellate or ciliate) group the photoreceptors of Coelenterata, Ctenophora, Chaetognata, Echinodermata, Protochordata and Vertebrata. He assigns to the second (rhabdome) group of photoreceptors those of Protozoa, flat worms, annelids, molluscs, arthropods, onichophora and rotifers. It is not possible to say at this time whether this zoological classification will prove correct. In some species of molluscs (e.g. the bicuspid scallop *Pecten*) photoreceptors develop at the expense of the growth of the membranes of the flagellum with which the photoreceptor cells of both the distal and proximal parts of the retina are equipped (BARBER, EVANS, and LAND, 1967). This applies to annelids as well; for instance, in Polychaeta *(Branchioma vesiculosum)* the membrane of the photoreceptor cell has a flagellate origin (LAWRENS and KRAUSE, 1965). Many more examples could be given. What strikes us as important, however, is that the photoreceptor cells of the eye, like those of other sense organs, have a common origin, i.e. they originate in a cell equipped with a flagellum or microvilli (VINNIKOV, 1964, 1965a, 1965b, 1966a, 1966b, 1967a, 1967b, 1968, 1969, 1970). Moreover, they also have in common the chemical nature of the photosensitive molecules that enter into the composition of the photoreceptor membranes of a wide variety of animals possessing both the "flagellate" and "rhabdome" type of eye. In both cases the photoreceptor membrane contains a visual pigment (rhodopsin), the molecules of which interact with photons, the photon being a quantum of light energy.

Thus, the process of evolution of the visual cell must be considered from several aspects: 1. as the molecular evolution of the visual pigment itself—rhodopsin—whether the photoreceptors have developed from modified flagella or from microvilli; 2. as the evolution of the subcellular organization of photoreceptor membranes of the visual cell among various types of animals; 3. finally, as the evolution of the retina and the eye as a whole, a subject not covered in this book.

## 2. Molecular Evolution of the Visual Pigment

The molecular evolution of the visual pigment, in fact, the origin of photoreception in animals, has links with photosynthesis in plants. Both photoreception and photosynthesis take place within a common, rather narrow band of electro-

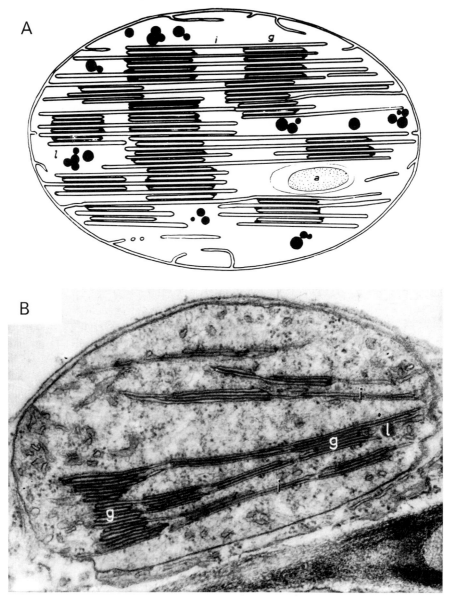

Fig. 26 A and B. A. Ultrastructural organization of a chloroplast. Diagram (BUVAT, 1963). B. electron micrograph (× 30,000). *g* lamellae; *i* inter-lamellar sectors; *l* extra-lamellar lipid globules; *a* starch grain

magnetic vibrations of wavelength 350—700 nm. There is also a striking similarity in the ultrastructural organization and the presence of common biological chemical substances in the photosensitive membranes of plants and animals.

Let us consider this statement in somewhat greater detail. The chloroplasts of plants are known to be small disk-like bodies measuring 1—10 μm which change their size and structure depending on the illumination (PARKER and SIEGENTHALER, 1966) (Fig. 26). They are covered with a sheath and inside is a system of ordered double membranes, or disks. The disks are surrounded by a granular matrix containing small vesicles. Following osmium fixation, light grains of starch are frequently observed between the disks. In contrast to lower plants, membrane disks in higher plants form thickenings or grains. Grains are stacks of disks of more or less the same size (about 1 μm in diameter). In the dark, the disks are oval in shape and the ratio of their axes is (4.4:2.9) 1.5 αα, whereas in the light they change shape and this ratio becomes (4.8:1.3) 3.7 αα (PARKER and SIEGENTHALER, 1966). The grains have a globular structure and consist of paracrystalline particles or quantosomes (PARK, 1966) that can be isolated as a separate fraction. Quantosomes were found to be particles flattened at the poles, resembling ellipsoids with axes 100—200 Å long and consisting of four or more subunits (PARK and BIGGINS, 1964).

Chloroplasts contain (calculated as dry matter) approximately 50% protein, 35% lipids and 7% pigments (DAVIES, GIOVANELLI, and REES, 1964). We think particular attention should be paid to their pigments. Chloroplast pigments belong to two basic groups, namely chlorophylls and carotenoids (Fig. 27). Chlorophyll is present in normal green leaves in much larger amounts than carotenoids, the ratio sometimes being as high as 5:1. Chlorophyll is a magnesium-containing porphyrin compound. In higher plants, chlorophyll *a* and chlorophyll *b* are distinguished. Carotenoids are yellow or red pigments of the aliphatic or alicyclic series. Among the large series of carotenoids, β-carotene is of special significance and also to some extent its isomer α-carotene. Carotenoids are formed from isoprene residues (usually eight). Series of conjugated double bonds form a chromophorous system of carotenoids. Hydrocarbon chains with conjugated double bonds are called polyenes. The $C=C$ bond in polyenes is 1.35 Å long (FREY-WYSSLING and MÜHLETHALER, 1965). The length of the polyene chain also depends on the configuration of the double bonds, which can be of *cis* or *trans* type (Fig. 28). With the addition of each $C_2$ group the chain is lengthened in the *trans* configuration by approximately 2.4 Å and in the *cis* configuration by approximately 2.0 Å. Thus, the *cis* configuration makes the chain considerably shorter. Carotenoids are usually all-*trans* chains so, considering that the chain is linear and consists of successive conjugated double bonds (~2.4 Å per bond) and two terminal half-rings about 3 Å in diameter, we can calculate that chains are usually of the order of 30 Å long. Carotenoids are capable of isomerization, i.e. they can change their configuration.

Both chlorophyll and carotenoids are believed to be located in grain membranes, where they are bound to proteins and lipids (Fig. 29). Photosynthesis occurs in the chloroplasts, and it is significant that it takes place in the morphobiological globular subunits of these membranes, namely in the quantosomes or their aggregates (PARK, 1966).

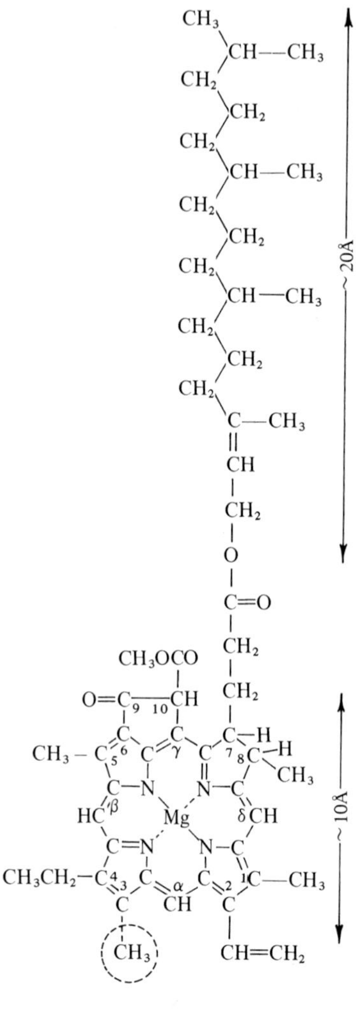

Fig. 27 I and II. Chemical structures of chloroplast pigments (FREY-WYSSLING and MÜHLETHALER, 1965). I chlorophyll; II β-carotene

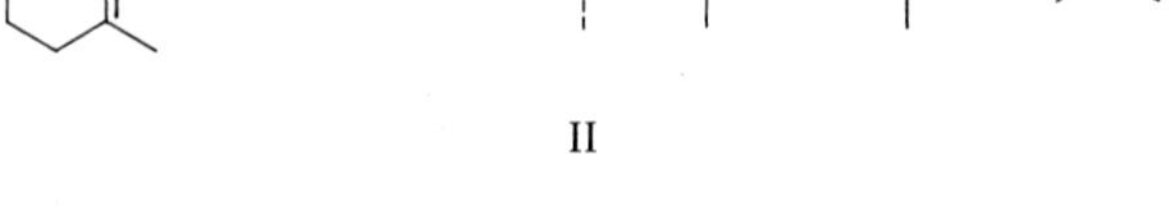

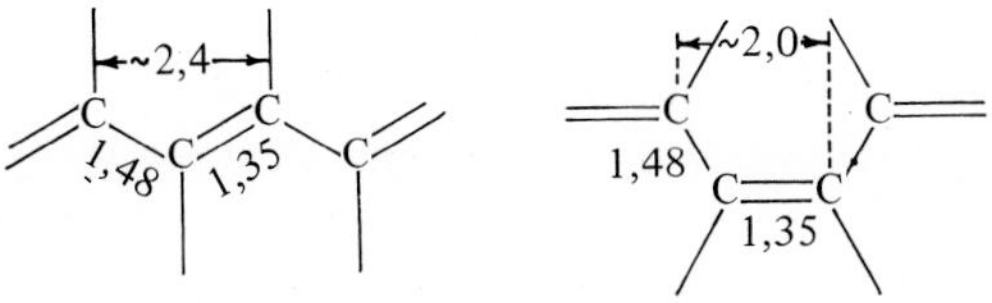

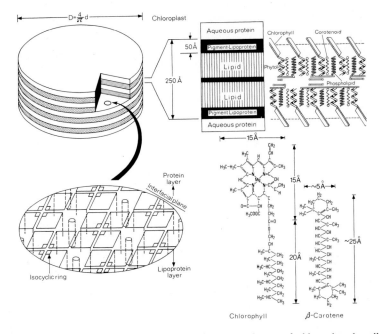

Fig. 28.  Increase in chain length depending upon the configuration of double bonds (FREY-WYSSLING and MÜHLETHALER, 1965). *1* trans-configuration; *2* cis-configuration

Fig. 29. Diagram of the molecular organization of the membrane of chloroplast lamellae. The water-soluble protein contains one cytochrome molecule for every 300—400 chlorophyll molecules (WOLKEN, 1963a)

The process of photosynthesis in plants is expressed by the empirically derived equation:

$$CO_2 + H_2O \xrightarrow{\text{light}} CH_2O + O; \quad \Delta \mathring{g} = 115 \text{ cal.}$$

This highly endoenergetic reaction is triggered by absorption of light energy. This energy accumulates in carbohydrates and other reduced compounds and can then be used in the form of ATP for the process of respiration and phosphorylation, or it can be directly converted into mechanical energy. The conversion of energy in chloroplasts is characterized by a very high rate.

In higher plants photosynthesis proceeds most effectively during light absorption by chlorophyll *a*. The role of chlorophyll *b* and other accompanying pigments has not been fully clarified. It is assumed that only energy absorbed by chlorophyll *a* can be used directly for photosynthesis, and that all other pigments transfer the energy they absorb to chlorophyll *a*.

The structural peculiarities of carotenoids (conjugated chains of alternating single and double bonds) lead us to believe that they are able to transfer electrons and therefore can participate in the transfer of electrons during photosynthesis (DINGLE and LUCY, 1965). Consequently, carotenoids in plants function both as photon receptors and as transmitters of the light energy absorbed by them. By way of idioadaptation in the process of evolution, this function of carotenoids was utilized by animals. Herbivorous animals, though unable to synthesize carotenoids, absorb them with their food and convert them to vitamin A (A$_1$ or A$_2$)[1]. Vitamin A is formed in the animal organism (liver) by breaking the carotenoid chain in half and adding water. Alpha- and β-carotenes differ in the structure of one of their terminal rings; because of this fact, two vitamin A molecules are obtained from β-carotene (diploid form) but only one from α-carotene.

The function of vitamin A in the organism is complex. For instance, we know that it is essential for the differentiation and maintenance of the structure of a ciliated cell. Differentiation of ciliated epithelium can be induced by the action of vitamin A on the stratified squamous epithelium. When the supply of vitamin A ceases the opposite transformation takes place and the ciliated epithelium is transformed into squamous epithelium (JACKSON and FELL, 1963). Apparently, vitamin A exerts a basic and direct effect on cell membranes; it also causes hemolysis of erythrocytes by dissolving their plasma membrane (DINGLE and LUCY, 1965). Addition of vitamin A to fibroblasts in tissue culture causes degranulation and swelling of the endoplasmic reticulum, the Golgi apparatus and the mitochondria. Isolated mitochondria also swell in the presence of vitamin A, but this swelling does not depend on respiration since it is inhibited by vitamin E (DINGLE and LUCY, 1965). Enzymes are liberated from lysosomes under the action of vitamin A. Vitamin A deficiency is accompanied by reduced synthesis of mucopolysaccharides (DINGLE and LUCY, 1965).

In the process of evolution, vitamin A came to occupy a very special place in the process of photoreception in animals, where it continues to perform in a very original way the same role of receptor and energy transmitter that its predecessors, the carotenoids, apparently performed earlier in the grains and quantosomes of plant chloroplasts. Some authors believe that vitamin A, being a carotenoid, undergoes a structural change on exposure to light and, by taking part in electron transfer, may be responsible for visual cell stimulation (JAHN, 1963).

Vitamin A accumulates in the pigment layer of the retina and undergoes oxidation, i.e. is converted into the aldehyde retinene or retinal (Fig. 30). It then enters into the composition of the photoreceptor membranes of the visual cells, where it is chemically bound to a special protein, opsin, a protein mutation developing only in animal visual cells. Thus, retinene acts in the rhodopsin molecule as a prosthetic group—i.e. chromophore—in relation to opsin, and the molecule of rhodopsin can be referred to as heterogeneous since it originates genetically from two different sources.

---

[1] Vitamin A$_1$ has been named retinol and vitamin A$_2$ 3-dehydroretinol (J. Amer. Chem. Soc., *82*, 5575—5584, 1960).

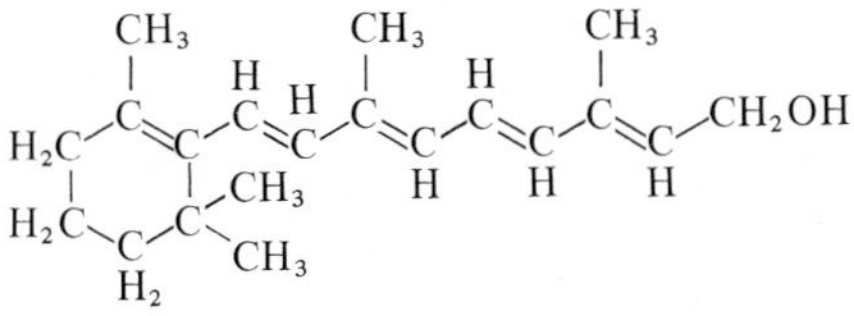

Vitamin $A_1$, $C_{19}H_{27}CH_2OH$
Retinene$_1$,  $C_{19}H_{27}CHO$:

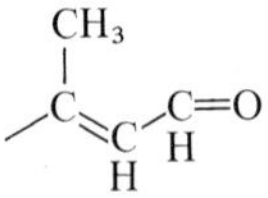

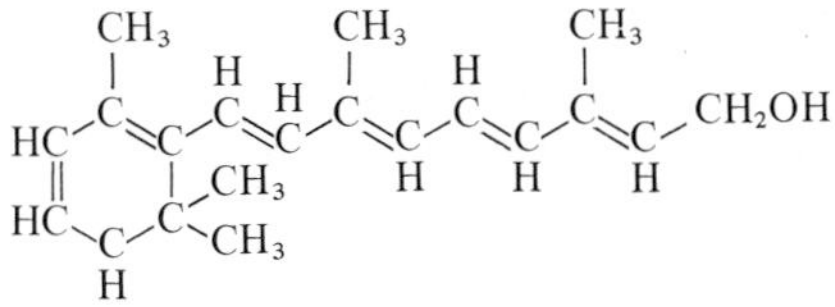

Vitamin $A_2$, $C_{19}H_{25}CH_2OH$
Retinene$_2$,  $C_{19}H_{25}CHO$:

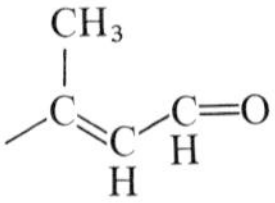

Fig. 30. Structural formulas of vitamin $A_1$ (retinol) and retinene$_1$ (retinal), and of vitamin $A_2$ (3-dehydroretinol) and retinene$_2$ (3-dehydroretinal) (WALD, 1960)

It should be emphasized that formation of a chemical bond between vitamin A aldehyde, retinal, and the protein molecule of opsin is possible only when the retinal is "twisted", i.e. is present in the *cis* form. This configuration, which is possible only in the dark, allows retinal to "slot itself" into an appropriate "recess" of the protein molecule (opsin); in the light, under the influence of photon energy, the chromophore "straightens", i.e. *trans* isomerization takes place, and as a result it no longer fits into the "recess" of opsin. The withdrawal of retinal is accompanied by the rupture of its bonds with opsin; this, as we shall see below, is the beginning of the stimulation of the visual cell. At the same time, bleaching of rhodopsin takes place. WALD (1960) has suggested that, should we reach the most distant planet and find there animals endowed with vision, the process would no doubt be based on a visual pigment containing a carotenoid chromophore of the vitamin A type.

## 3. Function of Rhodopsin

Let us now examine in greater detail the molecular structure of rhodopsin and its changes under the conditions of photoreception. Rhodopsin is the basic component of the photoreceptor membranes of visual cells. For example, in the outer segment of frog rod it comprises about 10% of the wet weight or 35% of the dry weight (HUBBARD, 1954a), and in the cattle rod 3.6% and 13%, respectively. Spectroscopic investigations have shown that frog rod contains $3.10^9$ and cattle rod $4.10^6$ molecules of rhodopsin (WALD et al., 1963). The diameter of the molecule is apparently close to 40—50Å (WALD, 1964; BLASIE *et al.*, 1965). According to HELLER (1969) the molecular weight of cattle rhodopsin is 27,707, while in the rat it is 27,769, and in the frog 28,029. According to the recent data the molecular weight of rhodopsin in the cattle rod is 40,000 (DAEMAN *et al.*, 1972). Rhodopsin was first isolated from the visual cells of the retina 100 years ago with the aid of bile salts (KÜHNE, 1878a, 1878b). According to KRINSKY (1958), rhodopsin is a lipoprotein which he calculated to have a molecular weight of 32,000, only 18,000 of which can be attributed to the protein moiety, i.e. opsin. The molecule of the visual pigment, named rhodopsin by KÜHNE (1878a, 1878b), regardless of the species of animal in whose photoreceptor cells it is found, consists of the chromophore 11-*cis*-retinene$_1$ (or retinene$_2$), the aldehyde of 11-*cis*-vitamin A$_1$ (or A$_2$) bound with the specific colorless protein, opsin. Formation of this complex results in its coloration.

Combinations of retinal or dehydroretinal and opsin constitute the visual pigments of photoreceptors in vertebrates (rods and cones). It should be pointed out that two forms of opsin can be distinguished in vertebrates: scotopsin (the opsin of rods) and photopsin (the opsin of cones) (WALD, 1960).

Rhodopsin exhibits two spectral absorption peaks: a protein peak in the ultraviolet region at 278 nm and a basic peak near 500 nm. The exact position of the absorption peak of the pigment in the visible region varies somewhat according to animal species. For example, in a number of species of freshwater fish the absorption peak is strongly shifted into the long-wave region, due to the presence of 3-dehydroretinal in the visual pigment. This pigment has been named porphyropsin (absorption peak at 522 nm). In migratory fish the visual pigment is a mixture of rhodopsin and porphyropsin (WALD, 1960). A gradual substitution of porphyropsin by rhodopsin has been observed in amphibia, e.g. during the development of photoreceptors in the tadpole. Special visual pigments are also found in cones: iodopsin (absorption peak at 562 nm) bound with retinal (WALD, 1960; BROWN and SMITH, 1954—1955), and cyanopsin bound with 3-dehydroretinal (absorption peak at 620 nm) (WALD and BROWN, 1953). In addition to the four visual pigments mentioned above, a large number of other pigments with different absorption peaks have been identified (DARTNALL, 1953, 1957; BRIDGES, 1962; DARTNALL and LYTHOGOE, 1964; HARA and HARA, 1965, 1967, 1968; HARA and TAKEUCHI, 1967; and others). The difference appears to be related to the molecular structural characteristics of opsins.

All light-sensitive proteins are chromoproteids with the polyene chromophore (retinal) bound to the protein. We have already pointed out that the attachment of opsin to retinal in the dark occurs only if the retinal is present in 11-*cis* configuration (Fig. 31). Even slight changes in the structure of the chromophore will prevent the formation of rhodopsin. For example, if the polyene chain is lengthened or the position of the terminal double bonds in retinene is changed, rhodopsin does not form. Owing to these characteristics of retinals, the polypeptide chains in opsin occupy a definite position and this contributes to the stability of the rhodopsin molecule as a whole. Disruption of the bond between retinene and opsin makes the opsin unstable (BOWNDS and WALD, 1965).

The bond between opsin and retinene is effected according to the protonated Schiff-base type by interaction of the aldehyde group in retinene with the amino group in one of the amino acids of the opsin (COLLINS, 1953; MORTON and

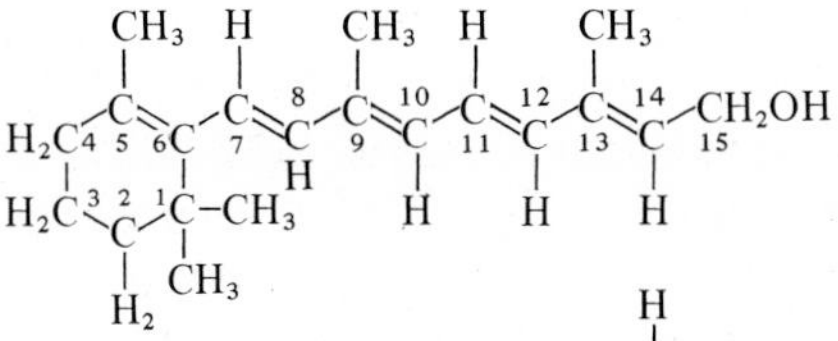

all-*trans* Vitamin A

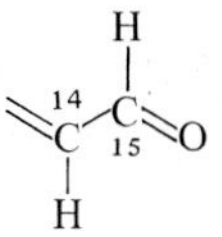

Retinene

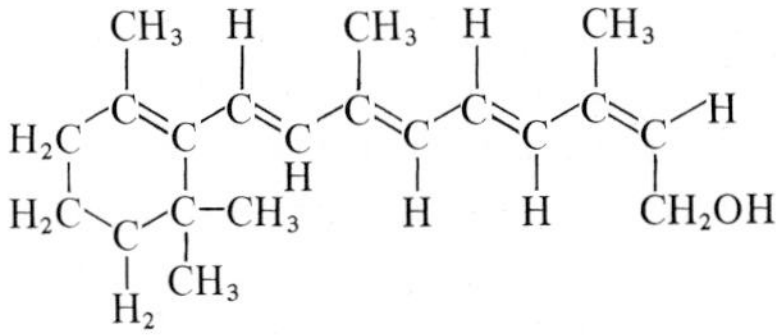

13-*cis* (*neo*-a)

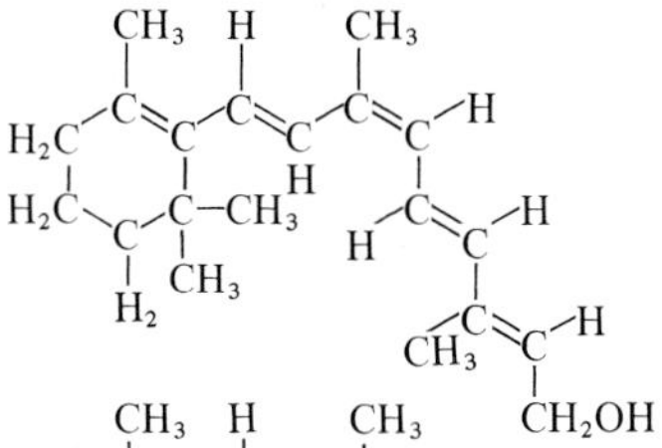

9-*cis* (*iso*-a)

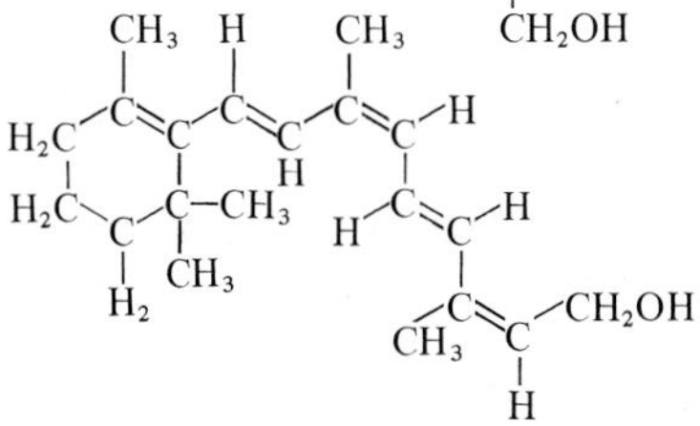

9,13-*dicis* (*iso*-b)

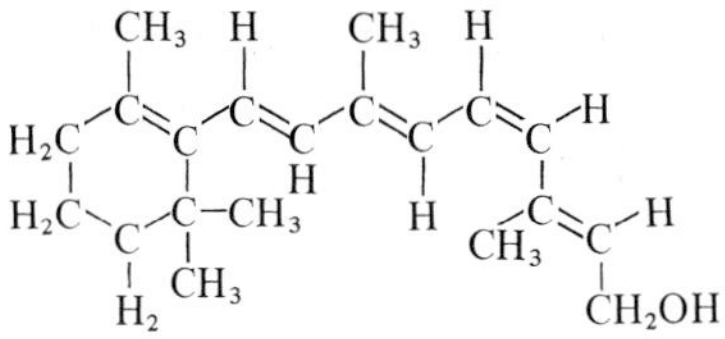

11-*cis* (*neo*-b)

Fig. 31. Geometric isomers of vitamin A and retinene (retinal). A similar series of structures, differing only by possessing an extra double bond in the 3, 4 position, represents vitamin $A_2$ (3-dehydroretinol) and $retinene_2$ (3-dehydroretinal). The upper four structures cannot combine with opsin; only the lowermost cis-isomer can combine with opsin in an unhindered manner and give rise to all visual pigments (WALD, 1960)

PITT, 1955; AKHTAR, BLOSSER, and DEWHURST, 1965; PESKIN and LOVE, 1965; ISHIGAMI, MAEDA, and MISHINA, 1966). It has been shown that opsin combines with retinal at the expense of the ε-amino group of lysine (HUBBARD, BOWNDS, and YOSHIZAWA, 1965). This bond, however, has a number of specific characteristics. For example, rhodopsin is stable over a wide pH range (4—10), which indicates stability of the proton in the nitrogen of the Schiff base and a very high pK (greater than 10) (BOWNDS and WALD, 1965).

Later reports have stated that in the dark retinal is bound in the Schiff-base linkage not with the ε-amino group of lysine in opsin but with the lipid phosphatidylethanolamine present in rhodopsin (ABRAHAMSON and WIESENFELD, 1969; DAEMAN and BONTING, 1968; DE PONT, DAEMAN, and BONTING, 1968; POINCELOT et al., 1969).

When opsin combines with retinal, a shift of the absorption peak into the long-wave region is observed; this seems to be connected with the presence of an additional bond, the nature of which has not yet been determined (DARTNALL, 1957; AKHTAR, BLOSSER, and DEWHURST, 1965).

Under the action of light, absorption of a photon by the rhodopsin molecule causes the heterogeneous molecule of rhodopsin to break down into retinal and opsin. The absorption of the photon results in the isomerization of the 11-cis form of retinal into the all-trans form; this is accompanied by a reduction of about 2 kcal/mole in the free energy. In turn, the opsin also undergoes a change in configuration (conformation). In this case, the pink color of rhodopsin rapidly turns yellowish and then becomes colorless. The disintegration of the molecule passes through a number of intermediate stages which are very unstable at room temperature (Fig. 32A). The first product formed, pre-lumirhodopsin, is stable at temperatures below − 140 °C. In this case, a significant shift of the absorption peak into the long-wave region is observed (500—543 nm), and also an increase in absorption by a factor of 1.13 (YOSHIZAWA and WALD, 1963). When pre-lumirhodopsin is illuminated by light of long wavelength (about 600 nm), a reverse transition into rhodopsin or isorhodopsin (9-cis-retinal + opsin) can be achieved. As regards the opsin, it apparently undergoes a very slight change in its configuration at this stage.

At temperatures above − 140 °C pre-lumirhodopsin is converted in the dark into lumirhodopsin, which is stable up to − 40 °C. Lumirhodopsin is also a chromoproteid, containing all-trans retinal and its absorption peak is shifted into the short-wave region (497 nm). The activation energy of this reaction ranges between 10 and 12.5 kcal (GRELLMAN, LIVINGSTON, and PRATT, 1962; PRATT, LIVINGSTON, and GRELLMAN, 1964). On the basis of the low heat and entropy of activation, it is possible to say that insignificant conformational changes in the protein portion of rhodopsin occur at this stage (ABRAHAMSON and OSTROY, 1967; ETINGOF, 1967).

The next stage involves the conversion of lumirhodopsin into metarhodopsin, which is stable at temperatures below − 15 °C (HUBBARD, BOWNDS, and YOSHIZAWA, 1966). The spectrum of metarhodopsin is slightly shifted into the short-wave region (max. 478 nm), as compared with lumirhodopsin. This stage is characterized by a considerably greater activation energy, almost equal to values for heat denaturation, thus indicating significant conformational changes in the protein at this stage (HUBBARD, 1958). At temperatures above − 15 °C, metarhodopsin-I is converted into metarhodopsin-II, entering into a tautomeric equilibrium with the latter. This transition is accompanied by a significant shift of the absorption peak into the short-wave region (380 nm). At the same time there is loss of hydrogen by the group with pK 6.4 (possibly the imidazole group in the histidine residue of opsin) (MATTHEWS *et al.*, 1963). Apparently this reaction is also accompanied by a considerable change in the configuration of the opsin.

Thus, the successive breakdown of rhodopsin leads to the appearance of increasingly stable products, the absorption peak of which gradually shifts into the short-wave region (except for pre-lumirhodopsin) (WALD, 1965).

Considerable conformational shifts in the opsin occur along with changes in the retinal. Conversions of iodopsin in cones in the light and in the dark generally coincide with conversions of rhodopsin (Fig. 32 B) (HUBBARD, BOWNDS, and YOSHIZAWA, 1966). The conformational shifts in opsin during rhodopsin conversion are indicated by data on changes in the electrical conductivity of rhodopsin solutions in the course of its bleaching (HARA, 1963, 1964), by directly observed changes in absorption in the ultraviolet region of the spectrum (TAKAGI, 1963) and by changes in the optical rotatory dispersion during rhodopsin bleaching (HUBBARD, BOWNDS, and YOSHIZAWA, 1966). Under the action of light the molecule of opsin "unfolds", and its radius changes from 23 Å to 25.5 Å (HELLER, 1968).

Data on the amino acid composition of the opsin are also available (ABRAHAMSON and OSTROY, 1967; HELLER, 1969).

According to HELLER (1962) the following amino acids enter into the composition of rhodopsin in different animals (in moles of acid per mole of rhodopsin):

|               | Cattle | Rat | Frog |
|---------------|--------|-----|------|
| Lysine        | 10     | 10  | 10   |
| Histidine     | 4      | 4   | 4    |
| Arginine      | 6      | 6   | 6    |
| Cysteine      | 5      | 6   | 6    |
| Asparagine    | 15     | 16  | 15   |
| Methionine    | 8      | 9   | 9    |
| Threonine     | 17     | 18  | 16   |
| Serine        | 12     | 13  | 17   |
| Glutamine     | 21     | 21  | 20   |
| Proline       | 13     | 14  | 14   |
| Glycine       | 16     | 16  | 15   |
| Alanine       | 20     | 19  | 18   |
| Valine        | 20     | 18  | 18   |
| Isoleucine    | 13     | 13  | 15   |
| Leucine       | 20     | 20  | 19   |
| Tyrosine      | 11     | 11  | 13   |
| Phenylalanine | 19     | 18  | 18   |
| Tryptophan    | 5      | 4   | 4    |
| Glucosamine   | 3      | 3   | 3    |
| Neutral sugars | 3     | 3   | 3    |

The liberated retinal is reduced to retinol, both in the retina of vertebrates and in the eye of invertebrates (WALD and HUBBARD, 1949; ARDEN, 1954; GOLDSMITH and WARNER, 1964), the reduction being effected with the aid of the enzyme retinene reductase (WALD and HUBBARD, 1949). The source of the hydrogen for the reduction reaction is not $NAD \cdot H_2$ as WALD and HUBBARD

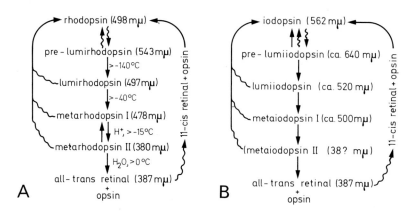

Fig. 32 A and B. Stages in the bleaching of the visual pigment. A. Bleaching of rhodopsin (MATTHEWS *et al.*, 1963). Photochemical reactions are denoted by wavy lines, thermal (dark) reactions by straight lines. B. Bleaching of iodopsin (HUBBARD *et al.*, 1965). The difference between the bleaching of iodopsin and rhodopsin consists in the reconversion (thermal) of pre-lumiiodopsin to iodopsin; moreover, metaiodopsin II has not yet been finally characterized

believed, but NADP·H$_2$ (FUTTERMAN, 1963). Vitamin A forms under light in the rat retina and disappears during dark adaption.

Resynthesis of rhodopsin in the retina occurs continuously both under light and in the dark by the reverse transformation of its nearest derivatives. Conversion of the all-*trans*-form of free retinal into a 11-*cis* isomer in light takes place with the aid of a special enzyme, retinene isomerase (HUBBARD, 1955, 1956). The course of this reaction in the dark is still not completely clear. It is assumed that in this case some special significance must be attributed to vitamin A, the conversion of which from the *trans* to the 11-*cis* isomer may take place during the etherification reaction (HUBBARD and DOWLING, 1962).

The renewal of proteins, including opsin, in the composition of disk membranes of cones and rods was investigated quantitatively by the radioautographic method under both the light microscope (DROZ, 1961, 1963) and the electron microscope (YOUNG, 1968, 1971; YOUNG and DROZ, 1968). A pulse of radioactive amino acid was given to an adult frog. The protein was synthesized in ribosomes of the ergastoplasm of photoreceptor cells in the region of what is called the myoid (Fig. 33). The newly synthesized protein, basically opsin, appeard to filter through the system of membranes of the Golgi apparatus. The label showed that a large portion of the protein in the rods had moved forward along mitochondria of the ellipsoid through the connecting cilium into the outer segment, where it was localized in the membranes of the basal disks. It was found that in the frog 36 disks are formed every day in red rods and 25 disks in green rods, an average of about 1.5 disks per hour (YOUNG, 1968, 1971). In cones, the new protein is distributed more or less uniformly throughout the entire outer segment, while new disks do not arise. The apical, "outworn" parts of outer segments, the phagosomes, can be found in the pigment epithelium where they are "dissolved" (YOUNG and DROZ, 1968).

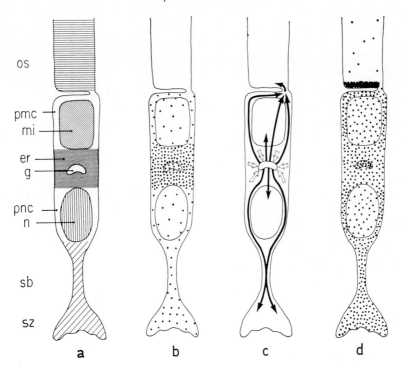

Fig. 33a—d. Diagram of protein biosynthesis in the rod of a frog (a—d), based on autoradiographic studies (YOUNG and DROZ, 1968). a Diagram of organization of frog's rod; *os* outer segment; *pmc* perimitochondrial cytoplasm; *mi* mitochondria; *er* ergastoplasm (myoid); *g* Golgi apparatus; *pnc* perinuclear cytoplasm; *n* nucleus; *sb* central process; *sz* synaptic zone. b Distribution of protein-bound radioactive label 10 min after injection of labeled amino acids; up to 80% of radioactivity is concentrated in the cytoplasm in the area of the so-called myoid; c Probable path of proteins (dark arrows) during their distribution in the cell, whereby the maximum radioactivity is observed in the area of basal disk membranes of the rod; d Distribution of labeled protein 8 hours after injection. At this stage, the labeled protein content in the basal disks is 20 times as great as in the ergastoplasm

The visual pigment is an integral component of the disk membranes of the outer segment, making up, as stated above, about 30% of their weight. It has been shown that, on the seventh day after introduction of labeled amino acids, the radioactive protein in the outer segments of the frog also includes rhodopsin (HALL, BOCK, and BACHARACH, 1968, 1969).

## 4. Development of the Visual Cell

It has been established with the light microscope that the development of the embryonic visual cell in the retina of the eye of vertebrates is associated with the flagellum or cilium and the adjoining basal bodies (LEBOUCQ, 1909; SEEFELDER, 1910; MANN, 1928; VINNIKOV, 1947). With the electron microscope it became possible to show how the membranes of outer segment disks in the photoreceptors of vertebrates arise as a result of the increasing folding and complexity of the plasma membrane of a cilium, but not by fusion or combining of vesicles (DE ROBERTIS, 1956; CARASSO, 1959; TOKUYASU and YAMADA, 1959; UENO, 1961; EAKIN, 1963; NILLSON, 1964a; GOVARDOVSKII and KHARKEEVICH, 1966a, 1966b).

One can detect the presence of remote phylogenetic connections between flagellate structures and photoreception, i.e. between locomotion and reception. Thus, among protists and members of the Phytoflagellata that exhibit photosynthetic activity, for example *Euglena* (WOLKEN, 1956), *Chromylina* (ROUILLER and FAURÉ-FRÉMIET, 1957), *Chlamydomonas* (SAGER and PALADE, 1957) and others, there is a spot located in the vicinity of the kinetosome of the flagella containing $9 \times 2 + 2$ fibrils; this spot consists of an accumulation of red pigment and is called the eyespot or stigma (Fig. 34). As is well known, a definite sensitivity to light together with the movement of the flagellum allows the protist to move to places where the intensity of illumination is optimal for the functioning of the chloroplasts. The stigma consists of ultramicroscopic vesicles or plates containing the carotenoid astacin which was first detected in the crab (Crustacea). Phytoflagellata exhibit a positive phototaxis in those regions of the spectrum which correspond to the absorption spectrum of the carotenoids.

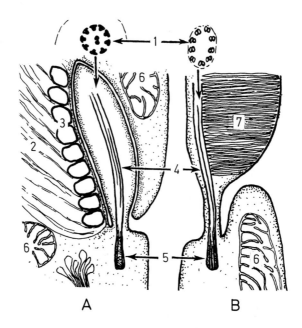

Fig. 34A and B. Structure of the stigma and rod in the retina of the eye (FAURÉ-FREMIÉT, 1961). A. Stigma (eye spot) of *Chromylina*. B. Connection between the outer and inner segments of the photoreceptor rod of vertebrates. *1* cross-sections of a *Chromylina* fibril bundle and a photoreceptor rod; *2 Chromylina* chloroplasts; *3* chambers of *Chromylina* eye spot; *4* fibril bundle; *5* basal body; *6* mitochondria; *7* disks of outer segment membrane (*3* and *7* contain a carotenoid pigment)

In *Chromylina* the pigment vesicles are formed along the ends of one of two large photosynthesizing plastids, namely chloroplast. Thus, the photosynthetic and photoreceptor functions are structurally connected in this protist. Thus we see that in protists, as well as in vertebrates and some other types of animals, light stimulation is transmitted with the aid of a flagellum or cilium; this was first pointed out by FAURÉ-FRÉMIET in 1961. This striking structural and functional analogy, however, is incomplete. In the retinal rod of vertebrates, for example, the photoreceptor membrane system is built into a cilium that has $9 \times 2 + 0$ fibriles; in *Chromylina* this system is bound to the plastid. It is difficult, however, to overestimate the importance of the fact that, both in protists and in the cells of multicellular organisms photoreception takes place with the aid of carotenoids bound to similar motile structures, namely flagella or cilia, of identical mechanochemical organization. It is clear that, from a biochemical and structural standpoint, photoreception had already evolved by natural selection in some protists, in which receptor and locomotor functions are already practically combined into a single system. It is possible that this organization was transmitted to multicellular organisms by autotrophic green or yellow-green flagellates (ERWIN and BLOCH, 1964; FREY-WYSSLING and MÜHLETHALER, 1965; IVANOV, 1968), or arose in certain types of animals in an independent or convergent manner.

Returning to the embryogenesis of the visual cell of vertebrates, it has since the advent of the electron microscope become possible to observe the development of all the complex structures of the visual cell. Thus, in vertebrates the outer segment disks develop at the expense of the plasma membrane coating the flagellum or cilium of the embryonic visual cell. According to data obtained in our laboratory on chicken embryos incubated for 8 to 10 days (GOVARDOVSKII and KHARKEEVICH, 1966a, 1966b) and on a 5 to 12 cm long ammocoete (GOVARDOVSKII, 1967), the future visual cells have an elongated shape and adhere tightly, attaching themselves with the aid of desmosomes to the pigment epithelium (Fig. 35). The connection to the pigment epithelium can vary, but it always remains a contact connection up to definitive stages. Numerous mitochondria are scattered through the entire cell but mainly around the nucleus. In the apical part of the cell is a centriole consisting of 9 pairs of tubules. Growing from the centriole is a flagellum or cilium with a diameter of 0.25 μm and a length of 1 μm, coated by a plasma membrane and penetrating deep into the pigment epithelium. The cilium consists of 9 pairs of peripheral fibrils; the two central fibrils are missing. At this stage, the future photoreceptors have a striking degree of ultrastructural organization, numerous, well-developed smooth and rough reticulum membranes and sectors of the Golgi apparatus. During the 12 to 13 days of incubation, the inner segment of the visual cell is formed. This region of the visual cell then becomes thicker, and all cellular mitochondria move into this region where they are later concentrated; these mitochondria can divide here at an intense rate by constriction (GOVARDOVSKII and TSIRULIS, 1969). The contiguous mitochondria together form an aggregate called the ellipsoid (Fig. 36) already detected under the light microscope. In birds, an oil droplet can be observed in the inner segments of rudiments of future cones; cells that do not contain this oil droplet apparently represent future rods. Thus, at this stage, there appears to be a difference between the

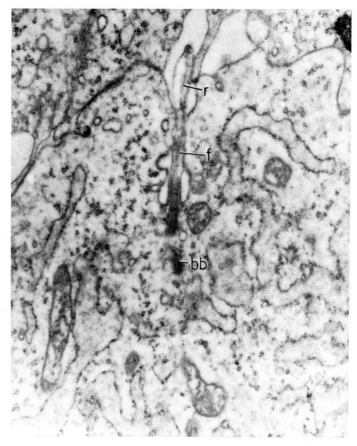

Fig. 35. Visual cell of a 10-day chick embryo (× 20,000) (GOVARDOVSKII and KHARKEEVICH, 1966a, 1966b). *f* flagellum; *r* fibrils; *bb* basal body

two types of visual cell. Oil droplets also develop in the inner segment of cones in reptiles, amphibians and ganoid fishes as well as birds. As in the photoreceptors of other vertebrates, in birds and cyclostomes (ammocoetes) the microvilli extend from the inner segment towards the pigment layer; these microvilli surround the flagellum and are later transformed into dendrites (Fig. 37). Their functional purpose is not clear. During this time, the number of cilium-carrying cells increases; cell length and the diameter of the distal end also increase to 1.5 and 0.35 μm, respectively. During these stages, connections begin to develop between the photoreceptor and bipolar cells; the intertwined and ramified processes of bipolar cells protrude into the basal part of the body of the photoreceptors directly below the nucleus; this is followed by the appearance of thickenings in the presynaptic membrane. The entire space between the nucleus and the cytoplasm becomes filled with synaptic vesicles. The long, axon-like processes of certain photoreceptors contain a cluster of microtubules, and between them are located vesicles resembling synaptic vesicles; the first synaptic plates appear at this stage. On the 19th day of incubation and during the first day of hatching the synapses appear fully differentiated (Fig. 38).

On the basis of a peculiar endoplasmic reticulum, a paraboloid develops in the cytoplasm (Fig. 39); it has the character of a reticulum, surrounded by glycogen granules about 150Å in diameter, soon increasing to 250Å. The sector corresponding to the myoid is located closer to the nucleus.

Development of the membrane of the outer-segment disks can be observed on the 13—15th day of incubation. The distal portion of the flagellum expands to a diameter of 1 µm and its plasma membrane forms numerous invaginations or folds (Fig. 40A). These invaginations form on different sides of the flagellum, and for this reason disk rudiments, both linked and unlinked to the outer membrane, can be observed on the same section. The rudiment of the outer segment is unsymmetrical in shape: flagellum fibrils branch out from basal bodies on one side, and no invaginations of the outer membrane are found on this side. From the start, the folds have a regular orientation perpendicular to the outer segment axis; the folds are about 120Å thick, approximately the same as the disks in differentiated photoreceptors. In the initial stage most invaginations of the plasma membrane form in the middle portion of the membrane. Later the outer segment rudiment rapidly lengthens, the number of folds increases, and folds arise along the entire length of the outer segment. In the ammocoete (see Fig. 40B) the development of photoreceptor disks also takes place as a result of growth of the plasma membrane of the flagellum, which acts as a "primer".

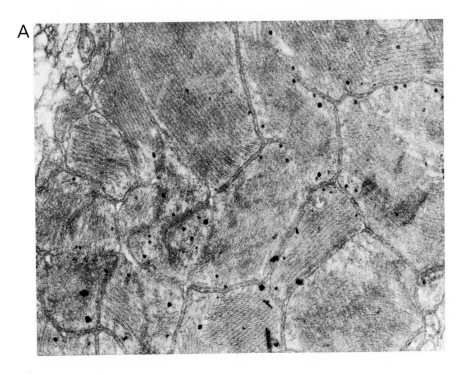

A

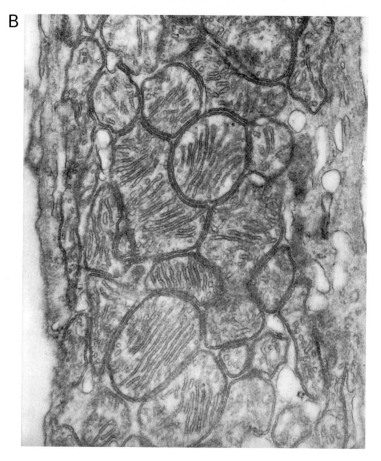

Fig. 36 A and B.  Mitochondria in the ellipsoid of (A) lamprey ( × 33,000) (GOVARDOVSKII and TSIRULIS, 1969), and (B) chicken ( × 45,000) (GOVARDOVSKII and KHARKEEVICH, 1965)

As noted above, in the definitive state formation of new rod disks is observed only at the base of the outer segment, and from here the disks, already in a finished form, move in a distal direction (YOUNG, 1968). The depth of the invaginations increases so that they occupy more than half the diameter of the outer segment, thereby forming disks. On the 18—19th day of incubation, the dimensions of the outer segment in many cells are the same as those of the segment in the adult animal. The disk membranes fill almost the entire cavity of the outer segment, but in chicks the final formation of this segment is delayed until long after hatching. At the same time, the rod disks lose their connection with the external plasma membrane, which persists only at the base of the outer segment. The connection of the cone disks with the external plasma membrane is preserved (Fig. 9B).

No differences whatsoever can be established in the structure of segment disks of rods and cones. With different fixation methods the disk membranes

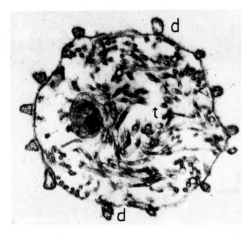

Fig. 37. Cross-section of the outer segment of a chick rod after hatching. Numerous tubules (*t*) can be seen, and the outer segment is surrounded by dendrites (*d*) ( × 55,000) (GOVARDOVSKII and KHARKEEVICH, 1967)

always exhibit constant structure and thickness (75 Å), both at the time of formation and during their subsequent development. The flagellar plasma membrane, which initially covers an area of 3 μm² in the chick embryo, increases to 4,000 to 8,000 μm² during days 4—5 of embryonic life, as a result of differentiation of the disk membranes (GOVARDOVSKII and KHARKEEVICH, 1966a, 1966b).

In our opinion, the increasing complexity in the organization of disk membranes, as well as their differentiation from the original plasma membrane of the flagellum in the embryonic visual cell, can be linked with the integration during these stages of the rhodopsin molecule into the structure of the membrane. During these stages rhodopsin can be extracted for the first time from outer segments and a retinogram can be obtained from the retina as a whole (COULOMBRE, 1961). If the above assumption is correct, the protein opsin must be synthesized in the photoreceptor cell during these early stages, while vitamin A from the liver reaches the pigment layer where it is oxidized into retinal (retinene). The combination of these molecules, i.e. the formation of the heterogeneous rhodopsin molecule in the original membrane ("primer") coating the flagellum is in our opinion what induces the appearance of folds, or disk membranes, in this membrane.

In order to verify this assumption, special experiments were set up in our laboratory. It has been shown that the embryonic retina of amphibians and birds can continue to develop for some time under tissue-culture conditions. Under such conditions typical photoreceptor cells can become differentiated to a certain extent in the growth zone (VINNIKOV, 1947). After a certain time, the photoreceptor cells lose their differentiated parts and begin to proliferate intensively. The extent and accuracy of their morphological differentiation obviously cannot be established with the light microscope. GOVARDOVSKII and KHARKEEVICH (1965), using the tissue-culture method and the electron microscope, followed the development of a chick embryo retinal receptor layer,

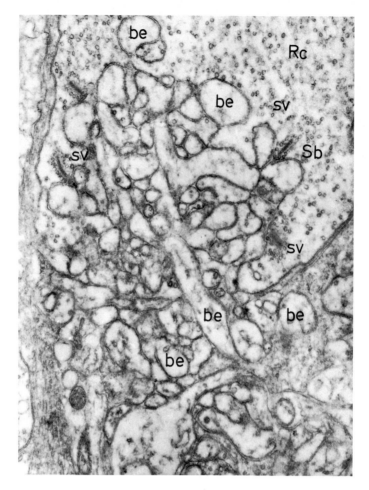

Fig. 38. Synaptic structures between photoreceptors and bipolars in a 1-day-old chick (× 30,000) (GOVARDOVSKII and KHARKEEVICH, 1965). *Sb* synaptic rods, surrounded by synaptic vesicles (*sv*); *be* bipolar terminals; *Rc* receptor cell

isolated on the 10th day of embryonic growth and separated from the pigment layer which supplies retinal. Under these conditions receptor cells developed, having a characteristic inner segment containing an accumulation of mitochondria, or ellipsoids, a flagellum with a cone-like extension grew out from the outer segment (Fig. 41). However, no folds developed in the disk membranes, i.e. there was no the outer segment. Rudiments of membranes or vesicles of irregular shape were observed only inside the matrix of the flagellum. Generally similar results were also obtained by other investigators under analogous culture conditions (HILD and CALLAS, 1967). In our view, the underdevelopment of the outer segment in tissue culture is probably due to disruption of the contact linkage between the embryonic photoreceptors and the pigment layer through which vitamin A is supplied. Vitamin A is necessary for synthesis of the aldehyde,

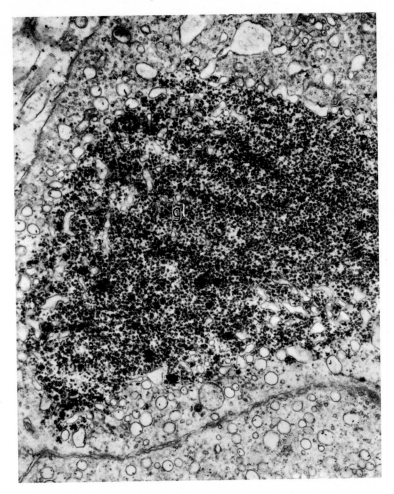

Fig. 39. Paraboloid of the frog's photoreceptor with extensive deposition of glycogen (*gl*) granules
(× 20,000) GOVARDOVSKII and KHARKEEVICH, 1965)

retinal, which enters into the composition of rhodopsin (Fig. 42). It is possible that the separation of the receptor and pigment layers disrupts the supply of components necessary for the formation of the heterogeneous rhodopsin molecule; consequently, processes involving the differentiation of outer-segment disk membranes cannot take place, although the primer (the plasma membrane of the flagellum) is available and the supply of the protein, opsin, synthesized by the cell itself, is also apparently maintained.

The above assumption can also be confirmed by special tests involving prolonged (10 months) vitamin-A deficiency in vertebrates (DOWLING and WALD, 1958, 1960; DOWLING and GIBBONS, 1961; EAKIN, 1964). When vitamin A is deficient in food, degeneration of disks in retinal rods and cones is observed (see Fig. 42), and the disk membranes are transformed into vesicles rather similar to those observed under tissue-culture conditions. The flagellum and its plasma membrane are preserved during prolonged vitamin-A deficiency, and when the supply of vitamin A is restored there is regeneration of the structure of the disk membranes, i.e. regeneration of the outer segment.

Thus, a comparison of observations on the development of embryonic photoreceptors under tissue-culture conditions and also of the changes induced in photoreceptors by vitamin-A deficiency in the organism reveals the structural significance of the formation of the heterogeneous rhodopsin molecule for the membrane in which it is localized, in this particular case the membrane of the photoreceptor disks. If some ingredient (for example, vitamin A) is not supplied from a known source, formation of the rhodopsin molecule and of the photoreceptor cell disk membrane, which is integrally linked to this molecule, is prevented.

In the course of development the rods are observed to have a recapitulation stage of cones (Fig. 9B), which is likely to testify, the fact that in vertebrates color vision precedes contour one. More complex structural differentiation of the rods seems to be connected to the peculiarities of their opsin.

A few words now about the development of photoreceptor structures in invertebrates, in particular insects, where photoreceptor membranes forming

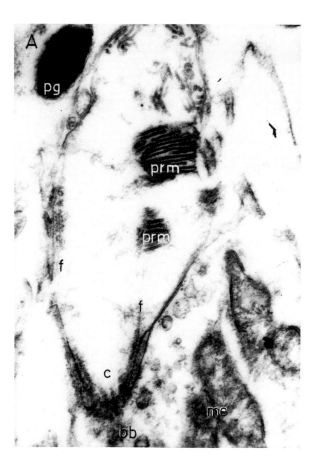

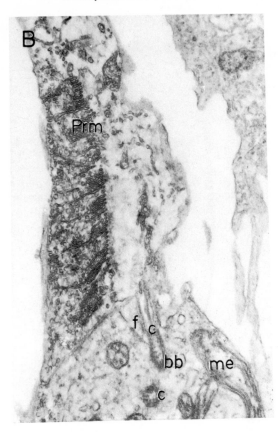

Fig. 40 A and B. Development of the outer segment of photoreceptors in (A) a chick embryo on the 13th day of incubation ( × 35,000) (GOVARDOVSKII and KHARKEEVICH, 1965), and (B) an 8.5 cm long ammocoete larva ( × 25,000) (GOVARDOVSKII and TSIRULIS, 1969). *Prm* laying of disk membrane; *pg* pigment granule; *f* fibril; *me* mitochondria of ellipsoid; *bb* basal body; *c* cilium

the rhabdomere develop as a result of the growth of microvilli. In the compound eye of the adult insect each ommatidium has on its distal end a group of four transparent cells, called the crystalline cone, which is coated with a transparent cornea. Located under this cone are several (usually 8) retinular cells forming the rhabdomere, a cluster of microvilli regularly oriented at right angles to the axis of the ommatidium. The proximal ends of the retinular cells extend in the form of axons into the nerve centers. Each ommatidium is surrounded by pigment cells separating it from neighboring ommatidia. In its embryonic growth stage, the compound eye of insects develops from an imaginal disk; the amount of ergastoplasm (rough reticulum membranes) in the cells of this disk increases sharply during the period of differentiation, i.e. of rhabdomere formation (WADDINGTON, 1964). The rhabdomere is formed by the development of microvilli on the lateral surface, facing the center of the future retinula, of embryonic retinular cells. For example, in *Drosophila* the first stage in the formation of rhabdomeres consists in the formation of microvilli of the plasma

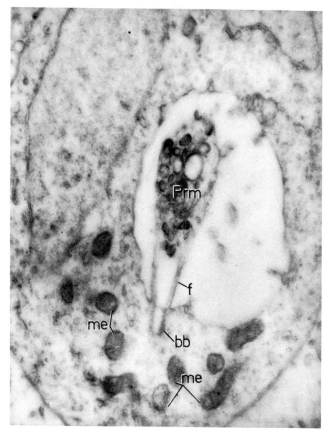

Fig. 41. Development of inner and outer segments of chick photoreceptors in tissue-culture conditions ( × 30,000) (GOVARDOVSKII and KHARKEEVICH, 1965). *me* mitochondria of ellipsoid; *bb* basal body; *f* fibrils; *Prm* vesicle-shaped rudiments of outer segment membranes

membrane (WADDINGTON and PERRY, 1960). At the same time, in the adjoining cytoplasm a large number of vesicles can be observed; according to WADDINGTON (1964), these vesicles move close to the base of the villi and attach themselves in some manner to them; this represents the substance of the rhabdomere, which is synthesized inside the cell but is not bound to the ergastoplasm. The vesicles may contain concentrations of vitamin A, as was recently established by autoradiography for the visual cells of molluscs (EAKIN and BRANDENBURGER, 1968). The visual pigments of insects are also built on the basis of vitamin A aldehyde or retinal. Retinal was discovered for the first time in bee-head extracts (GOLDSMITH, 1958), then in extracts obtained from the heads of orthopterans, coleopterans and lepidopterans (BRIGGS, 1961). Retinal is always found in the head of the insect, never in body tissues. In bees, retinal is bound to protein and forms a visual pigment with an absorption peak at 440 nm (GOLDSMITH, 1958). The visual pigment extracted from the eye of the oriental cockroach *Blatta orientalis* has an absorption peak near 500 nm, i.e. it coincides with that of rhodopsin (WOLKEN and SCHEER, 1963).

Unfortunately, no direct answer can yet be given concerning where retinal is localized in rhabdomere membranes and in membranes of outer-segment disks of photoreceptors in vertebrates; this problem can only be solved in an indirect way. For example, it has been established that an electrical response to light in the insect eye appears only with the start of differentiation of rhabdomeres (EGUCHI, NAKA, and KUWABARA, 1962). It has further been shown that the absorption spectrum of an individual rhabdomere, measured with a microspectrophotometer, is the same as that of cattle and squid rhodopsin (LANGER and THORELL, 1966). As we shall see liberation of retinal by the insect eye on illumination can be accompanied by a "swelling" of microvilli in the rhabdomeres (GRIBAKIN, 1969a, 1969b, 1969c).

Experimental vitamin-A deficiency in the fly *(Musca domestica)* reduces the sensitivity of the eye to light by a factor of about 100 as compared to the norm (GOLDSMITH, BARKER, and COHEN, 1964). As regards changes in structural organization, it has been shown that, if several generations of moths

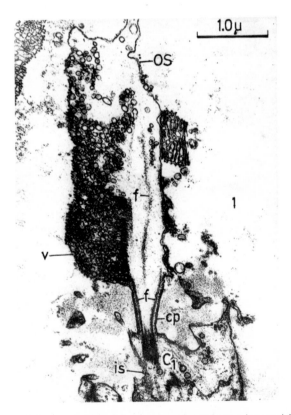

Fig. 42. Breakdown of the outer segment (conversion of membranes into vesicles) in the parietal organ of the turtle under conditions of prolonged vitamin-A deficiency (EAKIN, 1964). $C_1$ centriole; *cp* connecting pedicle of photoreceptor; *f* fibrils; *is* inner segment; *l* eye lumen; *OS* outer segment; *v* vesicles formed in the outer segment as a result of disk degeneration

(*Manduca sexta*) are fed a diet free from vitamin A and its carotenoid precursors, extensive histolysis of the retinular cells and tissues lining these cells is observed under the light microscope. These pathological changes were correlated with a strong deterioration of vision, although growth, metamorphosis and reproductive ability were not impaired in these insects (CARLSON *et al.*, 1967). Subsequent electron microscope studies showed that retinular cells develop in an abnormal manner under such diet conditions. However, adult moths exhibited a large increase in the number of microvilli instead of the expected degeneration. At the same time, the structure of the rhabdome was disrupted. Thus, at first sight vitamin-A deficiency resulted in an actual increase in photoreceptor surface and even in the preservation of light sensitivity. However, the moth does not exhibit a characteristic reaction to light, possibly due to disturbances in the conduction of nerve impulses in the visual centers (CARLSON *et al.*, 1968). Although the visual pigment is an integral part of the rhabdomere membranes in the visual cells of insects, in contrast to vertebrates, it is still unclear how its presence or absence affects the structural organization of the rhabdomere. New and careful investigations are required to clarify this point. However, according to SEVERTSOV (1967), the transformation of an embryonic cell into a visual cell is effected by means of an "extension" of the plasma membrane of the flagellum, which is converted into a stack of disk membranes in vertebrates or, in insects and a number of other invertebrates, a supplementary development of the plasma membrane in the form of microvilli which are converted into rhabdomeres. We believe the development of such an "extension" to be associated with the inclusion of the heterogeneous rhodopsin molecule into the cellular membrane.

## 5. Structural, Cytochemical and Functional Organization of the Visual Cell

### A. Photoreceptors of Vertebrates

A striking feature of photoreceptors in vertebrates is the general similarity of their structural, cytochemical and functional organization in members of all classes, from cyclostomes to primates and man (Fig. 43). As already noted, in addition to an outer segment having a rod- or cone-like shape, we can distinguish in the photoreceptor cell a connecting cilium with 9 pairs of fibrils, an inner segment containing the mitochondrial aggregate (ellipsoid with branching dentrites or microvilli), and a cylindrical elongated nuclear-plasma body, which is connected by means of peculiar synapses to the peripheral processes of bipolar and horizontal cells. The dimensions of photoreceptors vary widely in different vertebrates. Thus, the rod of a frog has a diameter of up to 5—6 μm, a length of 35 μm and a volume of $1.5 \times 10^{-9}\,cm^3$; in cattle the rod is considerably smaller: diameter 1 μm, length 10 μm and volume only $7.5 \times 10^{-12}\,cm^3$ (WALD, BROWN, and GIBBONS, 1963; WOLKEN, 1963a, 1966).

Electron microscope data have confirmed the laminar structure long ago postulated for the outer segments by SCHMIDT (1935, 1938). It was found that the outer segments consisted of a stack of twin membranes joined along their edges, known as disks. The thickness of a disk may be as much as 140Å, each of the membranes making up a disk being 70Å thick (Fig. 44).

Many investigators have found that membranes of rod disks are separated by an interval of variable width (SJÖSTRAND, 1953a; LASANSKY and DE ROBERTIS, 1960; NILSSON, 1964a). Others have found this interval also in cones (DE ROBERTIS and LASANSKY, 1958; COHEN, 1960, 1961a, 1961b, 1963a, 1963b). These differences in width are probably associated with the fixation conditions, the disk membranes in both rods and cones fitting tightly against each other (FERNÁNDEZ-MORÁN, 1961; BOROVYAGIN, 1962a, 1962b; ETINGOF, OSIPOVA, and GOVARDOVSKII, 1965). As already noted, the linkage of rod disks with their coating membrane can be detected only at the base of the outer segment. In cones, outer segment disks exhibit their connection with the plasma membrane along the entire segment, from base to top.

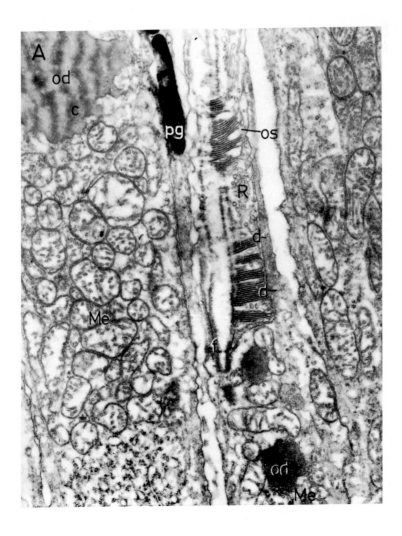

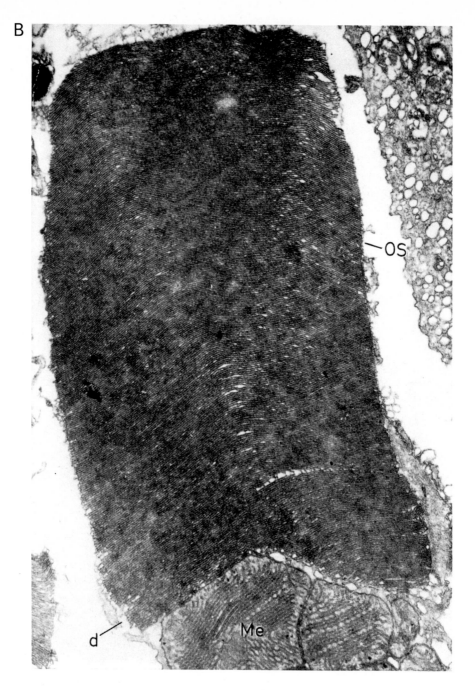

Fig. 43 A and B. Structural organization of photoreceptors in vertebrates. A. Rod and cone of chick retina (× 18,000) (GOVARDOVSKII and KHARKEEVICH, 1965). B. Outer segment and part of the inner segment of the lamprey photoreceptor (× 36,000) (GOVARDOVSKII, 1967). In the outer rod segment, fibrils of the flagellum can be observed over a distance of 5—6 μm. A dendrite (*d*) branches off from the inner rod segment; *od* oil drop; *c* cone; *R* rod; *pg* pigment granule in the processes of the pigment cell; *os* outer segment; *Me* mitochondria of the ellipsoid; *f* fibrils of the flagellum

Some outer segment disks are divided by radial incisions and have a festoon-like shape. The number of such incisions seems to depend on the size of the disks and ranges from one in the guinea pig (SJÖSTRAND, 1953a) to 5 to 10 in the frog (BOROVYAGIN, 1962a, 1962b).

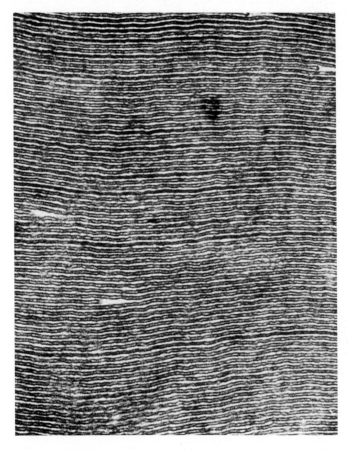

Fig. 44. Membranes of outer segment disks in photoreceptors of the lamprey ( × 86,000) (GOVARDOV-
SKII, 1967)

The number of disks varies in different animals. In the lamprey the outer segments of photoreceptors contain approximately 300 disks (GOVARDOVSKII, 1967); frog rods contain about 1,100 disks, and frog cones 750 (WALD, BROWN, and GIBBONS, 1963). Rods of cattle contain 180 disks (WOLKEN, 1936a). Computations performed by GOVARDOVSKII and KHARKEEVICH (1965) in our laboratory indicate that total surface area of the photoreceptor membrane of outer segment disks in hen cones lies within the range 5,000 to 8,000 $\mu m^2$. In *Necturus*, this area is approximately 70,000 $\mu m^2$ (BROWN, GIBBONS, and WALD, 1963).

Without dwelling on the description of the structural organization of membranes of outer segment disks, which does not differ greatly from that of other membranes (see Chap. I), we shall, however, examine in greater detail data on their chemical composition, particularly data on the special features of the localization of the visual pigment in such membranes. Modern investigative methods, in particular microspectrophotometry, have shown that the visual pigment molecule is oriented in outer-segment membranes in such a way that its chromophore, retinal, lies normal to the path of a light beam, i. e. perpendicular to the long axis of a rod. More precisely, 90 % of all rhodopsin molecules lie perpendicular, and the remaining 10 % parallel to the rod axis (WALD, BROWN, and GIBBONS, 1963). Thus, the rhodopsin molecule is oriented in the outer segment in such a way as to ensure a maximum absorption of the light propagating along the axis of the photoreceptor. This confirms the assumption made by SCHMIDT in 1935, that rod segments are endowed with dichroism, i. e. the absorption factor depends upon the direction of polarization of the incident light.

The use of the electron microscope allow us to obtain a more direct estimate of the structural localization of rhodopsin in disk membranes. Osmiophilic micellae of about 300Å diameter were detected in sections cut parallel to the plane of outer segment disks in *Necturus* rods. Such a micella could contain 50 molecules of the visual pigment porphyropsin. If we know the number of micellae present in one disk (about 30,000) and the number of disks (1,100), and assume that the micellae cover both sides of the disks, it is possible to calculate the total number of molecules present in one rod. The figure obtained is $1.75 \times 10^9$, which is in good agreement with spectrophotometric determinations (BROWN, GIBBONS, and WALD, 1963).

The number of molecules present in one rod of the frog can be determined from data on the dry weight of an outer segment, its rhodopsin content and its molecular weight (SIDMAN, 1957; WALD, 1961a, 1961b). This number can also be determined from microspectrophotometric data (WALD, BROWN, and GIBBONS, 1963). The relative reliability of these data is confirmed by the fact that an identical result was obtained from both sets of data, namely about $3 \times 10^9$ molecules per rod. We could therefore infer that rhodopsin molecules must cover the entire outer surface of disks on both sides (Fig. 45) (WOLKEN, 1961). At present rhodopsin is thought to localize on the inner surface of disks, also. According to immunological analysis data, combined with data obtained by electron microscopy and X-ray diffraction studies (BLASIE, DEWEY, and WORTHINGTON, 1966; DEWEY, DAVIS, and BLASIE, 1966; BLASIE and WORTHINGTON, 1969; DEWEY et al., 1969), rhodopsin molecules 40—60Å in diameter form on the disk surface a square lattice with a period of about 80Å. If this is so, only about 20—25 % of the disk area is occupied by these molecules, which contradicts the data obtained by WOLKEN (1961). According to the latest data, the rhodopsin molecules are localized inside the hydrocarbon chains of the fatty acids of the bimolecular lipid layer, i. e. penetrate through the disk membrane (DRATZ et al., 1972). Rhodopsine molecules have been proved to rotate in photoreceptor membrane (rotational diffusion) (BROWN, 1972; CONE, 1972). It is difficult to say at the present time what actually takes place, but there can be no doubt that, whatever the method of packing, rhodopsin constitutes an integral part of disk membranes.

The outer segment contains (calculated as dry weight) about 30% lipids and 60—70% proteins (COLLINS, LOVE, and MORTON, 1952; SJÖSTRAND, 1959a, 1959b; WOLKEN, 1961). Rhodopsin constitutes about half of all proteins found in the outer segment (WOLKEN, 1961). According to more recent data, opsin contributes as much as 92—95% of the total protein of the photoreceptor membrane (BOWNDS and GAIDE-HUGUENIN, 1970). The study of the distribution of lipids in membranes of disks is making rapid progress just now.

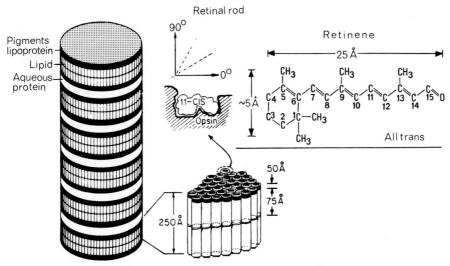

Fig. 45. Outer segment (rod) of photoreceptor. Schematic model showing the molecular structure of retinene and how it combines with opsin to form rhodopsin (HUBBARD and KROPF, 1959)

During exposure to light and consequent breakdown of the rhodopsin molecule the disk membranes undergo morphological changes. The structure of the membranes changes and their total surface shrinks. The distance between disks in outer segments of vertebrate photoreceptors may vary, as well as the length of microvilli in some invertebrates (FERNÁNDEZ-MORÁN, 1961; ETINGOF, OSI-POVA, and GOVARDOVSKII, 1965; GRIBAKIN, 1969b). Prolonged and intense light exposure may result in a complete breakdown of photoreceptor disk membranes in vertebrates and of microvilli in some invertebrates (RÖHLICH, 1967; RÖHLICH and TAR, 1968). Thus, the state of the membranes of photoreceptor cells is changing all the time, depending upon the function of the membrane. As already noted, the membranes "pulsate" or "beat" (KAVANAU, 1966). In the first place, the structural shifts enumerated above are associated with the dynamics of the molecular transformations of rhodopsin that take place under the action of light.

Numerous data have been obtained on the enzyme composition of outer-segment disk membranes in photoreceptors. Thus, it was shown that outer segments of photoreceptor cells in the frog retina are capable of aerobic respiration; this respiration is intensified upon addition of fructose diphosphate and succinate and is inhibited in the presence of cyanide (HUBBARD, 1954a). It was also established that the breathing of "light" segments is generally weaker than that of "dark" segments (HANAWA, KIMURA, and HOSOYA, 1955; HANAWA, 1956; HANAWA and KUGE, 1961). The activity of cytochromoxidase was detected in outer segments by histochemical methods (NIEMI and NERENMIES, 1961a, 1961b). These data were confirmed in our laboratory by biochemical methods (ETINGOF and SHUKOLYUKOV, 1963; ETINGOF, 1966). Monoaminoxidase was detected in outer segments by a histochemical method (SHANTHAVERAPPA and BOURNE, 1964). Outer segment disk membranes of cattle contain alcohol dehydrogenase, lactate dehydrogenase and enzymes of the pentosophosphate shunt: dehydrogenases of glucose-6-phosphate and phosphogluconate (FUTTERMAN and KINOSNITA, 1959). The presence of ubiquinone, one of the components of the respiratory chain, was established in outer segments of photoreceptors (PEARSE, 1957, 1961, 1965). Some investigators, however, believe that oxygen absorption by outer segments is associated with the presence of iron in these segments and does not have an enzymic character.

The activity of adenosine triphosphatase (ATPase), which is activated by Na, K and Mg ions (Fig. 46), has been demonstrated in outer segments of photoreceptors by both histochemical and electron microscopic methods (SCARPELLI and CRAIG, 1963; MCCONNEL and SCARPELLI, 1963) and also by biochemical methods (SEKOGATI, 1960; BONTING and CARAVAGGIO, 1963; BONTING et al., 1962, 1964). A number of investigators suggest that rhodopsin itself may be endowed with ATPase activity (MCCONNEL and SCARPELLI, 1963; FRANK and GOLDSMITH, 1965; OSTROVSKII and FEDOROVICH, 1965; OSTROVSKII, FEDOROVICH, and DZHANSKAYA, 1965). The site of location of ATPase has been established: it is found on the periphery of the disks between the twin membranes of cones in the outer segment and in the mitochondria of the ellipsoid (Fig. 46). ATPase has also been found in synaptic layers. There are reasons to assume that its activity in the outer segment increases under illumination (MCCONNEL and SCARPELLI, 1963; SCARPELLI and CRAIG, 1963; OSTROVSKII and FEDOROVICH, 1965).

Regardless of whether rhodopsin acts at the same time as ATPase or whether ATPase coexists with it, the presence of ATPase in disk membranes explains a number of energy characteristics exhibited by outer segments of photoreceptors. In the first place, it is possible to suppose that the activity of $Mg^{++}$-ATPase sets off mechanochemical process involving shortening of cones in light and elongation of cones in the dark, and elongation of rods in light and shortening of rods in the dark. This phenomenon, combined with the movement of pigment granules discovered 100 years ago, has been given the name of retinomotor phenomenon (BOLL, 1877; KÜHNE, 1878a, 1878b). Its functional significance has not been clarified up to the present, although no-one doubts that it reflects the phenomenon of photoreceptor adaptation to light and darkness. The mechanism of the retinomotor phenomenon was thought to be connected with the hypothetical ability of a special sector of the photoreceptor cytoplasm, called the "myoid", to undergo contraction. The electron microscope, however, has

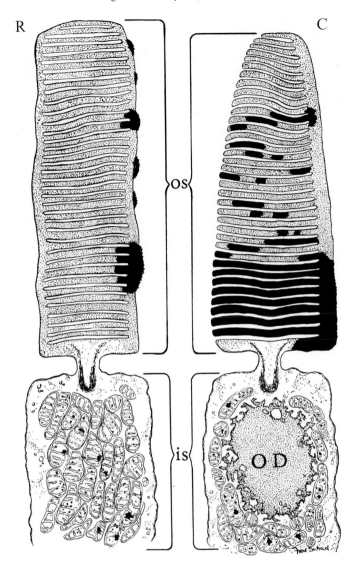

Fig. 46. Diagram showing the distribution of the enzymic activity of nucleoside triphosphatase in the outer segments (*OS*) of rods (*R*) and cones (*C*) of the frog (SCARPELLI and CRAIG, 1963). *OD* oil drop; *is* inner segments. In rods, the enzyme is localized at the periphery of disks, and in cones in the disk membranes, especially in the basal region. Insignificant enzyme deposits are observed in the mitochondria of the ellipsoid. No enzymic activity is observed in the oil drop

shown that elements of the endoplasmic reticulum and of the paraboloid are located in the myoid region; no structures are found there. The striated rootlets and tubules, which may branch out from the basal body of the flagellum, are located higher, and although they exhibit location sites of ATPase (MATSUSAKA,

1967), it is doubtful whether they themselves perform any motor function that is not inherent to the inner and outer segments as a whole. In addition, we cannot exclude the fact that the elongation or shortening of the photoreceptor is associated with the 9 pairs of flagellar fibrils located in the region of the connecting cilium, where they may extend over $\frac{2}{3}$ of its length. Although the presence of ATPase in these cilia has not yet been proved, neither can it be excluded if their structural organization is taken into account. Thus, along with disk membranes, fibrils of the photoreceptor flagellum also apparently take part in the outer segment contraction processes that occur in light and darkness (VINNIKOV, 1964, 1965a, 1965b, 1966a, 1966b, 1969).

Finally, in view of the presence in the outer segment of a high activity of $Na^+$- and $K^+$-ATPase, comparable in magnitude to the activity of brain ATPase and the electric organs of the electric eel (BONTING, CARAVAGGIO, and HAWKINS, 1962; BONTING and CARAVAGGIO, 1963), we can assume that its function in membranes of the receptor cell is analogous to the function of ATPase in the nerve cell (HODGKIN, 1965; DUNCAN, 1967; OSTROVSKII, FEDOROVICH, and GOLUBEV, 1967). It can take part, from an energy standpoint, in the active transport of Na and K ions across the cellular membrane under the action of light. Thus, it was shown in our laboratory that, under the effect of illumination or of vitamin A, an increase is observed in the number of $K^+$ (and to a somewhat lesser extent of $Na^+$) ions escaping from the photoreceptors into the supernatant fluid, obtained from the fraction of isolated photoreceptor segments (ETINGOF, SHUKOLYUKOV, and LEONT'EV, 1964). On the other hand, other workers' data show that $Na^+$ ions in this case enter the outer segments (BONTING and BAGHAM, 1967). Recently, in our laboratory, GOVARDOVSKII (1970, 1971), using KOMNICK'S (1962) electron microscopic and histochemical method for the determination of Na ions, has shown that the distribution of the reaction product (granules of Na pyroantimonate) is completely different in the frog retina adapted to the dark for 1—3 hours and from retina exposed to normal room illumination (Fig. 47). Na ions are not found in rod and cone outer segment membranes of dark-adapted frogs, whereas copious deposits of reaction products are found in outer segments of light-adapted rods. The Na pyroantimonate granules are located inside the disks on the inner-membrane surfaces, but not in the interdisk spaces.

When the frog retina was frozen and the $Na^+$ reaction was carried out by substituting water, to prevent ion losses and ion redistributions caused by diffusion, it was found that the bulk of $Na^+$ reaction product granules was located inside the disks. These facts fit in with the data discussed above on the development of disks, which constitute essentially closed "islands" in the extracellular medium, which is, of course, usually rich in sodium. The intervals between the disks, which correspond to the cellular cytoplasm, exhibited a high content of $K^+$ which is in general characteristic for cytoplasm. Consequently, the rod outer segment can be considered as a sort of battery, consisting of an extracellular substance (the disk contents) separated by the space between the disks (the cytoplasm). Thus, rods consist of structures effecting a multiple repeating cation concentration gradient, apparently maintained by ATPase. Because $Na^+$ and $K^+$ concentration gradients are present in these structures, we can also assume the existence of a potential difference in the system disk—inter-disk cytoplasm.

In cone outer segments, granules of the reaction product cannot·be detected either in the dark or in the light. On the basis of these tests, we can assume that Na ions bound to outer-segment disk membranes are liberated under the action of light (GOVARDOVSKII, 1969). Liberation of Na ions must result in the escape of Na from the cell, which is in agreement with the data obtained by ETINGOF, SHUKOLYUKOV, and LEONT'EV (1964) and others. As will be shown below, the results described above probably reflect the bioelectrical pheno-mena which have recently been shown to occur in photoreceptors.

Thus, the outer segment of the photoreceptor in vertebrates is truly a mobile antenna, in which physiological processes and reception of light energy are associated with a chain of dynamic molecular and ionic changes. Molecular transformations of the visual pigment in disk membranes can be considered as a trigger mechanism for the excitation of photoreceptors and the accompanying mechanochemical phenomena, and also for biopotentials, as we shall explain later.

What is the nature of the inner segment in photoreceptors, and, most impor-tantly, of its mitochondrial aggregate, the ellipsoid? What part does it play

A

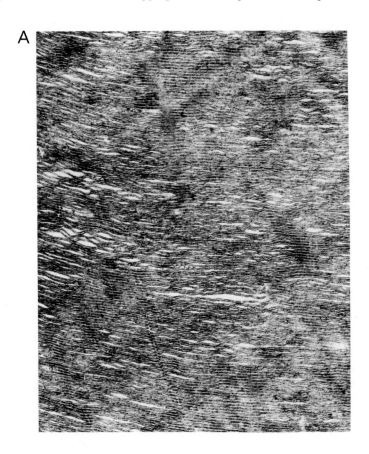

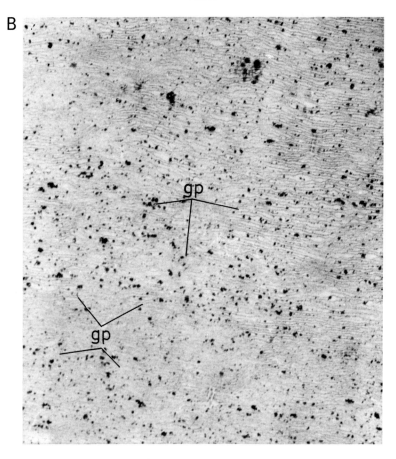

Fig. 47 A and B. Distribution of Na$^+$ in the outer-segment disks of frog photoreceptor rods (A) in the state of dark adaptation and (B) after adaptation to indoor light ( × 60,000) (GOVARDOVSKII, 1969). *gp* granules of Na pyroantimonate

in the functional performance of the visual cell under the action of light? Electron microscopic studies carried out in our laboratory (LUKASHEVICH, 1966; GOVARDOVSKII and TSIRULIS, 1969) have shown that in the lamprey, frog, chick and cattle under dark-adaptation conditions, mitochondria of the ellipsoid are characterized by large dimensions and a circular shape; they fit tightly against each other, making contact through their surface membranes (see Fig. 36). Apparently, such a tight arrangement of the mitochondria is necessary to ensure the efficiency of their overall performance. In the lamprey, the cristae of tightly packed mitochondria of the ellipsoid are sometimes folded. The orientation of the cristae with respect to the photoreceptor axis can differ in different mitochondria. The area occupied by the membrane system of mitochondrial cristae is just as large as that of the outer-segment disk system, perhaps larger. Dense granules, which are strongly stained by lead and have a diameter of 350—500 Å, can be detected in the mitochondria. These granules are very similar to the glycogen granules found in the mitochondrial membranes of rat photoreceptors (ISHAIKAVA and YEN FEN PEI, 1965). In birds, mitochondria of the ellipsoid are located directly under the outer segments in rods and under the oil droplets in cones. In the ellipsoids of certain cones, the mitochondria are packed very tightly and have a relatively regular shape. Ellipsoids of rods are characterized by the loose arrangement and irregular shape of their mitochondria. In mammals, the mitochondria of cones are usually oriented along the long axis of the cell. The orientation of rod mitochondria is expressed in a particularly distinct manner. Mitochondria of cone ellipsoids contract in the light yet along with the contracted mitochondria, separate partially or fully swollen mitochondria can be observed. It should be noted that, like the isolated cells with modified mitochondria, the ellipsoid mitochondria retain their original structure in most cones of a previously illuminated retina.

When the retina is illuminated, the rods exhibit completely distinct shifts such as are frequently encountered in the structure of mitochondria. These changes under the action of light are expressed in a considerable swelling of practically all ellipsoid mitochondria. However, along with a large number of rods with swollen mitochondria, there are still some rods in which no significant changes whatsoever can be observed after illumination. The reaction of mitochondria in the ellipsoid of photoreceptor rods and cones of cattle is illustrated in Fig. 48.

A histochemical study under the light and electron microscope of the location site of oxidative enzymes in photoreceptor ellipsoids of members of all vertebrate classes has shown the presence of the activity of succinate dehydrogenase and maleate dehydrogenase belonging to the Krebs aerobic cycle, of lactate dehydrogenase belonging to the anaerobic cycle, and of alcohol dehydrogenase (LUKASHE-VICH, 1962). Illumination of animals for 15—30 minutes with a steady or flickering light causes changes in the shape of the ellipsoidal mitochondria (rounding and swelling) and also, as a rule, a distinct increase in succinate dehydrogenase activity. These results agree with the histochemical data obtained by a large number of other investigators, which have demonstrated the high succinate dehydrogenase activity of ellipsoids in photoreceptors of mammals and changes of this activity under illumination conditions (FRANCIS, 1953a, 1953b; WISLOCKI and SIDMAN, 1954; HELLSTRÖM, 1956; COGAN and KUWABARA, 1959; PEARSE, 1961; ERÄNKÖ, NIEMI, and MERENMIES, 1961; KARPENKO, 1962; OSTROVSKII, 1961a, 1962; NASU, APPONI, and VIALE, 1962; ENOCH, 1963, 1964). From these data we can conclude that the ellipsoid, which occupies a central position in the visual cell, is the main source of ATP. The ellipsoid appears to be capable of transporting ATP along the photoreceptor in the direction of the outer segment, as well as in the opposite direction. It can be assumed that expansion of ATP from this center is a necessary condition for the fulfillment of energy processes responsible both for the perception of a photon and for the initiation of a stimulation of the visual cell and its transmission to the synapse where, by the way, mitochondria are generally absent. As we have seen, ATPase activity is always observed in all enumerated sectors of the visual cell. Naturally, the presence of such an energy center by no means excludes the possibility of a local process of ATP generation in the photoreceptor membranes proper

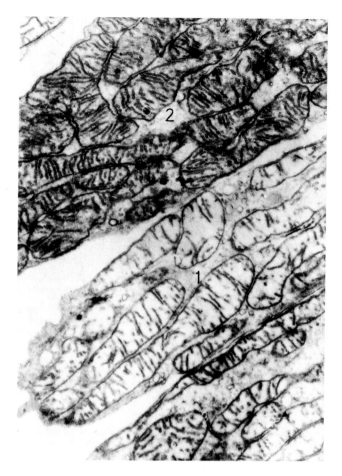

Fig. 48. Reaction to light of ellipsoid mitochondria in photoreceptors of the bull ( × 25,000) (LUKASHE-VICH, 1966). *1* Swollen mitochondria of the rod ellipsoid; *2* unchanged mitochondria of cones

(GREEN, 1964; ETINGOF, SHUKOLYUKOV, and ZHUCHIKHINA, 1967). Thus, the mitochondrial aggregate, i. e. the ellipsoid of the visual cell, not only looks after the development of outer-segment disk membranes during embryogenesis and further ontogenesis, but along with the outer segment, also determines the ability of the cell to function as a photoreceptor. Consequently, the ellipsoid can be considered as the energy center of the cell.

A few words now about the oil droplet consisting of lipids, which is present in the photoreceptor inner segment of birds (see Fig. 43A), reptiles, amphibia and ganoid fishes. This oil droplet is located directly under the outer segment and can be colorless, or given a red, yellow or yellow-green color by the presence of carotenoids. In the chick, it was possible to extract three carotenoids of corresponding colors, of which the red one, or astacene, has been reliably identified. Already in 1939, WALD had made the assumption that the oil droplet acts as a light filter and is thus responsible for color perception. This hypothesis has now been confirmed experimentally (ORLOV, 1963; ORLOV and MAKSIMOVA, 1964). Under the electron microscope, the oil droplets of the chick can be subdivided into three types, reacting differently to fixation (GOVARDOVSKII, 1967). The first type is distinctly osmiophilic, homogeneous in its electron density, and is located nearest to the so-called outer limiting membrane of the retina. The second type has a distinctly less osmiophilic character and is located somewhat higher with respect to the outer limiting membrane. The third type includes light oil droplet located at the highest level; their lipid content probably did not undergo fixation and was extracted during passage through alcohols.

Located under the oil droplet and the ellipsoid is the hypothetical myoid region; the paraboloid is also located in this region (Fig. 39). At least three types of structures, presumably containing glycogen, have been found in the paraboloid region. Small ribosome-like particles, arranged in the form of characteristic rosettes, were detected by CARASSO (1960) in amphibian photoreceptors. EICHNER and THEMANN (1963), while studying the localization of glycogen in cockerel retina under the electron microscope, found rather large (200—250Å) granules bound to a characteristic endoplasmic reticulum, which consists of a dense arrangement of sinuous tubules 600—800Å in diameter. An identical structure was described in photoreceptors of the turtle (YAMADA, 1960) and in the double cones of the pigeon (COHEN, 1963a). In the PAS-positive region of rat rods granules about 300Å in diameter and forming compact clusters were detected.

The granules could be removed by digestion with saliva prior to osmium fixation (ISHIKAWA and YEN FEN PEI, 1965). According to data obtained in our laboratory (GOVARDOVSKII, 1967), all three types of structures can be detected in the paraboloid of the chick.

What is the function of the paraboloid? Under the light microscope and with histochemical methods glycogens and enzymes bound to them were discovered in the paraboloid region (GOUREVITCH, 1951, 1954; RABINOVITCH, MOTA, and YONEDA, 1954; SIDMAN and WISLOCKI, 1954; WISLOCKI and SIDMAN, 1954; SAXEN, 1955; MATSUSAKA, 1956; EICHNER, 1958; CARASSO, 1960; EICHNER and THEMANN et al., 1962, 1963). A study of glycogen distribution in the retina of animals under different illumination conditions has shown that light stimulation is always accompanied by a fall in glycogen content and that the original amount is restored after the animal has been kept in the dark for a long period of time (GOUREVITCH, 1951, 1954; SCIMIZU and MAEDA, 1952; EICHNER, 1958; EICHNER and THEMANN, 1962, 1963). Although the electron microscope enables the distribution of glycogen to be determined more precisely within the limits of the visual cell, where it can be observed in the form of electron-dense granules 150—300Å in diameter, the fall in glycogen content observed in the retina of illuminated animals under the light microscope is not clearly visible in electron micrographs (EICHNER and THEMANN, 1963). The electron microscopic data show that an increase takes place under the action of light in the granular component of the cytoplasm in the paraboloid region of photoreceptors. At the same time there is an increase in the number of vacuoles in the myoid portion, which can be associated with glycogen resynthesis (YAMADA, 1960; BOROVYAGIN, 1962a, 1962b). Thus, we believe that cytochemical processes associated with glycogen exchange are also taking place in the paraboloid during the functioning of photoreceptors.

As already noted, in the ellipsoid region dendrites develop from microvilli and branch off from the plasma membrane of the inner segment of photoreceptors (Fig. 37). Dendrites originate in the ellipsoid region and surround the base of the outer segment over a distance of 4—5 µm to form a sort of palisade, being equidistant from each other. They may enter into the mouth of the spiral-shaped grooves located on the surface of the outer rod segment. The length of a dendrite does not exceed several microns, and its diameter is 0.2—0.5 µm. The function of dendrites is not clear. According to BROWN, GIBBONS, and WALD (1963), dendrites can transmit to outer segments the metabolic products of mitochondria, including ATP. In *Necturus*, fibrils and vacuoles are found in the cytoplasm of dendrites. As we have pointed out, dendrites should be considered as specialized microvilli, which nearly always surround a flagellum.

Located under the paraboloid is a part of the cytoplasm, which, though essentially still considered as a "myoid", is immediately adjacent to the nucleus and the cytoplasm surrounding this nucleus. This part has a relatively low structural differentiation; located here are elements of the smooth and rough reticulum, individual ribosomes and elements of the Golgi apparatus. Mitochondria are absent. We have mentioned already that electron microscopic studies with labeled amino acids have shown that protein, including opsin, is synthesized in the ergastoplasm and is condensed in the region of the Golgi apparatus. From here, protein is distributed to other parts of the cell, first through the region of the ellipsoid and the connecting cilium into the outer segment, and then in the opposite direction toward the synapse (Fig. 33). It is still not quite clear how RNA and protein undergo a change in this region during the functioning of the photoreceptor cell. Qualitative histochemical data indicate that the RNA content of the cytoplasm of photoreceptors falls during illumination (DE VINCENTIS, 1949, 1953; KHAN VAN KIEN, 1955; MATSUSAKA et al., 1956).

More definite results are available with respect to nuclear RNA, the content of which varies under different illumination conditions. The nucleus of photoreceptor cells is located below the outer limiting membrane or partially above it. The chromatin of the nucleus is distributed in a fine granular form more or less uniformly through the karyoplasm, forming thickenings in the region of one or two nucleoles. Under the light microscope, DNA can be observed in photoreceptor nuclei in the form of large granules up to 1.5 µm in diameter adhering tightly to each other (BRODSKII, 1959, 1966; SVANIDZE, 1963). The nucleus has a two-layer membrane containing numerous pores. The outer membrane has in many places passages linking it with membranes of the endoplasmic reticulum. However, the passage of the granular content of the nucleus into the cytoplasm has not been observed.

According to UTINA and BYZOV (1965) and BYZOV (1966), under constant illumination the amount of RNA in nuclei of frog rods and cones increases by 30—70% as compared to dark conditions; under flickering light, this increase is even greater. Consequently, for photoreceptors the reaction to changes in the duration and intensity of illumination is associated with a higher expenditure of energy than the reaction to constant illumination (BYZOV, 1966).

Also very instructive are the variations in the RNA content of the neural cells of the retina in light and in darkness, which we shall not discuss here (BRODSKII, 1966; BYZOV, 1966).

The narrow cytoplasmic body of the photoreceptor, or central process, which soon expands slightly, forms a very complex synaptic structure (see Fig. 38). This structure contains recesses into which intrude several dendritic processes of bipolar cells, as well as digitiform processes of adjacent photoreceptors and, according to recent data, also the processes of horizontal cells (YAMADA and TSHIKAVA, 1965; BOROVYAGIN, 1966). The synapse of visual cells was first described by SJÖSTRAND (1953a, 1953b, 1958, 1961) and then by DE ROBERTIS and FRANCHI (1956).

The cytoplasm of the synaptic region of photoreceptors is filled with synaptic vesicles of diameter 300—400 Å, which are thought to contain a mediator, probably acetylcholine. The presynaptic membrane of the photoreceptor frequently forms what are called synaptic rods or synaptic ribbons, double folds 2—3 μm long and several tenths of a μm wide.

The plate of ribbons is always surrounded by a cluster of vesicles. There is a greater concentration of synaptic vesicles in rods than in cones. It has been calculated that sections of the synaptic zone of rods in monkey and man contain about 190 to 250 vesicles per $\mu m^2$ and cones about 170. We have already pointed out that the same synaptic structure also characterizes synapses of the central nervous system. Mitochondria are usually absent in the body of the photoreceptor and in its synaptic region, although one or two giant mitochondria can be observed in the synapse of the white rat and, in the cat, a group of mitochondria (LADMAN, 1958; VILLEGAS, 1960, 1964; PEASE, 1962). In birds, according to GOVARDOVSKII (1967), interesting structural characteristics are noted in the synapses of double cones; the two together form a larger synapse in which the synapse of one cone, probably the main one, partially encompasses the synapse of the other cone, probably the accessory one. Some processes of bipolar cells are in contact simultaneously with both components of the synapse. A long axon-like process intruding into the synapse of one the neighboring single cones branches off from the body of the main component in the vicinity of the synapse, extending downward and to the side. Microtubules run along the length of this process.

In the lamprey, synaptic ribbons and an extraordinarily large number of synaptic vesicles can be found in the synaptic region of photoreceptors, whereas the number of bipolar cell processes is relatively small compared to photoreceptor synapses in birds. Thus, the structure of photoreceptor synapses in vertebrates, from lamprey to man, remains practically unchanged.

How does the structure of the synapse change when subjected to functional effects? In a study of synaptic vesicles in the synaptic photoreceptor region of rabbits kept in the dark for from 24—26 hours up to 9 days, it was found that the size of the vesicles decreases in proportion to the time the animal remains in darkness. Under illumination, synaptic vesicles are seen to pass through the synaptic membrane, and accumulate in the postsynaptic cytoplasm (DE ROBERTIS and FRANCHI, 1956; DE ROBERTIS, 1958). An increase in the number and size of synaptic vesicles under the effect of flickering light was also noted in synaptic terminals of frog photoreceptors (BOROVYAGIN, 1962a, 1962b). However, contradictory data are also available, indicating that no changes are observed in the number and size of synaptic vesicles, either in the dark or under illumination (MOUNTFORD, 1964).

Cytochemical data reveal the activity of acetylcholinesterase in the synaptic zone of photoreceptors (KOELLE et al., 1952; FRANCIS, 1953a, 1953b; GEREBT-ZOFF, 1959; ERÄNKÖ, NIEMI, and MERENMIES, 1961; OSTROVSKII, 1961a, 1961b). This enzyme can also be found in other zones of the retina, for example in the inner plexiform layer. Biochemical studies have revealed the presence in the retina of large amounts of acetylcholine (LEPLAT and GEREBTZOFF, 1956), cholinacetylase (HEBB and WAITES, 1956) and cholinesterase (WECKER and FISCHER, 1939; ANFINSEN, 1944). Cholinesterase appears in the retina in the course of postnatal development; the appearance of acetylcholinesterase has been associated with the first electric potential recorded from frontal lobes during electric stimulation (RAVIOLA and RAVIOLA, 1960; LIEBERMAN, 1962). At the same time, OSTROVSKII (1961b, 1964) was unable to detect any shift in the activity of acetylcholinesterase in the retina of animals subjected to stimulation by flickering light. All that can be said is that photoreceptor synapses are structures with a chemical transmission that apparently takes place with the aid of a cholinergic mechanism. Thus, the visual cell is characterized by a complex (mosaic) organization; it consists of a whole series of subcellular and molecular components, and it is the interaction of these components, following the primary molecular reaction of rhodopsin, that leads to stimulation of the visual cell.

## B. Biopotentials of the Visual Cell

Relatively recently it has become possible to identify in the overall reaction of the retina to light, or electroretinogram (ERG), those structures which constitute the source of its separate components. This applies also to photoreceptors.

Against the background of the cytophysiological and cytochemical processes occurring in the visual cell, starting, with the molecular transformation of rhodopsin in light, the receptor potential of the visual cell seems to have special significance (BROWN and MURAKAMI, 1964a, 1964b; BROWN, WATANABE, and MURAKAMI, 1965; CONE, 1964; BAUMANN, 1965; PAK and CONE, 1964; BORTOFF and NORTON, 1965a, 1965b; PAK, LETTVIN et al., 1965; OSTROVSKII et al., 1967). According to the length of the latent period, we can distinguish two types of receptor potentials: an "early" potential, recorded 25 to 50 μsec after the start of the light stimulus, and a "late" potential with a latent period of the order of 5 to 7 msec. The early receptor potential consists of two components, a negative and a positive one; this potential is stable and is evoked in response to strong flashes of light. The appearance of both components of the early receptor potential coincides with the absorption spectrum of rhodopsin. While the contour of the absorption spectrum does not depend upon the intensity of the flash and the state of adaptation, the amplitude of the early receptor potential is proportional to the number of rhodopsin molecules stimulated and is restored during the course of dark adaptation at a rate which coincides with the regeneration time of rhodopsin. It is assumed that this potential arises during the transition stage of pre-lumirhodopsin into lumirhodopsin or of lumirhodopsin into metarhodopsin I (PAK, 1965; PAK and EBREY, 1965). It was found in our laboratory (GOVAR-DOVSKII, Vision Res., 1974, in press), that the cone early receptor potential is generated by the visual pigment molecules enclosed within the outer segment disks. In rod early receptor potential is generated by the rhodopsin molecules fitted into the envelope membrane of the outer segment.

In regard to the late receptor potential, it was concluded after prolonged arguments that this potential indeed arises in the receptor cell. It is observed in both rods and cones; in rods, however, the potential decays slowly and yields a long trace potential, whereas in cones it decays rapidly and the more intensive the stimulus the later is the trace potential observed (BROWN and MURAKAMI, 1964a, 1964b). It is assumed that the early receptor potential acts as a trigger for the late one; the latter arises a long way from the outer segment, and the early potential apparently reaches this segment by traveling along the 9 pairs of peripheral fibrils of the connecting cilium or along the outer membrane of the cell and is transmitted through the synapse to the nearest neurons of the retina (BROWN, WATANABE, and MURAKAMI, 1965).

Recent progress achieved in the intracellular recording of potentials from photoreceptors, and based on studies carried out in Tomita's laboratories (TOMITA, 1965; TOMITA et al., 1967; TOYODA, NOSAKI, and TOMITA, 1969) has shown that the electrical response to light in the carp, proteus and gecko consists in a hyperpolarization of several millivolts lasting during the entire period of illumination. This hyperpolarization is caused (or is accompanied) by an increase in the resistance of the photoreceptor membrane; however, some species show depolarization.

The mechanism of the generation of an electrical response was studied on the PIII component of the isolated retina of the frog (SILLMAN, ITO, and TOMITA, 1969a, 1969b), pigeon (ARDEN and ERNST, 1969) and rat (ARDEN and ERNST, 1969; PENN and HAGINS, 1969). The action of light decreases the sodium permeability of the outer segment membrane and consequently induces hyperpolarization of the cell. This implies passive movement of sodium ions along an electrochemical gradient, since suppression of the sodium-potassium pump by ouabain does not affect the response when the difference in sodium concentration outside and inside the cell is maintained by appropriate changes in the extracellular medium. PENN and HAGINS (1969) found that approximately 60,000 ions are transferred across the photoreceptor membrane as a result of the absorption of one light quantum. These authors believe that such a flow is quite sufficient for the transmission of information from the outer segment to the photoreceptor synapse. It was shown earlier that the necessary change in the permeability of the membrane can be caused, in theory, by a single event of molecular scale, for example, by a change in the conformation of a protein molecule (HAGINS, 1966).

How can the molecular conversions of rhodopsin at one or another stage of its decomposition lead to the appearance of a potential in the visual cell? In this respect, three different theories exist: an enzymic theory, a solid-state theory, and an ionic theory. The first starts from the hypothesis that rhodopsin is a proenzyme, which is activated by a photon, and that this is followed by the exposure of a catalytic center that in the dark is covered by a chromophore group (WALD, 1960). This theory also assumes that the mechanism responsible for the increased nervous activity of the outer segment is associated either with rhodopsin itself, which apparently possesses ATPase properties, or with ATPase bound to rhodopsin (OSTROVSKII, 1965; OSTROVSKII and FEDOROVICH, 1965; OSTROVSKII, FEDOROVICH, and GOLUBEV, 1967; DUNCAN, 1967).

The second theory is based on the concept that the outer segment has a quasicrystalline structure, approximating to the structure of a solid body (WOLKEN, 1964). In a solid body, under the effect of photon energy, the excited state is propagated from one rhodopsin molecule to another without the further action of light. So far, there is no direct experimental proof in support of this theory (HAGINS, ZONANA, and ADAMS, 1962).

The third theory is based on a number of known facts, which could also be demonstrated with the aid of the electron microscope. This theory is based on data that suggest that $Na^+$ enters the outer segments and $K^+$ leaves them during illumination in obedience to the same rules which have been established for nerve stimulation (BONTING and BAGNHAM, 1967). It is assumed that rhodopsin undergoes photolysis under the action of light. The all-*trans* isomer of retinal, which is liberated during this process, reacts with the amino groups of phosphatidylethanolamine or phosphatidylserine, present in rod disk membranes to form a Schiff-base linkage. The blocking of the amino group in the phospholipid makes the membrane more negatively charged, which greatly increasing the permeability of the membrane for actions.

This induces a receptor potential, which activates a cholinergic mechanism in the synapse. In the restoration phase, retinal is liberated from the phospholipid, isomerizes again into the *cis* form, and combines with the opsin. The ionic gradient is restored at the expense of $Na^+ = -K^+ = ATPase$ (BONTING and BANGHAM, 1967). Unfortunately, this detailed model is at variance with the experimental data on the direction of the ionic gradient (GOVARDOVSKII, 1971), as well as on changes of permeability of disk membranes in the light (ARDEN and ERNST, 1969).

It is difficult to say which of these three theories is most nearly correct. They may all reflect to some extent different stages in the initial process of stimulation of the visual cell and the appearance of biopotentials, which are preceded by conformational shifts of rhodopsin. In our opinion, the main weakness of these theories is that intracellular structural components are completely disregarded. For instance, the inner segment, with its ellipsoid and paraboloid endowed with enormous energy power and undergoing structural changes during illumination, must contribute along with the outer-segment membranes to the act of stimulating the visual cell. Under illumination conditions a change takes place in the RNA content of the cytoplasm and the nucleus, and also probably in the protein content, by analogy with other receptor cells. Finally, a change also occurs in the structure of the synaptic zone of the photoreceptor cell. All of the above-mentioned changes, including the biopotentials, together characterize the stimulation of the visual cell. This stimulation proceeds in increasing degree from the outer segment, is in all probability much intensified with the aid of the ellipsoid in the inner segment, and after transformation in the nuclear-cytoplasmic section, is converted in the synapse region into excitation of other units of the retina. The consecutive association of these processes is obvious; however, a great deal of effort will be required to clarify the nature of this association.

## C. Insect Photoreceptors

The compound eye of an insect is the system formed by a number of units called ommatidia. An ommatidium has a dioptric system (corneal lens and crystalline cone) and a photoreceptor apparatus or retinula (Fig. 49). The retinula consists of some (eight, as a rule) primary sensory visual cells with their axons ending in the first optic ganglion. The axial region of the retinula is occupied

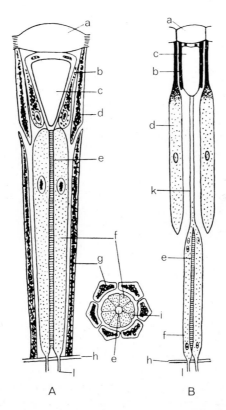

A                    B

Fig. 49 A and B. Schematic structure of the ommatidium of (A) photopic and (B) scotopic eye (MAZOKHIN-PORSHNYAKOV, 1965). Center-cross-section of the ommatidium of the photopic eye at the rhabdome level. *a* corneal lens (crystalline lens); *b* main pigment cells (corneagenic); *c* crystalline cone; *d* iris (outer) pigment cells; *e* rhabdome; *f* visual cells; *g* retinal (basal) pigment cells; *h* basal membrane; *i* reduced visual cell; *k* filiform portion of visual cell; *l* central process of visual cell

by a rhabdome, a group of rhabdomeres belonging to a visual cell. A rhabdomere of a visual cell can be considered by analogy with the outer segment of the photoreceptor cell of vertebrates. However, unlike the outer segment, which consists of a stack of photoreceptor membranes (disks), the rhabdomere consists of a number of tightly packed tubules or microvilli (Fig. 50A). Both cases exhibit a much expanded area of the surface of the cell plasma membrane, which forms some kind of light-absorbing periodic structure and contains the visual pigment. According to the calculations of GRIBAKIN (1969b), in the retinula of the bee the average surface area of one microvillus is $7.5 \times 10^{-2}\,\mu m^2$, while the surface area of the entire photoreceptor membrane of the microvilli belonging to one visual cell comprises about $3,800\,\mu m^2$. Thus, the surface area of the photoreceptor membrane of the visual cell in the bee is fully comparable with that of vertebrates. At the same time, it should be pointed out that the utilization of the volume of the photoreceptor structure is approximately twice as efficient in the bee as in vertebrates. This condensation of the photoreceptor structure may be one of the advantages presented by the rhabdomeric organization of the eye.

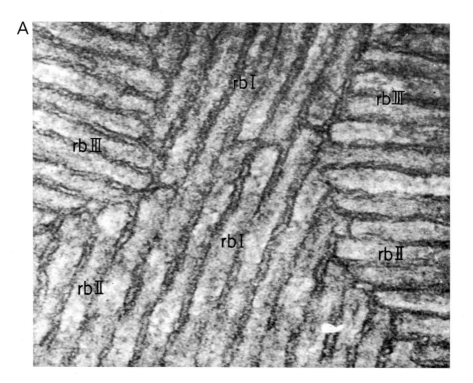

Fig. 50A and B. Structural organization of the rhabdome and retinular cells of the bee (GRIBAKIN, 1967b). A. distal area of the retinula, seen in cross-section ($\times$ 5,000); B. Ventral portion of rhabdome ($\times$ 160,000); *frc* I—III visual cell types; *rb* I—III rhabdome types; *rb* rhabdome; *m* mitochondria; *gp* pigment granules; *opc* outer pigment cell; *d* desmosome; *hec* main endoplasmic cistern

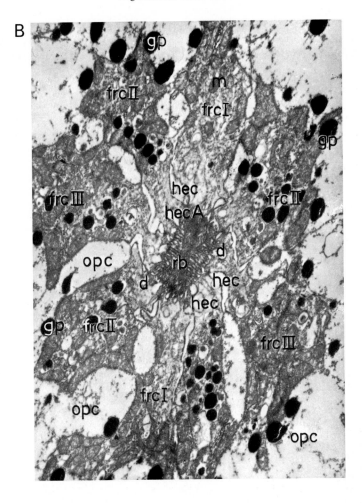

Since the time of EXNER (1891), the complex eyes of arthropods are usually assigned to one of two types—superpositional or appositional—depending upon how the image is formed. However, subsequent research has shown that there exist other and possibly greater differences between these two types of eyes (see, for instance: GOLDSMITH, 1964; MAZOKHIN-PORSHNYAKOV, 1965; POST and GOLDSMITH, 1965). Superposition eyes are found in insects living in conditions of poor lighting (mostly of a nocturnal mode of life), whereas appositional eyes occur in day-active insects. The superposition eye is characterized by a very high light sensitivity (and great total light power) and a low adaptation rate; at the same time, migration of granules of the screening pigment plays an important role in the process of adaptation (as a result of pigment migration, the sensitivity of the superposition eye may vary, for instance by a factor of $10^2$) (POST and GOLDSMITH, 1965). The apposition eye is characterized by a high adaption rate, absence of pigment migration with a change in illumination, and a considerably lower overall light sensitivity. POST and GOLDSMITH (1965)

therefore proposed to change the terminology and subdivide the compound insect eyes into two types according to their optical adaptation characteristics, calling them the scotopic and photopic eye types. This classification, in our opinion, is certainly a better reflection of the progress made in the study of insect vision in recent years (Fig. 49).

Thanks to rather numerous electron microscopic studies (FERNÁNDEZ-MORÁN, 1956; DANEEL and ZEUTZSCHEL, 1957; GOLDSMITH and PHILPOTT, 1957; WOLKEN, CAPENOS, and TURANO, 1957; YASUSUMI and DEGUCHI, 1958; WOLKEN and GUPTA, 1961; GOLDSMITH, 1962; GRIBAKIN, 1967a), the general ultrastructural organization of the retinular cell is quite well known (Fig. 50A, B).

In the photoreceptors of vertebrates the structure which absorbs light (i. e. the outer segment) is to a marked degree dissociated from the body of the cell, whereas in arthropods the rhabdomeres run parallel to the bodies of the retinular cells. This may well account for the more rapid action of insect eyes compared to the eyes of vertebrates (in bees, the flicker fusion frequency attains up to 300 flashes per second).

The distal region of the cell (nearest to the crystalline cone) usually contains the greatest number of mitochondria and granules of the screening retinular pigment, e. g. fly *(Lucilia)* (TRUJILLO-CENOS, 1965); bee (GRIBAKIN, 1967a). The distal region most frequently contains membranes of the rough endoplasmic reticulum, which is directly involved in protein synthesis (PORTER, 1961). Such a saturation of important organoids in the distal region of the cell probably indicates intensified energy activity in this region. This hypothesis is supported by the fact that, in the apposition eye, the plane of the image (and consequently the region of maximum illumination) is situated in the distal region of the retinula (EXNÉR, 1891; DE VRIES and KUIPER, 1958). Electron microscopic studies show that the microvilli of rhabdomeres are connected with the central portion of the cell by a system of radial "fibers" or bridges (Fig. 51) (GRIBAKIN, 1969a). These cytoplasmic bridges pass through a large cytoplasmic cistern (the principal endoplasmic cistern, according to GRIBAKIN), which extends parallel to the rhabdomere, running alongside of it throughout the entire length of the visual cell (about 250 µm in the bee). It is possible to trace the transition of the membrane surrounding the principal cistern into the membrane of the endoplasmic reticulum canals. This cistern extends all the way up to the origin of the axon. An approximate calculation shows that in the bee the volume of the principal endoplasmic cistern in the visual cell is in the dark-adapted eye about 150—250 µm$^3$, whereas the volume of the rhabdomere is 75—150 µm$^3$ (GRIBAKIN, 1969a). It is also possible to observe mitochondria bordering on the membranes of the endoplasmic reticulum; this indicates intensive local energy processes associated with ATP consumption. Thus, the cistern and the endoplasmic reticulum probably differ in their ion content from the cytoplasmic matrix; this may be associated with an active transfer of ions and transmission of neural stimulation inside the visual cell. The nucleus of the retinular cell is usually elongated along the length of the cell; in some insects (for instance, the wax moth) it is capable of shifting its position longitudinally along the cell with changed illumination (POST and GOLDSMITH, 1965).

In the proximal region of the retinular cell numerous protoneurofibrils, typical for an axon, can be seen under the electron microscope; the mitochondria are usually shifted into the peripheral region, which is also characteristic for

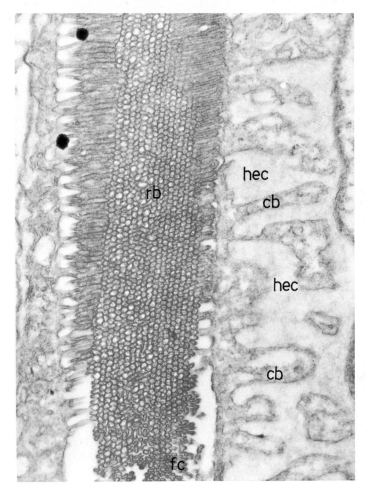

Fig. 51. Longitudinal section of the bee rhabdome (×20,000) (GRIBAKIN, 1967a). *fc* visual cell; *rb* rhabdome; *hec* main endoplasmic cistern; *cb* cytoplasmic bridges

an axon, and the rhabdomere gradually disappears in this region. The proximal end of the rhabdome, which is an optical waveguide (see, for instance, GOLDSMITH, 1964), is usually closed by an "optical plug" (GRIBAKIN, 1967a, 1974) consisting of thickenings of the interretinular fibers filled with granules of screening pigment. Such a "plug" apparently prevents light from penetrating into higher sections of the visual tract, where light (and particularly ultraviolet radiation) could disrupt the function of cells in optical centers.

At the present time, discussions are in progress as to which is the functional unit of the compound eye, the ommatidium or the individual retinular cell (see e. g. GOLDSMITH, 1964). The second hypothesis is favored by the fact that cells of the compound eye differ not only in their spectral sensitivity and in their reaction to the position of the polarization plane of incident light (GOLD-SMITH, 1964; MAZOKHIN-PORSHNYAKOV, 1965; SHAW, 1966, 1967) but also in their morphological characteristics (Fig. 52). For example, electron micrographs

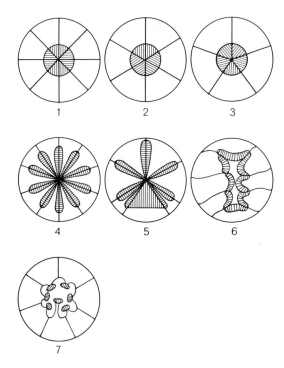

Fig. 52. Orientation of rhabdomere microvilli in various insect species (GRIBAKIN, 1979a). *1* bee *Apis mellifera*; *2* dragonfly *Anax junius*; *3* grasshopper *Dissoseria*; *4* silk worm *Bombyx mori*; *5* tropical butterfly *Epargyreus*; *6* tropical butterfly *Erubus odora*; *7* flies *Musca, Lucilia, Drosophila,* and *Calliphora*

obtained by FERNÁNDEZ-MORÁN (1958) show that the retinula of the superpositional (or scotopic) eye of the tropical night butterfly *Erebus odora* contains seven rhabdomeres, one of which has a much larger cross-sectional area than the others. It is likely that the cell forming this rhabdomere also has maximum light sensitivity (as compared to the remaining cells making up the retinula). It has been demonstrated (GRIBAKIN, 1967b, 1974) that the retinula of the apposition (or photopic) eye of the bee *Apis mellifera* contains three types of cells which differ in cross-sectional area of rhabdomeres, diameter of microvilli, and also depth at which the nucleus is located (Fig. 50, Fig. 53). As we shall see, these types of cells perceive light radiations of different wave lengths, i. e. they are responsible for the color vision of the bee.

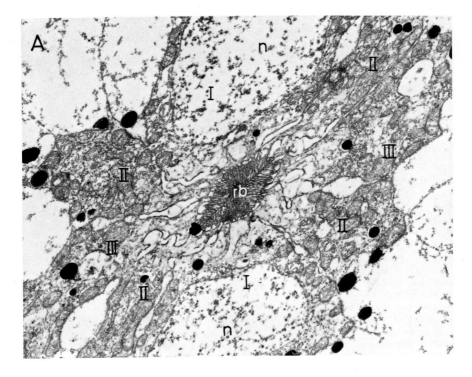

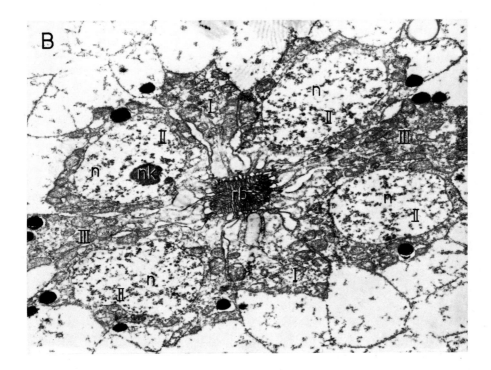

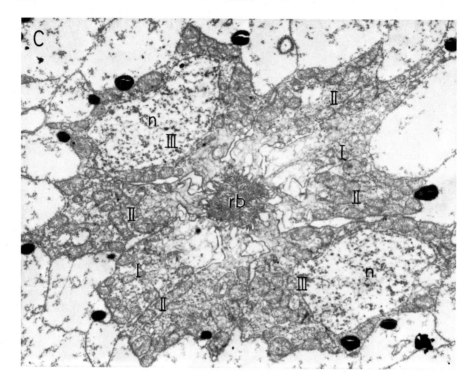

Fig. 53 A—C. Cross-section of bee retinula in the nuclear region. Types I (A), II (B) and III (C) ( × 5,000) (GRIBAKIN, 1970). *I—III* visual cells of different types; *n* nucleus; *nk* nucleolus; *rb* rhabdome

Even with the electron microscope, it is still not possible to visualize the paths of the synthesis of the visual pigment in the cell or to study its localization. Moreover, the study of the visual pigments of insects is greatly complicated by at least two factors: 1. the structures containing the visual pigment are situated in the center (more exactly, in the bottom) of each retinula, and this makes it difficult to obtain rhabdomere fractions with the methods currently used by biochemists for obtaining fractions of retinal outer segments in vertebrates; 2. the study of isolated specimens of the eye is complicated by the presence in every ommatidium of a pigment sheath and an optical "plug" closing the proximal end of the rhabdome. Nevertheless, a large number of interesting data have been obtained concerning the visual pigments of insects. Their visual pigments have considerably lower molecular weight (3,000 to 4,000) than visual pigments of vertebrates 40,000 (DAEMEN *et al.*, 1972), and therefore the diameter of the visual pigment molecule in insects must be considerably smaller, about 20Å as compared to 40—50Å in vertebrates. There is evidence that the vision of many insects (and perhaps all insects) is based on retinal; this substance has been found in bees, domestic flies, certain orthoptera, dragonflies, beetles, and butterflies (GOLDSMITH, 1958; WOLKEN, BOWNESS, and SCHEER, 1960; BRIGGS, 1961). GOLDSMITH (1958) was able to extract the visual pigment from the bee's compound eye, not with detergents but with a simple phosphate buffer;

after illumination, the solution of the visual pigment was bleached, releasing retinal. GOLDSMITH and WARNER (1964) have clearly proved that the visual system of the working bee is built on the basis of vitamin A (retinol): in the dark, vitamin A is oxidized to retinal, and in the light retinal is converted into vitamin A. GOLDSMITH and WARNER have also found that in the bee vitamin A is present only in the head, or more precisely, in the eyes. They do not think there are any metabolic reserves of vitamin A or retinal in either the head or the body of the bee.

The nature of the localization and orientation of the visual pigment molecules (more exactly, of the dipole moments of these molecules) in the rhabdomeres of the compound eye of insects is still unclear in many respects. Moreover, until relatively recently, there was no direct proof in general that the rhabdomere is a light-receptive structure (i. e. that the visual pigment is present in the rhabdomere).

Thanks to the work of LANGER (1960, 1965) and THORELL (LANGER and THORELL, 1966), it was shown that rhabdomeres do contain visual pigment. LANGER and THORELL, studying individual rhabdomeres in the compound eye of the white-eyed mutant of the fly *Calliphora* (utilization of the white-eyed mutant made it possible to avoid the interfering effect of the screening pigment), showed that:

1. The absorption spectrum of an individual rhabdomere conforms well with a) the well-known curve of DARTNALL (1953); b) the absorption spectrum of cattle and squid rhodopsin; c) the spectrum sensitivity curve measured from the electroretinogram; d) the sensitivity spectrum curve obtained by recording intracellular potentials.

2. The absorption spectra of rhabdomeres are not identical. Six of the seven rhabdomeres present in the same retinula have absorption peaks at 500 nm, while the central one has a peak at 460 nm, which probably corresponds to the "blue-sensitive" and "green-sensitive" receptors of BURKHARDT (1962).

3. After prolonged light exposure, the magnitude of the absorption peak at 500 nm decreases; this is probably the result of a partial bleaching of the visual pigment, as occurs in vertebrates.

4. An inherent property of rhabdomeres is dichroic light absorption; the dichroic ratio in *Calliphora* is 4:3, i. e. 1.33.

The last fact is probably of the greatest interest, since it brings us close to the problem of orientation of visual pigment molecules in the rhabdomere microvilli and, in our opinion, deserves a closer examination.

First let us recall that all animals possessing the rhabdomere type of retina (arthropods and cephalopods) are capable of orienting in the environment in the polarization plane of light (see, for instance, the review by JANDER and WATERMAN, 1960; also MOODY and PARRISS, 1961; TASAKI and KARITA, 1966; and others). In 1950 AUTRUM and STUMPF advanced the hypothesis that an individual visual cell can act as analyzer of polarized light; shortly afterwards, with the progress of electron microscopy, it became possible to identify the peculiarities of the structure which performs this function, i. e. the rhabdomere (FERNÁNDEZ-MORÁN, 1956; GOLDSMITH and PHILPOTT, 1957). Numerous studies were published confirming the reaction of the individual visual cell in arthropods to the rotation of the polarization plane of incident light in the fly *Lucilia* (BURKHARDT and WENDLER, 1960), the fly *Calliphora* (AUTRUM and ZWEHL, 1962a), the crab *Carcinus maenas*, and the locust *Locusta* (SHAW, 1966, 1967). It became clear that if the retinular cell is capable of analyzing linearly-polarized light, the immediate analyzer of such light must be the rhabdomere. In turn, the rhabdomere can act as analyzer of plane-polarized light only if the absorption coefficient is dichroic (DE VRIES, SPOOR, and JIELOF, 1953; STOCKHAMMER, 1956). Filter mechanism of polarized light perception in insect eye was suggested in our laboratory by GRIBAKIN (1973). In 1961, MOODY and PARRISS, who discovered that the octopus is capable of distinguishing the plane of light polarization, attempted to estimate the magnitude of the dichroism of the rhabdomere. Their calculation was based on the assumption that the visual pigment is a structural element of the membrane of rhabdomere microvilli, as it is in vertebrates (BROWN, GIBBONS, and WALD, 1963). MOODY and PARRISS believed (again in analogy to vertebrates) (WALD, BROWN, and GIBBONS, 1963) that the dipole moments of the visual pigment molecules lie in the plane of the microvilli membrane but have a random orientation in this membrane. As a result of a rather simple analysis, MOODY and PARRISS obtained the following expression for the relative absorption of a single microvillus:

$$E(e) = \tfrac{1}{2}\pi\sigma r l(1+e_z)^2, \tag{1}$$

where $E$ is the relative light absorption, $\sigma$ is the surface density of the visual pigment molecules in the membrane of the microvillus (number of molecules per unit surface area of the microvillus membrane), $r$ is the radius of the microvillus, $l$ is the length of the microvillus, $e$ is the unit electric vector, having components along the 3 coordinate axes, $e_x, e_y, e_z$, respectively. (In the calculations of MOODY and PARRISS, it was assumed that the direction of the microvillus axis coincides with the axis $z$.)

If light propagates along the axis $y$, which is parallel to the optical axis of the ommatidium, then it has two components of the electric vector $-e_x$ and $e_z$. The dichroism of absorption is determined by the ratio of relative absorptions for the two components $e_x$ and $e_z$, and in the case of experiments with rotation of the polarization plane for two positions of the vector $e$, i.e. when it is parallel to the axis $z$ (or to the microvillus axis, which is the same) $-E_{||}$, and when it is perpendicular to this axis $-E_\perp$.

Obviously, when $e$ is parallel to axis $z$, we obtain $|e| = e_z = 1$, and Eq. (1) yields

$$E_{||} = \tfrac{1}{2}\pi\sigma r l(1+e) = \pi\sigma r l. \tag{2}$$

Accordingly, when $e$ is perpendicular to the axis $z$ (i.e. when $e$ is parallel to axis $x$), we have:

$$e = e_x = 1, \quad \text{and} \quad e_z = 0;$$

then:                                                                                (3)

$$E_\perp = \tfrac{1}{2}\pi\sigma r l.$$

The coefficient of dichroic absorption (which by definition is greater than unity) is determined by the ratio between the greater relative absorption $(E_{\parallel})$ and the smaller one $(E_{\perp})$:

$$\frac{E_{\parallel}}{E_{\perp}} = \frac{\pi \sigma r l}{\frac{1}{2}\pi \sigma r l} = 2, \tag{4}$$

and this is indeed what MOODY and PARRISS obtained.

However, the value of the dichroic ratio obtained by LANGER and THORELL (1966) is less than 2, namely $4:3$. This may be due to the fact that not all visual pigment molecules are situated in the plane of the membrane, which is the case for the membranes of outer-segment disks in vertebrates (WALD, BROWN, and GIBBONS, 1963). GRIBAKIN (1969a) proposed a correction in the calculations of MOODY and PARRISS as follows: the dipole moments of some of the visual pigment molecules must be considered as being oriented perpendicular to the surface of the membrane. Let $\sigma_s$ be the surface density of molecules with dipole moments lying in the plane of the membrane, and let $\sigma_r$ be the surface density of molecules with dipole moments oriented perpendicular to the surface of the membrane (let us call them radial dipole moments, since they are directed along the radii of the microvilli). The total surface density of the visual pigment molecules is then $\sigma = \sigma_s + \sigma_r$. Hence different positions of the polarization plane of the light wave (i.e. different orientations of the vector $\mathbf{e}$, which is perpendicular to the polarization plane and lies in the so-called plane of vibration will yield different relative absorptions of molecules entering $\sigma_s$ and of molecules entering $\sigma_r$. Thus, for $\mathbf{e}$ parallel to the $z$ axis, we obtain:

$$E_{s\parallel} = \pi \sigma_s r l \quad \text{and} \quad E_{r\parallel} = 0.$$

($E_{r\parallel}$ is equal to zero, since $\mathbf{e}$ is parallel to the $z$ axis and therefore perpendicular to $xoy$, the plane parallel to which lie the radially oriented moments).

For $\mathbf{e}$ perpendicular to the $z$ axis, we obtain:

$$E_{s\perp} = \frac{1}{2\pi \sigma_s r l},$$

since the calculations of MOODY and PARRISS are valid for $\sigma_s$.

Moreover,

$$E_{r\perp} = \pi \sigma_r r l,$$

which can also be easily obtained by the calculation method of MOODY and PARRISS. The dichroic ratio will then be defined as:

$$\delta = \frac{E_{s\parallel} + E_{r\parallel}}{E_{s\perp} + E_{r\perp}}. \tag{5}$$

If the fraction of molecules having radially oriented dipole moments is equal to $n$, where $n < 1$, then:

$$\left. \begin{array}{l} \sigma_r = n\sigma \\ \sigma_s = (1-n)\sigma \end{array} \right\}. \tag{6}$$

and

$$\delta = \frac{E_{s\parallel} + E_{r\parallel}}{E_{s\perp} + E_{r\perp}} = \frac{\pi \sigma_s r l + 0}{\dfrac{1}{2\pi \sigma_s r l} + \pi \sigma_r r l} = \frac{\sigma_s}{\dfrac{1}{2\sigma_s} + \sigma_r} \tag{7}$$

expressing (7) by (6), we obtain:

$$\delta = \frac{(1-n)\sigma}{\dfrac{1}{2(1-n)\sigma} + n\sigma} = \frac{2(1-n)}{1+n}. \tag{8}$$

Hence, $n=(2-\delta)/(2+\delta)$. Substituting here the value for $\delta=\frac{4}{3}$, as given by LANGER and THORELL for *Calliphora*, we get $n=0.2$. Thus, in *Calliphora* 20% of pigment molecules are oriented perpendicular to the surface of the membrane. Of course, these conclusions cannot be extrapolated to other species with a rhabdomeric type of retina unless the dichroic ratio is known. Moreover, BURK-HARDT and WENDLER (1960), also working with *Calliphora*, found that when the plane of polarization is rotated through 90° the electrical response of a single retinular cell varies by 15%. A similar variation in the magnitude of the cell response was obtained by the above authors by doubling the light intensity. The dichroism of a rhabdomere in such a cell must therefore have a value of the order of 2, if we assume that the electric response of the cell depends only upon the number of quanta absorbed by the visual pigment of the rhabdomere.

Similar results were obtained by KUWABARA and NAKA (1959) on the fly *Lucilia*. They showed that rotating the polarization plane through 90° decreases the electrical response of the cell by about 20%. Unfortunately, these authors did not measure the change in light intensity which induces the same lowering of response, as did BURKHARDT and WENDLER. Nevertheless, even on the basis of the lower response value (20% in the case of KUWABARA and NAKA, as compared to 15% in the case of BURKHARDT and WENDLER), we can still state that the dichroism of rhabdomeres in *Lucilia* is small. Experiments on the locust by SHAW (1966) showed that rotating the polarization plane of light through 90° reduces the response in the retinular cell by 0.1—0.7 logarithmic unit, or a factor of 1.25—5. The average value cited by SHAW for the locust is 0.37 logarithmic unit, or a factor of about 2.3. Such a large variation in the value of the cell response may indicate a stronger dichroism in locust rhabdo-meres as compared to those of Diptera so that the dipole moments of visual pigment molecules must be to a certain degree oriented along the axes of microvilli. Rhabdome microvilli in the eye of the crab *Carcinus maenas* must possess very strong dichroism since, when the polarization plane is rotated by 90°, the response of the retinular cell varies by 0.89 logarithmic unit, or a factor of 7.7 (SHAW, 1966).

Dichroism of rhabdomeres can also be deduced from experiments performed by GIULIO (1963), who illuminated longitudinal sections of the compound eyes of various flies (*Calliphora erythrocephala, Calliphora vomitoria, Musca domestica*) with linearly-polarized light, incident perpendicular to the optical axes of the ommatidia. In this case, GIULIO recorded the overall electroretinogram (ERG) and obtained ERG's of different amplitudes at different positions on the polariza-tion plane. However, it is difficult to make a quantitative evaluation of his experimental results because of inadequate data.

SHAW (1967) revealed an interesting coincidence between the ultrastructural organization of the rhabdome and the value of the electrical response of the cell. He succeeded in inserting two microelectrodes into different retinular cells in the same retinula of a locust and found that, upon rotation of the polarization plane of light, the maximum responses of the cells are shifted by 60° relative to each other. This agrees with the electron microscopic data of HORRIDGE and BARNARD (1965), according to which microvilli in the locust rhabdome are oriented in three directions with 120° angles between them.

Further experiments to find out how insects (and arthropods, in particular) are able to distinguish the polarization plane of light will unquestionably be of great importance, not only for the study of this phenomenon, which is interesting in itself, but also for an understanding of those molecular mechanisms upon which stimulation of the visual cell is based in general.

From this point of view, it would be very important to know what changes occur in the ultrastructure of the rhabdome and in the retinular cells proper under the effect of light. However, there is very little experimental material available in this field. HORRIDGE and BARNARD (1965) showed that, following illumination, the ultrastructure of the locust retina undergoes certain changes ("palisade movement") although the rhabdome remains unchanged. EGUCHI and WATERMAN (1967) showed that, under illumination, the number of lamellar bodies increases in the visual cells of the eye of the crab *Libinia*, the process of pinocytosis is intensified in the cell region adjacent to the rhabdome, a change takes place in the configuration of the endoplasmic reticulum membrane, the number of ribosomes increases, etc. Statistical processing of a large number of electron micrographs allowed EGUCHI and WATERMAN to propose valid criteria for the detection of cells with different degrees of light adaptation. In particular, they were able to demonstrate that cells with variously oriented microvilli are actually stimulated in a different way by polarized light; this can be considered as a clear confirmation of the hypothesis of AUTRUM and STUMPF (1950). The most important structure of the visual cell, the rhabdome, showed absolutely no changes in the process of adaptation to light. However, data obtained in our laboratory show that, upon illumination of the compound eye of the working bee, substantial changes can be observed in the rhabdome. It is thus possible to make a definite statement on the operation of retinular cells, as we explain below.

In conclusion, it is interesting to compare certain features of the insect compound eye with the eye of vertebrates. Both types of eye utilize a much ramified surface area of the photoreceptor membrane to increase the probability of light quanta absorption; the methods used to create such a surface are, however, different: disks in one case and microvilli in the other. In vertebrates and apparently also in insects, the visual pigment is the structural element of the photoreceptor membrane. These organisms, so different in their phylogenesis, use the same substance as the chromophore group of the pigment, namely vitamin A aldehyde, or retinal. Both types of eye should be able to distinguish colors, although they do not always. The most serious defect of the compound eye is "myopia" (i. e., a low angular resolution power), but this seems to be fully compensated for by its rapid action and ability to distinguish the polarization plane of light, and by an extension into the ultraviolet region of the range of light perceived. From the fact that vision in both vertebrates and insects (including arthropods in general and cephalopod mollusks) is based on vitamin A, we may assume that the molecular mechanisms of vision are more or less identical in all these animals, whereas peculiarities in the physiology of vision are mainly due to differences in the ultrastructural organization of the photoreceptor cells. The structural organization and functional shifts in the insect retinula will be examined in greater detail in the section devoted to color vision.

## D. Photoreceptors of Cephalopod Molluscs

The eyes of cephalopod molluscs are characterized by their huge dimensions. In the cuttlefish the body length is only 10—20 times the diameter of its eye, and in *Lycotenthis diadema* only 10 times (CHUN, 1910). The diameter of the eyeball of *Architeuthis* is, for instance, 40 cm. In $1 mm^2$ of the retina of *Scaergus* up to 26,000 visual cells are present, in the octopus about 64,000, in *Sepia* 105,000, and in *Loligo* 162,000 (AKIMUSHKIN, 1963a). The eyes of cephalopod molluscs have a noninverted retina, a vitreous body, a crystalline lens, an iris and pupil, and a cornea; Octopoda also have eyelids.

Over a hundred years ago BABUKHIN (1864) carried out the first histological study of the retina in cephalopods. Later, the retina was studied with the light microscope by GRENACHER (1886), HENSEN (1885), SCHULTZE (1869) and others. It was established that the retina consists of bipolar cells, oriented parallel to the direction of the light ray. The apical portion of these cells forms outer and inner segments, which contain a light-sensitive pigment, rhodopsin, and a nerve fiber branches off from the basal portion. The retina in the squid is 0.5 mm thick. The ratio of the length of the outer segment to that of the inner segment is 2.1:1. In the retina, the following have been described with the aid of the electron microscope (Fig. 54): an inner limiting membrane, a layer of outer segments or rods; a layer of bases of rods, located between the outer and inner segments, containing the pigment and the nucleus of so-called epithelial cells; a layer of inner segments with visual cell nuclei and myeloid bodies; a reticular layer and a layer of optic nerve fibers. Visual cells of the squid and octopus were studied under the electron microscope (WOLKEN, 1958; MOODY and ROBERTSON, 1960; MOODY and PARRISS, 1961; ZONANA, 1961; NISHIOKA, HAGADORN, and BERN, 1962; YAMAMOTO et al., 1965; and unpublished data obtained in our laboratory). It was found that the outer segment consists of tubules, or microvilli. The inner segment contains the above-mentioned "myeloid" bodies, developing apparently from endoplasmic reticulum membranes, and the visual pigment of cephalopods, retinochrome (HARA and HARA, 1967, 1968).

The outer segments, or rods are 0.3 μm long. The apices of the outer segments are separated from the vitreous body by an inner limiting membrane, which has an amorphous structure and a thickness of 5 μm. The apex of the outer segment is thought to be attached to the inner limiting membrane. The plasma membrane of the outer segment forms microvilli oriented perpendicular to the light beam. The ensemble of microvilli constitutes the rhabdome (Fig. 55A, B). The microvilli are about 1.1 μm long and 0.1 μm in diameter. According to our data, in cross-sections microvilli of the visual cell have an irregular annular shape. Each microvillus is in contact with six other microvilli (Fig. 55 B); a microtubule is located at the center of each microvillus. Two types

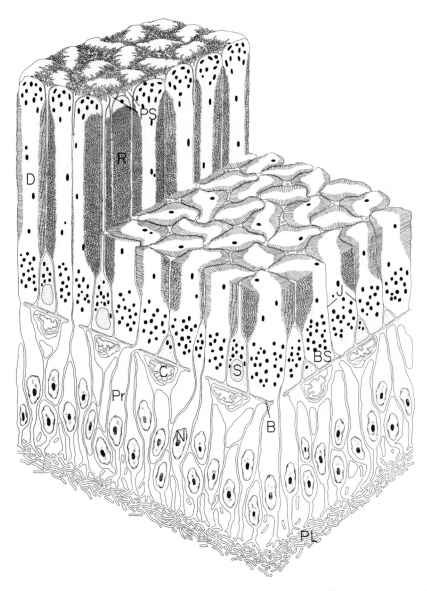

Fig. 54. Schematic three-dimensional reconstruction of the octopus retina (YAMAMOTO et al., 1965). *B* basement membrane; *BS* basal portion of receptor (visual) cells loaded with numerous pigment granules; *C* blood capillaries; *D* distal segments of the visual cells carrying rhabdomeres (*R*) on their lateral surfaces; *J* junction of plasma membranes between two adjoining basal portions; *N* nucleus of the visual cell; *PL* plexiform layer of the retina; *Pr* proximal segment of the visual cell; *PS* tips of the supporting cells (*S*). The glial fibers and the limiting membrane, which covers the ventral (upper in this diagram) surface of the retina, are not depicted

of outer segments are found: circular (type 1) and elongated like ellipsoids (type 2). In the squid, each segment of type 1 is usually surrounded by four segments of type 2. In cross-sections, it is calculated that in each 1,000 cells there are 690 segments belonging to type 2 and 310 to type 1. Some transitional forms are also present. The extracellular substance is located between the segments. Microvilli of adjacent segments are not in contact with each other, since there are no microvilli at the contact point on one of the adjacent segments, and only the plasma membrane is preserved. Microvilli on two neighboring rhabdomes

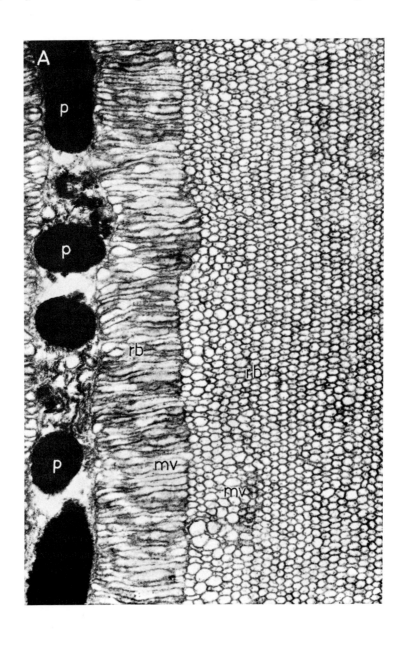

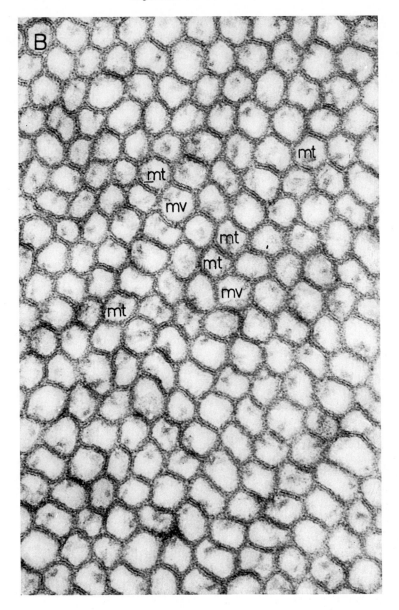

Fig. 55 A and B. Structural organization of the rhabdomere in the squid retina, as seen in (A) longitudinal section (× 50,000) and (B) cross-sections (× 160,000). The microvilli (*mv*) in each rhabdome (*rb*) of adjacent segments, containing pigment (*p*), are mutually perpendicular. In the center of each microvilli (*mv*) in the squid rhabdome is a microtubule (*mt*). (× 160,000 Original)

are always orthogonal (Fig. 55A). In each segment the microvilli lie parallel to each other.

The proximal portion of the visual cell of the squid and the octopus contains, in addition to a nucleus, numerous mitochondria, an endoplasmic reticulum, ribosomes, multivesicular bodies and elements of Golgi's apparatus. The most important structure in the proximal segment comprises the "myeloid" bodies, consisting of a myelin-like system of membranes, up to 50 in number, and having a sequence period within the range 160 to 250Å. Small vesicles or cisterns of irregular shape may be located between the membranes. The myeloid membranes have the usual three-layer structure and are about 150Å thick; myeloid bodies of similar structure have been discovered in cells of the pigment layer of the retina in vertebrates (PORTER and YAMADA, 1960), where their origin and function are as yet obscure. In the basal portion of the distal segment can be found round or oval granules of the screening pigment, mitochondria and elements of the endoplasmic reticulum (YAMAMOTO et al., 1965).

One of the curiosities of the evolution of vision in cephalopod molluscs (Decapoda and Octopoda) is the presence of a dual system of light-sensitive pigments: rhodopsin and retinochrome (HARA, HARA, and TAKEUCHI, 1967; HARA and HARA, 1968). Rhodopsin is localized in the rhabdomere of the visual cell and acts as a visual pigment. It was discovered and isolated in the nineteenth century (KROHN, 1839—1842; KRÜKENBERG, 1882). It has been known for a relatively long time that in cephalopods rhodopsin does not break down completely under the effect of light, but only undergoes the isomerization associated with early stages of molecular transformation. It was assumed that under the action of light metarhodopsin would be reconverted into the original rhodopsin:

$$\text{rhodopsin} \underset{}{\overset{\text{light}}{\rightleftharpoons}} \text{metarhodopsin}$$

(HUBBARD and ST. GEORGE, 1957—1958). Retinochrome is localized in the region of the retina lying directly under the rhabdomeres and is most probably bound to the membranes of myeloid bodies situated in the proximal segment of the photoreceptor cell (HARA and HARA, 1967). The absorption maximum of rhodopsin in various species of cephalopod molluscs is between 475 and 500nm, whereas the absorption maximum of retinochrome is between 480 and 512nm (HARA and HARA, 1968). Although the absorption spectra of these photopigments are very similar, they differ considerably in their characteristic changes under the effect of light. For example, rhodopsin is not bleached at 20°C and acid pH, since a mixture of rhodopsin and acid metarhodopsin is formed, whereas retinochrome is bleached regardless of pH, just like the rhodopsin of vertebrates (HARA and HARA, 1967; HARA, HARA, and TAKEUCHI, 1967). Both rhodopsin and retinochrome are chromoproteids, containing retinal as a chromophore. Nevertheless, they differ substantially in the stereoisometric configuration of their chromophore: rhodopsin binds the 11-*cis* form of retinal, whereas retinochrome binds the all-*trans* form. Under the effect of light, the chromophore of retinochrome undergoes a conversion from the all-*trans* form to the 11-*cis* form. The reverse changes take place in rhodopsin, which is then present as opsin, i.e., part of the visual pigment. It has been shown that the specific function of retinochrome consists in the catalysis in visible light of the isomerization of retinal from the all-*trans* form to the 11-*cis* configuration (HARA and HARA, 1968).

The products of the light reaction of retinochrome can regenerate the original pigment by attaching the all-*trans*-retinal to the protein component of retinochrome (HARA and HARA, 1968). The photoisomerization of rhodopsin proceeds in the opposite direction to the isomerization of retinochrome; functionally the two pigments complement each other, although the processes of their photoisomerization are mutually opposed. In vertebrates, as we have seen, the isomerization of retinal is indispensable for the regeneration of the visual pigment and is achieved partly with the aid of the catalytic effect of retinal isomerase (HUBBARD and ST. GEORGE, 1957—1958). In cephalopods such isomerization is associated with the specific function of another auxiliary pigment, namely retinochrome (Fig. 56). Thus, the discovery of retinochrome made it possible to explain the presence of the light-sensitive pigment in the photoreceptors of cephalopod molluscs.

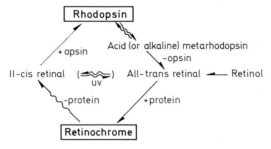

Fig. 56. Schematic representation of the function of the dual system of photopigments (rhodopsin and retinochrome) in cephalopods, in connection with the isomerization of their chromophore, retinal (HARA and HARA, 1968)

The characteristics of the organization of rhabdomeres of cephalopods and the presence of visual pigment as a structural component in these organisms led to the discovery of the important fact already mentioned, that the octopus is able to distinguish the polarization plane of light (MOODY and PARRISS, 1961). Molecular calculations made it possible to compare the dichroism displayed by rhabdomere microvilli of the octopus with that of insects.

Interesting electrophysiological data obtained on the retina of cephalopod molluscs make it possible to compare, in many respects, their vision with that of insects (BYZOV, 1966). A layer-by-layer analysis of electroretinograms (ERG) shows that two components with different properties can be distinguished in the ERG of the octopus: a relatively rapid and brief potential deflection at a depth of 250 to 300 µm (distal component), and a gradually increasing deflection (generator potential), flattening out into a plateau which persists throughout the period of illumination and gradually falls after the light has been switched off (trace potential) in the 325 to 350 µm layer (proximal component) (BYZOV, 1966). Two analogous components of the retinogram were obtained in the squid by BYZOV (1966). BYZOV thinks that the distal component does not arise in the rhabdomere layer, but rather at the level of the nucleus-containing portion of photoreceptor cells, where the myeloid bodies containing retinochrome are situated (HARA and HARA, 1968). The proximal component arises in the neuroglia region, where axons of visual cells are located. Byzov's data go far to clarify the results obtained in a study of the electroretinogram of the octopus (TASAKI, NORTON, and FUKUDA, 1963; TASAKI, OIKAWA, and NORTON, 1963). In the squid and the octopus, after exposure to bright light, the proximal component has a very long trace potential. These facts suggest that the process of dark adaptation in these animals lasts for dozens of minutes.

Whereas there is no doubt that the electrical reaction of visual cells, and in particular the generator potential, is the result of changes in the permeability of the cell membrane, the mechanism of the preceding link (the reactions occurring at the moment when light is absorbed by the visual pigment) is still not clear. In other words, we do not know what triggers the stimulation of the visual cell and is associated with changes in rhodopsin and retinochrome, on the one hand, and the appearance of a potential, on the other hand. What happens at this moment is still essentially unclear, even in the case of the much-studied visual cells in vertebrates and the well-studied eye of *Limulus*.

Experiments carried out with colorimetric methods have shown that neither the squid *Ommastrephes sloanei pacificus* nor the octopus *Octopus dofleini* appears to possess color vision (ORLOV and BYZOV, 1961); this is probably associated with the absence of corresponding molecular protein variations of their visual pigments. The cuttlefish *Sepia officinalis* is thought to have color vision, since its integuments contain yellow, orange and brown chromatophores which undergo selective contraction, depending upon the nature of the illumination (KUHN, 1950). However, such chromatophores are present in the integuments of both the octopus and the squid.

## E. Color Vision in Vertebrates and Insects

The presence in vertebrates of two types of photoreceptors, differing in the shape of their peripheral processes, led as long ago as the 1860's to the conclusion that one type, the rods, comprises receptors of a monochromatic visual system, while the other type, the cones, includes receptors of a color visual system (SCHULTZE, 1866). However, it soon became clear that cones should be further subdivided into three types, and that each of these types responds to perception of its "own" primary color. Even in 1802 YOUNG pointed out the existence of three simple colors, perceived by us as sensations of red, green and purple; there are three binary combinations of these colors, namely yellow, consisting of red and green; crimson, consisting of red and purple; and blue, consisting of green and purple; the seventh color in this series is white, formed by mixing all three colors.

In fact, whereas in vertebrates, color perception is associated with cones that are morphologically similar whatever their color perception, in insects, and specifically in bees, three morphologically different types of cells have been discovered in our laboratory (GRIBAKIN, 1967b, 1969b, 1969c). Hence, in the more "ancient" animal forms, insects, the difference in the function of photoreceptors has already found cytological expression, whereas in "younger" forms, vertebrates, these functional differences are still restricted to the molecular level of organization.

The presence in one retina of cones with a different spectral absorption selectivity was confirmed in birds, turtles and lizards; their colored oil droplet, as noted above, apparently acts as a light filter ensuring the relative "monochromaticity" of a given cone (ORLOV, 1963; ORLOV and MAKSIMOVA, 1964).

Basically, however, it was found that the matter can be reduced to differences in the light sensitivity of the visual pigment present in cones. Thus, RUSHTON (1959) found in the fovea of human retina two light-sensitive pigments with absorption peaks at 540 and 590 nm. Analogous data were obtained by WEALE (1959). STILES (1959, 1964) obtained three distinct spectral curves with absorption peaks at 440, 540 and 590 nm; this, in his opinion, corresponds to the three types of photoreceptor. By the method of "partial bleaching" with colored light it was possible to obtain on the retina of the enucleated human and monkey eye two absorption peaks at 533 and 565 nm (BROWN and WALD, 1963). Finally, the presence was demonstrated in the human retina of three types of cones: blue-sensitive ($\lambda_{max} = 445$—447—450 nm); green-sensitive ($\lambda_{max} = 525$—535—540 nm), and red-sensitive ($\lambda_{max} = 555$—570—574 nm) (MACNICHOL, 1956; BROWN and WALD, 1964; MARX, DOBELLE, and MACNICHOL, 1964; WALD, 1964). Finally, three spectral types of cones were demonstrated in goldfish by a direct microelectrode technique (TOMITA, 1965).

According to WALD (1964), the data thus obtained suffice to explain the various forms of color blindness: thus, in protanopics the red-sensitive receptors do not function, in tritanopics it is the blue-sensitive, and in deuteranopics the green-sensitive and red-sensitive receptors are combined into a single mechanism. For convenience in comparison, GRIBAKIN and GOVARDOVSKII (1966) have summarized the results obtained by various authors in table form (Table 1).

Table 1.   Types of color receptors in vertebrates (GRIBAKIN and GOVARDOVSKII, 1966)

| Subject | $\lambda_{max}$ (nm) | | | Method | Literature reference |
|---|---|---|---|---|---|
| | Blue-sensitive | green-sensitive | red-sensitive | | |
| Man | — | 540 | 590 | Reflectometry | RUSHTON, 1965 |
| | — | 540 | 600 | Reflectometry | WEALE, 1959 |
| | 440 | 540 | 590 | Chromatic adaptation | STILES, 1959, 1964 |
| Man, Monkey | — | 535 | 565 | Differential bleaching of enucleated eye retina | BROWN and WALD, 1963 |
| Man | 450 | 525 | 555 | Absorption spectra of single cones | BROWN and WALD, 1963 |
| | 430 | 540 | 575 | Chromatic adaptation | BROWN and WALD, 1963 |
| | 447 | 540 | 577 | Absorption spectra of single cones | MACNICHOL, 1956 |
| | 450 | 540 | 567 | Study of color vision defects | LOBANOVA, RAUTIAN, and SPERANSKAYA, 1963 |
| Goldfish (Carassius auratum) | 455 | 530 | 625 | Absorption spectra of single cones | MARX, DOBELLE, and MACNICHOL, 1964 |

In view of the immutability of the structure and function of retinal, the exceptionally great variety of visual pigments (DARTNALL and LYTHGOL, 1964) must be attributed to the structural peculiarities of the protein portion of the visual pigment, namely opsin.

Insects may be endowed with a monochromatic, dichromatic and even a trichromatic system of color vision. Monochromatic vision, i.e. the absence of color vision, has been found, for example, in the termite *Anacanthotermes ahngerianus* (MAZOKHIN-PORSHNYAKOV et al., 1967). In some cases, only a specific part of the compound eye is endowed with monochromatic vision (e. g., the dragonfly *Libellula quadrimaculata*) (MAZOKHIN-PORSHNYAKOV, 1965). However, members of the most highly organized insect orders, such as Hymenoptera, have trichromatic color vision. The spectral sensitivity of individual cells in the compound eye of the drone and the working bee was studied electrophysiologically by AUTRUM and ZWEHL (1962b, 1963, 1964); they established the presence of three types of cells having spectral sensitivity maxima at 330 nm (ultraviolet radiation receptors), 543 nm (yellow-green radiation receptors), and 430 nm (blue radiation receptors), respectively (Fig. 57).

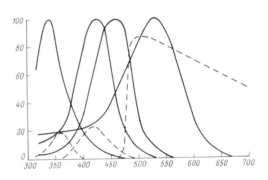

Fig. 57. Spectral sensitivity response of visual cells in the compound eye of the worker bee (solid line) (AUTRUM, 1965, 1968) and transmission curves (broken line) of the light filter system for selective light adaptation (GRIBAKIN, 1969c). The length of the light line (in nm) is plotted along the abscissa, and the relative sensitivity of the visual cell, or filter transmission factor, is plotted along the ordinate

Color vision in insects is believed to be effected by different visual pigments, although so far only one pigment with an absorption peak near 440 nm has been detected in bees (GOLDSMITH, 1958). In this respect, additional biochemical studies are required. In our laboratory, GRIBAKIN (1967a, 1967b, 1969b, 1969c) in electron microscope studies has found three types of retinular cells in which the structural organization of the rhabdome microvilli changes according to the wavelength of the radiation acting upon these cells (see Fig. 53).

The four quadrants into which the retinula rhabdome of the bee is subdivided can be clearly seen in cross-section to fall into two pairs. One pair of diametrically opposed quadrants converges at the center in such a way that a distinct contact line is formed between the quadrants; this line is up to 0.5—0.8 μm long, or

0.3—0.5 percent of the diameter of the rhabdome. The other pair of quadrants accordingly cannot make contact. This nonequivalent subdivision of the rhabdome is maintained throughout its length. In the quadrants that are in contact with each other two rhabdomeres are clearly visible, and these are denser than the other six rhabdomeres. The visual cells, to which these higher-density rhabdomeres belong, are diametrically opposite in the retinula. Distal regions of cells with denser rhabdomeres are generally characterized by a smaller number of granules of retinular screening pigment (Fig. 53A, type-I cells).

More proximal sections show that the nuclei of cells with dense rhabdomeres lie at the same level but are distally more remote from the nuclei of the remaining cells of the retinula (Fig. 53A, B). Slightly more proximal and at the same level four nuclei are found together (Fig. 53B). These nuclei belong to two cells with microvilli pointing in the same direction as in the cells with denser rhabdomeres, and two cells with microvilli at right angles to them. If we make a section through the retinula, we find that cells having nuclei in the second layer alternate.

Lying still deeper are nuclei of the third "layer" (Fig. 53C); these nuclei belong to cells with microvilli oriented at right angles to those in cells with dense rhabdomeres. GRIBAKIN (1967b) was able to find all three types of cells within the limits of a single retinula; they differed both in the arrangement of their nuclei and in the density of their rhabdomeres. He classifies as type-I cells the two cells possessing denser rhabdomeres and containing the most distally located nuclei. The axons that branch out from these cells are larger than those found in other cells. The cross-sectional area of these axons is approximately three times that of the other six axons in the retinula. Classified as type-II cells are the four cells of the retinula with nuclei located in the middle layer. The two cells of the retinula with nuclei located in the proximal layer are classified as type-III cells. Thus, whereas type-I cells differ from the other cells in the retinula by the position of their nuclei, rhabdomere density, and axon thickness, cells of types II and III differ from each other only in the position of their nucleus.

GRIBAKIN (1967b) was able to demonstrate that the higher density of rhabdomeres in type-I cells is associated with the fact that they are formed by thinner microvilli (about 370 Å in diameter), whereas rhabdomeres in type-II and type-III cells are formed by microvilli of about 500 Å diameter. Further, rhabdomeres of type-I cells occupy in the ventral portion of the compound eye an area equal on the average to 18 % of the rhabdome cross-sectional area, approximately 10 % of this area being occupied by the rhabdomeres found in each of the remaining types of cells (Fig. 58). Finally, calculations have shown that the total surface area of microvilli membranes in type-I cells is almost three times the surface area of microvilli membranes in either of the other types of cells.

The first attempts to study the topography of the three types of cells within the compound eye of the bee have shown that type-I cells occur in every retinula and in the dorsal portion of the eye, although here the relative area occupied by their rhabdomeres is smaller (GRIBAKIN, 1967b). Under conditions of selective light adaptation, significant ultrastructural changes affecting both the rhabdomere and the cytoplasm were found in visual cells of a particular type. However, changes undergone by the rhabdomeres of visual cells containing visual pigment proved to be the most convenient and distinct criteria for judging the extent of the reaction of a visual cell toward irradiation.

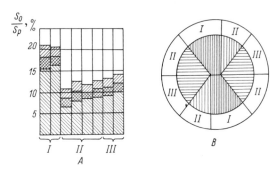

Fig. 58A and B. Schematic rhabdomere area ratios (GRIBAKIN, 1969a). A. Ratio between the cross-sectional area of the rhabdomere ($Sp$) and the rhabdome section area ($So$) for different types of cells (based on measured data from 27 rhabdomeres); B. diagram of the bee rhabdome in the state of light adaptation. Roman figures denote the types of cells

Selective adaptation to long-wave (yellow-green) light ($\lambda_{max} \geqq 480$ nm) results in swelling, shortening, and finally destruction of microvilli in rhabdomeres of type-II and type-III cells in a whole complex of adjacent ommatidia over large sectors of the faceted eye of the bee. Under stronger illumination, large light vacuoles appear in the region where the microvilli branch out (Fig. 59). Thus, the action of light causes vacuolation of the space in the vicinity of rhabdomeres. Another aspect of this process is the probable passage of part of the material that previously constituted the photoreceptor membrane and the matrix of microvilli into the cytoplasm of the visual cell (GRIBAKIN, 1969b, 1969c). An increase in the number of ribosomes is observed in the cytoplasm. The nuclei remain practically unchanged. The changes detected in rhabdomeres of type-II and type-III cells have an identical character along the entire length of the rhabdomeres. Thus, long-wave light ($\lambda_{max} \geqq 480$ nm) affects only type-II and type-III cells.

Selective adaptation to ultraviolet radiation ($\lambda_{max} = 365$ nm) resulted in shortening and drawing off of microvilli in rhabdomeres of type-I cells. The rhabdomeres of ommatidia then acquired a characteristic butterfly appearance over large sectors of the faceted eye (Fig. 60) (GRIBAKIN, 1969b, 1969c, 1969d). As a result of the shortening of microvilli, the space they formerly occupied is taken by the cellular cytoplasm, which forms wedges in the rhabdomere of type-I cells, whereas type-II and type-III cells remain unchanged and similar to the control cells, i.e. in a state of dark adaptation. Thus, ultraviolet radiation ($\lambda_{max} = 365$ nm) affects only type-I cells.

Selective adaptation to blue light ($\lambda_{max} = 420$ nm) led to a swelling of microvilli without significant destruction in two (out of the four) cells of type II and in ommatidia located closer to the central zone of the eye (40th to 50th horizontal rows of ommatidia) (Fig. 61). These cells belong to the same quadrants as type-I cells, i.e. the orientation of their microvilli is the same as that of type-I

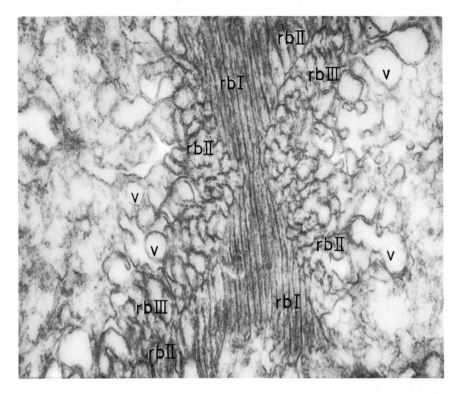

Fig. 59. Changes of microvilli in rhabdomeres (*rb*) of type-II and -III cells as a result of adaptation to long-wave light ($\lambda_{max} = 480$ nm). Rhabdomeres of type-I cells are intact ($\times 55,000$) (GRIBAKIN, 1969a, 1969b). *rb I, rb II, rb III* rhabdomes of type-I, -II, and -III cells; *v* vacuoles

cells. The swelling of microvilli in these cells is of similar character to the reaction of type-II and type-III visual cells towards long-wave radiation. Thus, visual cells capable of perceiving blue light are found in the 40th to 50th horizontal rows.

Thus, tests performed in our laboratory by GRIBAKIN (1969b, 1969c) have shown that, under conditions of selective adaptation of the bee's compound eye to light of different structural composition, three morphologically different types of cells present in the same retinula also possess a different function. Each of these types is specialized for the perception of radiation of a definite spectral composition. Type-I cells are photoreceptors reacting mainly to ultraviolet radiation (GRIBAKIN's 340 receptors). Type-II and type-III cells in the ventral portion of the eye are receptors of long-wave radiation (GRIBAKIN's 530 receptors). Finally, in regions closer to the center of the eye (40th to 50th rows of ommatidia) two of the type-II cells are receptors of the radiation emitted by the blue part of the spectrum (GRIBAKIN's 430 receptors). According to GRIBAKIN's calculations, 340 receptors make up 25% of the total number of visual cells, 530 receptors slightly over 50%, and 430 receptors less than 25% of the total number of photoreceptors. Thus, in insects (bee), in contrast to vertebrates, some conformity can be established between the electrophysiological and structural organization of the visual cells.

The shortening or drawing-off of rhabdomere microvilli, under the effect of light, leads essentially in all three types of cells to a reduction in the surface area of the photoreceptor membrane. This reduction may be the result of the liberation, due to illumination, of retinal and its reduction to vitamin A in

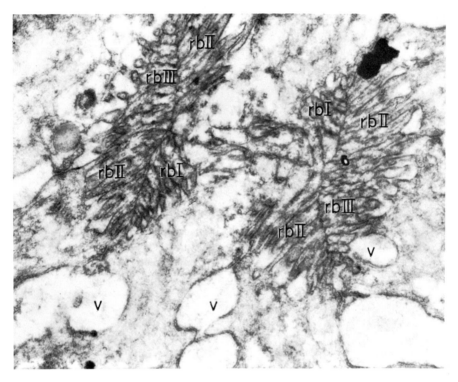

Fig. 60. Changes of microvilli in rhabdomeres of type-I cells after adaptation to ultraviolet light ($\lambda_{max} = 365$ nm) ($\times 35,000$) (GRIBAKIN, 1969a, 1969b). Designations as in Fig. 59

the visual cell. Under analogous conditions in vertebrates, as we have seen, a change takes place in the period between disks in the outer segments. It appears that in both insects and vertebrates the changes undergone by the visual pigment induce changes in the structure and chemical character of the membrane, and that this is reflected in corresponding shifts of the ultrastructural organization of the membrane. Thus, although in vertebrates, color vision has not yet found morphological expression at the cellular level, it is as clearly expressed as in insects at the molecular level, a result of the presence of different types of pigments.

Recording biopotentials in the bee yields an electroretinogram (ERG) which is essentially associated only with visual cells; this was found to be a multicomponent ERG (AUTRUM, AUTRUM, and HOFFMANN, 1961; MAZOKHIN-PORSHNYAKOV, 1965; BYZOV, 1966). The response of a cell to brief illumination is represented by a large positive plateau (20—30 mV) with an initial peak-shaped "transient" of the same sign. Visual cells of insects generate slow (generator) potentials associated with a depolarization of the cellular membrane. Variation of the ionic conductivity of the cellular membrane is, of course, considered to be the cause of the electrical reaction of the insect visual cell. How is this process connected with the transformation of the visual pigment? At present,

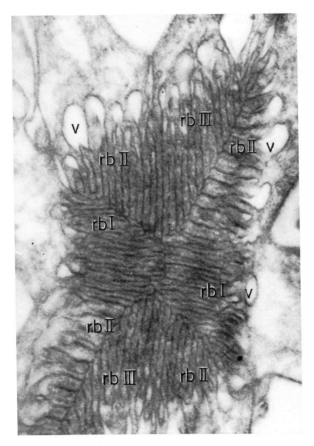

Fig. 61. Reaction of two type-II cells towards blue light ($\lambda_{max} = 420$ nm) ($\times 35,000$) (GRIBAKIN, 1969a, 1969b). Designations as in Fig. 59

it is not easy to answer this question. Some investigators think the rhabdomes can be considered as the source of slow (generator) potentials (BURKHARDT and AUTRUM, 1960), while others maintain that no electrical current whatsoever can be detected in rhabdomes, except for stray current "flowing in" from other layers (BYZOV and ORLOV, 1962; BYZOV, 1966). In this respect, additional studies on insects and vertebrates are needed.

# 6. Conclusion

We have examined the molecular, structural and functional organization of vision in representatives of the three phyla: vertebrates, arthropods, and molluscs, which have been investigated most extensively in this respect. The parallel nature of the evolution of visual pigments in these animals is striking; it is always associated with vitamin A (retinol), a derivative of the light-sensitive carotenoids found in the chloroplast grains of plants, together with chlorophyll. Animal visual cells, by virtue of a special protein mutation known as opsin, ensured the formation of the heterogeneous rhodopsin molecule. The opsin molecule exhibits a number of variations, which differ in molecular weight, in size, and consequently also in structure (the retinochrome protein in cephalopod molluscs?). the chromophore, that is, the molecule of oxidized vitamin A, on the other hand, does not change. The molecular conversions of the visual pigment in light and darkness follow a similar course, although certain variations do occur. On the basis of these observations, we believe that the molecular evolution of the visual pigment was determined by its origin and was completed at an early stage of the formation of the visual cells of multicellular animals, maybe even already in protists (cf. the eyespot of Diflagella).

The appearance of the membrane structures of the visual cells in which the visual pigment molecules are localized is associated with an increase in their receptor (light-sensitive) surface area. This process is effected by means of growth and differentiation of the plasma membrane of the visual cell, which is equipped with a flagellum (cilium) or microvilli. In the case of vertebrates, it is the plasma membrane of the flagellum which expands by forming folds, while in insects and cephalopod molluscs the plasma membrane of the microvilli undergoes a similar process. The important fact is that in both cases, in the disk membrane as in the microvilli, we find a similar picture of visual pigment localization in space. The chromophore molecule is always oriented in a plane perpendicular to the direction of the light beam. The visual pigment is a structural part of the disk membranes in vertebrates and of microvilli in invertebrates. In embryogenesis the parallel formation and supply of opsin and retinal and their combination in the form of rhodopsin lead to the subsequent differentiation and development of efficiently functioning photoreceptor membranes. The absence of one component of this heterogeneous molecule, for example, vitamin A, is sufficient to prevent the development or cause the degeneration of disk membranes in vertebrates.

As we have said, intensive studies are in progress on the molecular changes undergone by the visual pigment, localized in the disk membranes or microvilli of photoreceptors. The energy of one photon is sufficient to initiate the breakdown of the rhodopsin molecule that induces stimulation of the visual cell, which thus receives information on the light energy supplied by the environment. Under illumination a change takes place, not only in the general structure of the cell but also in the supramolecular organization of the receptor membrane (for example, in insects its surface may be reduced). It is becoming increasingly clear that color vision is associated primarily with the structural peculiarities of opsin. The cones of vertebrates, however, have an identical cellular structure whatever the radiation perceived, so that the differentiation of color perception must be attributed to the molecular organization level. In more ancient phyla, for example in bees, the molecular differences in visual pigments have led to the appearance of three morphologically different types of cells, capable of perceiving respectively ultraviolet, yellow-green, and blue.

We believe that the conformational changes undergone by the opsin molecule in vertebrates are transmitted in some way to neighboring molecules and to other structures of the photoreceptor cell, resulting in the general stimulation of the cell. Changes can be detected in these structures by cytochemical and biochemical methods and are expressed in receptor biopotentials; this is the means by which the visual cell transmits the encoded information through synapses to central neurons. A significant energy intensification for these processes is achieved by means of the universal ATP–ATPase mechanism.

However, up to the present it has not been possible to answer the following question: In what sequence are the changes by the rhodopsin (opsin) molecule transmitted to the remaining subcellular structures of the visual cell? As explained, the cell undergoes a number of structural, cytochemical, and biochemical changes, starting with the disks, the ellipsoid, the glycogen in the paraboloid, and the nucleic acids in the nucleus, and ending with the synaptic vesicles in the synapse region. It is difficult to believe that the entire process of visual cell stimulation is limited to its surface membrane. If this were so, it would be hard to understand why natural selection during the process of evolution had created all the complex structural variations of the visual cell. A great deal of effort will be required to produce a coherent picture of stimulation and total excitation of the visual cell, which would embrace processes originating in the outer photoreceptor membranes and terminating in their axons or synapses.

As a result of numerous studies conducted by various investigators, and in the first place by WALD (1960, 1968), it can be said that vision above all most fully demonstrates the processes involving the interaction of energy supplied from outside with a specific molecule entering into the composition of the receptor membrane. Vision is unlike any other kind of perception in that it enables us to follow with the utmost clarity the mechanism that triggers perception at the molecular level. This mechanism involves a change in the molecular conformation of rhodopsin; during this change, the wavelength or energy of a photon is encoded. The encoded information is transmitted in the form of receptor biopotentials at the supramolecular level as a result of a change in the polarization of the disk membranes or microvilli; it is transmitted at the subcellular level of organization of the photoreceptor cell as a result of the integration into the overall stimulation process of all cell organoids and associated biochemical processes.

Chapter V

# Taste

## 1. Introduction

The ability to recognize food by contact and differentiation, permitting the utilization or rejection of certain substances, was of decisive importance in the evolution of animals. The chemical compounds that make up the food consumed by animals, whether herbivorous, carnivorous or omnivorous, are responsible for its taste—salty, acid, sweet or bitter. It is the combined effect of gustatory substances and the synchronous function of the olfactory organ, and of warm, cold and tactile receptors that is responsible for overall taste sensations.

LOMONOSOV (1752—1757) distinguished seven different taste sensations: 1. acid, as in vinegar; 2. caustic, as in grain alcohol; 3. sweet, as in honey; 4. bitter, as in tar; 5. salty, as in salt; 6. pungent, as in wild radish; 7. sour, as in unripe fruit. As LOMONOSOV said, it will not be possible to explain which of these tastes are simple and which are complex until we gain a knowledge of the "nature of origins."

We can state that substances having a salty or sour taste are the simpler ones; historically, they have been connected with the environment and perception of these substances is more primitive. This perception is related to what is called the "general chemical sense". Sweet and bitter substances enter into the composition of most foodstuffs, but their perception is more complex.

In multicellular, highly organized animals, taste perception is effected by means of special receptor cells. In vertebrates, these cells are secondary sensory cells and their receptor surface consists of microvilli. In invertebrates (insects) they are primary sensory cells and their peripheral process is a modified flagellum. It was long ago discovered that salty, sour, sweet and bitter sensations can be induced in man, not only by subjecting receptor cells to sweet, bitter, acid and salty factors but also by artificially stimulating these cells with an electric current. This fact alone should lead us to expect that gustatory receptor cells include some sort of molecular structure, which brings about, under the effect of both adequate and inadequate excitation, the perception of sweetness, bitterness, acidity, or saltiness, as the case may be. A special "sweet-sensitive" protein has recently been isolated from gustatory receptor cells located in the anterior portion of the mammalian tongue, and a "bitter-sensitive" protein was extracted from cells of taste buds located in the posterior portion of the tongue. We know that in mammals the highest sensitivity for sweetness is in the front part of the tongue, and the highest sensitivity for bitterness in the back part of the tongue. Thus, with respect to sweet and bitter stimuli, we are beginning to discover the molecular mechanism of their perception. This mechanism seems to be somewhat similar to the mechanism of light perception.

In this chapter we shall attempt to examine the problem of taste reception in vertebrates and insects in the light of new findings which bring us closer to an understanding of its cellular and molecular mechanisms.

## 2. Chemical Basis of the Action of Gustatory Substances and Theories of Taste

BRONSHTEIN (1950) divides gustatory substances into three groups: 1. substances closely related in chemical structure and causing identical or similar gustatory sensations; 2. substances closely related in chemical structure but having different tastes; 3. substances with a different structure but similar tastes.

The first group includes certain optical isomers. For example, D- and L-α-alanine both have the same sweet taste; D- and L-β-aminobutyric acids also have the same taste. The following isomers have a similar taste! D- and L-phenylglycine, o-, m-, and p-nitroanisoles, o-, and p-nitrophenols, and o- and p-hydroxyphenylacimides. A bitter taste of different strength is exhibited by o-, m- and p-nitrocinnamic acids. Dissociated inorganic and organic acids and acid salts have an acid taste. Many salts possess a salty or bitter-salty taste. Sugars like glucose, saccharose, galactose and lactose all have a sweet taste.

The second group includes a number of stereoisomers. For example, the amino acid D-valine has a weak bitterish-sweet taste, L-valine and D-leucine have a sweet taste, L-leucine has a bitter taste; D-asparagine has a sweet taste and L-asparagine has no taste, while α-alanine is sweet and β-alanine is tasteless. There are many other examples of such compounds.

The third group includes, for example, tetramethyl ammonium iodide (and tetraethyl ammonium iodide), formaldehyde (and acetamide), diphenylurea (and creatinine). Many alkaloids, for example quinine, and strychnine, nitro derivatives of benzene, and many inorganic acids and salts have a bitter taste. A sweet taste is exhibited, in addition to polysaccharides, by glycol, glycerol, resorcinal, phloroglucinal, methylchloride, ethylchloride, chloroform, glycine, dulcin, nitrobenzene, saccharin, etc.

The ability of a number of compounds to produce a certain similar taste sensation has been associated with similar intramolecular rearrangements of the specific chemical groups present in these compounds, occurring on contact with particular receptive protein molecules located in the gustatory receptor cells (BEIDLER, 1961a, 1961b; SHALLENBERGER and ACREE et al., 1967).

### A. Chemical Basis of the Action of a Saline Stimulus

The salty taste of NaCl is also an inherent property of other chlorides (K, $NH_3$, Ca, etc.); from this we can conclude that the free anion $Cl^-$ rather than the cations $Na^+$, $K^+$, $NH_4^+$ or $Ca^{++}$ is responsible for a saline taste. At the same time, however, we cannot exclude the significant role of cations. Thus, NaCl in a weak concentration has a saline taste, NaBr a bitterish-salty taste, NaI a saltish-bitter taste, and $Na_2SO_4$ a salty-bitter-acid-sweetish taste. Hence we are led to believe that the Na ion imparts to solutions of all these salts their characteristic brackish taste. According to BEIDLER (1961a, 1961b), cations play a predominant role during stimulation with salts, while anions exert a weak inhibitory effect. Thus, both anions and cations help to create a saline stimulus (GAUDA, 1912). It is assumed that the taste intensity of salts depends upon the cations $Na^+$, $K^+$, $Rb^+$, $Cs^+$, etc., while the character of the taste depends on the anions $Cl^-$, $Br^-$, $I^-$, etc. (KIONKA and STRÄTZ, 1922). It was further found that salts of low molecular weight have a saline taste, while those with a high molecular weight have a bitter taste (MAYBEE, 1939).

What concentration of salt can stimulate a gustatory receptor cell? In adults, a salt concentration of 0.02% in distilled water is sufficient for this purpose. In rats, this threshold is close to that for humans, being 0.055%. The threshold concentration for a NaCl solution lies between 0.009 and 0.002 $M$ (PFAFFMANN, 1941).

## B. Chemical Basis of the Action of an Acid Stimulus

Acids occur in the composition of numerous gustatory substances. As we know, the property common to all acids is their ability to ionize in aqueous solution into anions and a hydrogen cation (proton). Acids are either weak or strong, strong acids having a higher degree of ionization.

For example, $HCl \rightleftarrows H^+ + Cl^-$, but in this ionization reaction not all molecules are dissociated. In dilute solutions the degree of dissociation is greater than in concentrated solutions, although the absolute concentration of $H^+$ will be greater in concentrated solutions. Weak acids are ionized to a lesser degree, and their solutions contain a relatively large number of undissociated molecules; for example, $CH_3COOH \rightleftarrows CH_3COO^- + H^+$. In this case, only an insignificant fraction of the $CH_3COOH$ molecules is dissociated.

An acid stimulus is associated with the action of hydrogen ions on gustatory receptor cells. The effect of $H^+$ is proportional to its concentration. This fact can be confirmed by means of rather simple tests. For example, HCl is perceived as acid from a dilution of n/800, whereas at the same concentration ionized $NaCl \rightarrow Na^+ + Cl^-$ is practically tasteless. It follows that an acid taste stimulus is associated with $H^+$ (KAHLENBERG, 1900). As BEIDLER (1967) pointed out, $H^+$ ions attach to the taste receptor membrane, increasing its surface charge, which hinders the addition of more $H^+$ ions.

A generation after KAHLENBERG threshold concentrations were determined for various buffer solutions, (ROSENBAUM, 1925) for example:

$$Na_2HPO_4 \quad \text{and} \quad NaH_2PO_4 \qquad \text{at pH} \quad 6.4;$$
$$K_2HPO_4 \quad \text{and} \quad KH_2PO_4 \qquad\qquad\quad 6.2;$$
$$CH_3COOH \quad \text{and} \quad CH_3COONa \qquad\quad 5.9;$$
$$CH_3COOH \quad \text{and} \quad CH_3COOK \qquad\quad\ 5.6;$$
$$CH_3COOH \quad \text{and} \quad (CH_3COO)_2Mg \qquad 5.3;$$

On the basis of this fact, we can conclude that an acid stimulus arises at different pH values, depending both upon the concentration of $H^+$ ions and the total concentration of the solution.

At the same time, we should note that, although an acid taste stimulation is associated mainly with $H^+$, both anions and undissociated molecules, which act as a reserve by constantly supplying fresh ions, play a distinct role in this stimulation, as pointed out by MONCRIEFF (1946) and BRONSHTEIN (1950). The possible significance of the anion of the dissociated acids, of the undissociated molecule and of the lipid solubility of weak acids was discussed in detail by BEIDLER (1967). Threshold values for an acid stimulus equal n/800 HCl (MONCRIEFF, 1946).

## C. Chemical Basis of the Action of a Sweet Stimulus

A sweet stimulus is produced by a large number of organic compounds, which are not as a rule ionized. MONCRIEFF (1946) postulates that perception of a sweet stimulus as a gustatory stimulus by animals began at a later date in the course of evolution then did the perception of saline and acid stimulis. The sweet substances most frequently encountered are sugars, glycerol and saccharin. Sugar (saccharose) and glycerol have a definite similarity; they are polyatomic alcohols of the following formulas:

Glycerol $CH_2OH \cdot CHOH \cdot CH_2OH$

$$\text{Saccharose} \quad CH_2OH \cdot CH \begin{array}{c} CHOH—CHOH \\ \diagdown \\ O——CH \end{array} CHOH \begin{array}{c} CH_2OH \\ \diagup \\ O \end{array} C \begin{array}{c} CHOH—CHOH \\ | \\ O——CH \cdot CH_2OH \end{array}$$

A striking feature of the above formulas is the recurrence of the $CH_2OH$ group.

Saccharin, which is not assimilated in the organism, has a completely different structure:

Saccharin
(O-Sulfobenzimide)

$$\begin{array}{c} CH \\ CH \diagup \diagdown \\ | \qquad C \cdot CO \diagdown \\ CH \qquad \| \qquad NH \\ \diagdown \diagup C \cdot SO_2 \diagup \\ CH \end{array}$$

The presence of an aromatic benzene ring, as we shall see later, can also impart a bitter stimulus. In fact, many bitter glucosides found in nature contain a benzene ring; when this ring is removed, these compounds acquire a sweet taste.

Attempts to clarify the nature of the chemical basis of a sweet stimulus have led to the assumption that, for a substance to act as a sweet stimulus, it must contain molecules of a glucophore and auxogluc, by analogy with the chromophore and auxochrome upon which the theory of color is based (OERTLY and MYERS, 1919). The following six glucophores were found:

1.    $-CO-CHOH-[H]$

2.    $CH_2OH \cdot CHOH-$

3.    $-COOH \cdot CHNH_2-$

4.    $-CH_2ONO_2$

5. 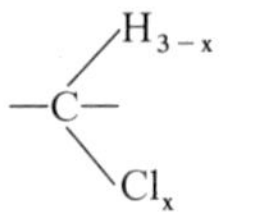    $-\overset{\diagup H_{3-x}}{\underset{\diagdown Cl_x}{C}}-$

6. 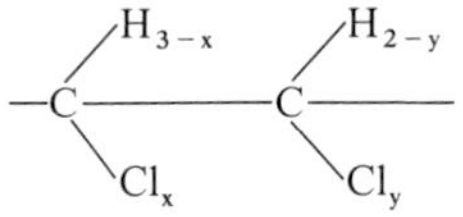    $-\overset{\diagup H_{3-x}}{\underset{\diagdown Cl_x}{C}}-\overset{\diagup H_{2-y}}{\underset{\diagdown Cl_y}{C}}-$

Thus, the CO—CHOH-group must combine with at least one hydrogen atom in order to become a glucophore.

The following auxogluc groups of a normal polyhydric alcohol were also found:

1. $H-$
2. $CH_3-$
3. $C_2H_5-$
4. $CH_3-CH_2-CH_2-$
5. $(CH_3)_2CH-$
6. $CH_2OH-$
7. $CH_3-CHOH-$
8. $CH_2 \; H-CH_2-$
9. $C_nH_{2n+1}O_n-$

The most simple of these groups is $CH_2OH-CHOH-$.

In order to have a sweet taste, a substance must contain both glucophore and auxogluc groups. In this respect, the following compounds constitute a typical example:

|  | *glucophore* | *auxogluc* |
|---|---|---|
| Glycol | $CH_2OH-CHOH-$ | $H-$ |
| Glycerol | $CH_2OH-CH \; H-$ | $CH_2OH-$ |
| Glucose | $-C \; -CH \; H-$ | $CH_2OH-$ |
| Glycine | $OOH-CHNH_2-$ | $H-$ |
| Chloroform | $-CCl_3$ | $H-$ |
| Ethyl nitrate | $-CH_2ONO_2$ | $H_3-$ |

Although this theory does not explain the nature of the sweet stimulus imparted by saccharin and a number of other sweet substances, it serves as a starting point for the further development of concepts on the molecular foundations of sweet stimulation in general. The dimensions of the glycol molecule and the large size of pyranose and furanose rings were utilized by SHALLENBERGER and his coauthors in explaining the sweet stimulation of various sugars (SHALLEN-BERGER, 1963, 1964; SHALLENBERGER, ACREE, and GUILD, 1965; SHALLEN-BERGER and ACREE, 1967).

The intensity of the sweet taste varies in inverse proportion to the degree to which the OH group of glycol is bound within the molecule. Apparently, adjacent OH groups in the glycol must be present in a state of unstable conformation. Adjacent OH groups, if present in an anti-conformation, are located too far from each other to induce a sweet sensation. Other OH groups seem to be involved in intramolecular hydrogen bonds which inhibit the reaction of a glycol with the sweet-sensitive protein in the taste cell. The stereo properties of the sweet and non-sweet stimulating units of a glycol are illustrated in the following diagram:

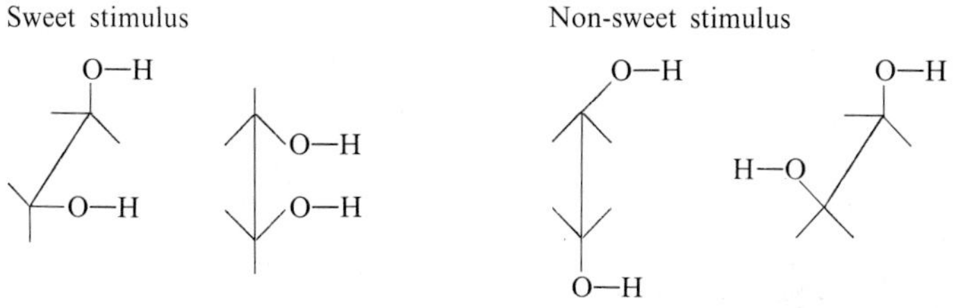

Sweet stimulus                    Non-sweet stimulus

Thus, SHALLENBERGER and ACREE (1967) reached the conclusion that a sweet stimulus in a sugar is associated with the establishment of hydrogen bonds between the glycol and the receptor site of the "receptor" molecule located on the receptor taste cell. The sweet stimulating property of a glycol is associated with a bifunctional structure consisting of two components: AH and B. These components are universal and are inherent in many substances having a sweet taste. In the system AH and B, A and B are electronegative atoms, separated by a distance greater than 2.5Å and less than 4Å; this distance is apparently equal to 3Å. $H^+$ is a hydrogen ion linked to one of the electronegative atoms by means of a covalent bond. A and B are usually either oxygen or nitrogen, but sometimes one of them is carbon or chlorine, or is an unsaturated center. The AH proton is a donor, while the B proton is an acceptor. SHALLENBERGER and ACREE give the following examples of sweet stimulators and of their AH and B systems:

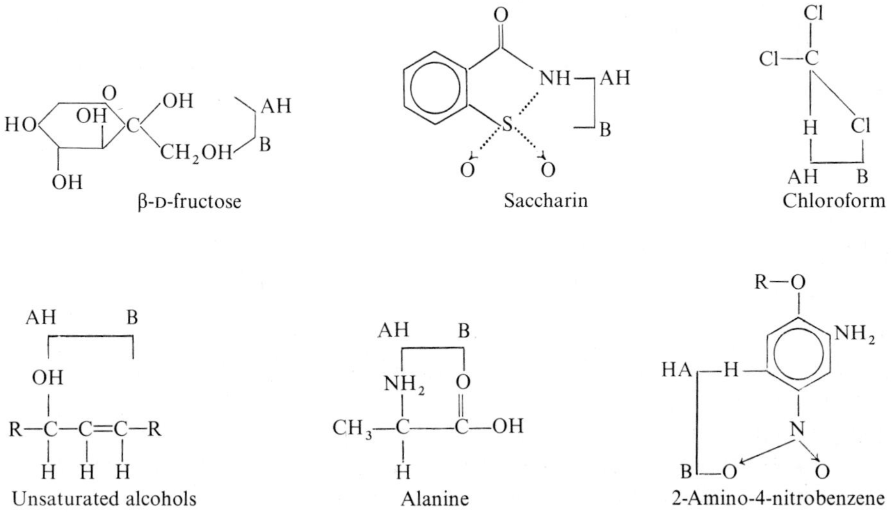

β-D-fructose                    Saccharin                    Chloroform

Unsaturated alcohols                    Alanine                    2-Amino-4-nitrobenzene

Thus, not only sugars but also saccharin, chloroform, unsaturated alcohols, alanine and 2-amino-4-nitrobenzene were all found to be similar in that the electron density at a specific point of their molecule determines its ability to act as a sweet stimulus.

It is conceivable that the receptor substance in the taste cell is also a bifunctional unit of similar nature to the AH—B system of sweet substances. The interaction between the sweet-sensitive protein of the taste cell and the specific group of the taste stimulus includes two simultaneous hydrogen bonds:

$$
\begin{array}{ll}
\text{Receptor site of} \\
\text{sweet-sensitive} \\
\text{protein}
\end{array}
\left[
\begin{array}{l}
\text{—A—H ...... B} \\
\\
\text{—B} \quad \text{...... H—A}
\end{array}
\right]
\begin{array}{l}
\text{Specific group} \\
\text{of the sweet substance}
\end{array}
$$

SHALLENBERGER and ACREE assume that this interaction is not a proton transfer or an electrostatic interaction, but is realized by means of London dispersion forces (WIEBERG, 1964).

Consequently, the AH—B system necessary for a sweet stimulus is universal and common to all sweet substances, regardless of chemical class and structure. This system must always correspond to the spatial location and possibilities of the hydrogen bonds in the sweet-sensitive protein of the taste cell.

In order to induce a sweet sensation, in other words, to allow the interaction described above to take place, it is sufficient to use, for example, $10^{20}$ molecules of sugar (0.5%), a 0.7% saccharose solution or a $\sim 0.001\%$ saccharin solution.

# D. Chemical Basis of the Action of a Bitter Stimulus

The nature of the bitter stimulus of gustatory substances has been least studied. Whereas NaCl has a typically salty taste, CsCl has a bitter taste, while KI also frequently has a bitter taste. Thus, with increasing molecular weight, salts have an increasingly bitter taste. The same relations seem to exist between sweet and bitter factors. It is interesting that magnesium, the last member of this group in which beryllium (a sweet salt) is the first member, and calcium, one of the latest members of the group, have a bitter taste. Other well-known bitter substances are free bases, for example, alkaloids. Picric acid contains three $NO_2$ groups which apparently are responsible for the bitter taste of its molecule (MONCRIEFF, 1946). The bitter stimulus is frequently associated with

the group $\begin{array}{c} NO_2 \\ \diagdown \diagup \\ C \\ \diagup \mid \\ CH_2OH \end{array}$ . With many organic compounds the lower members of

a homologous series are sweet, while the higher members are bitter. The symmetry of the structure often leads to the appearance of a bitter taste or destroys an existing sweet taste (FERGUSON and LOWRENCE, 1958).

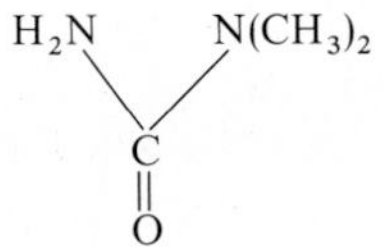

$$H_2N \diagdown \qquad \diagup N(CH_3)_2$$
$$\underset{O}{\overset{C}{\|}}$$
Sweet

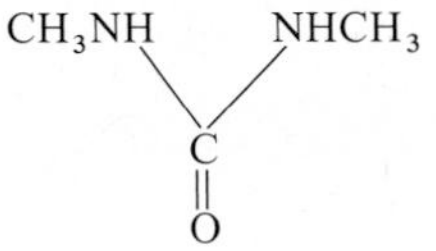

$$CH_3NH \diagdown \qquad \diagup NHCH_3$$
$$\underset{O}{\overset{C}{\|}}$$
Bitter

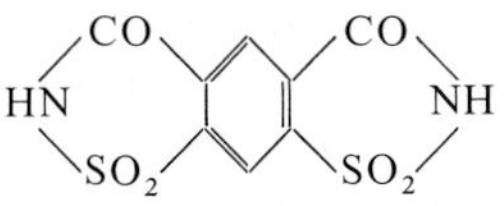

$$HN \diagup \overset{CO}{\diagdown} \quad \overset{CO}{\diagup} \diagdown NH$$
$$\diagdown SO_2 \diagup \qquad \diagdown SO_2 \diagup$$
very bitter

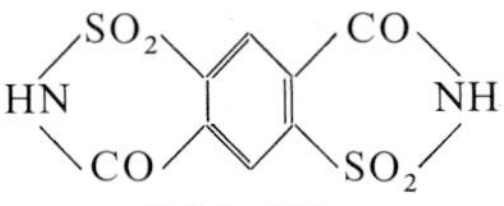

$$HN \diagup \overset{SO_2}{\diagdown} \quad \overset{CO}{\diagup} \diagdown NH$$
$$\diagdown CO \diagup \qquad \diagdown SO_2 \diagup$$
slightly bitter

Introduction of a phenyl group into the structure frequently makes a sweet-tasting compound bitter or tasteless (FERGUSON and LOWRENCE, 1958).

| Sweet | Bitter |
|---|---|
| $CH_3$—CHOH—$CH_2OH$ | $C_6H_5$—CHOH—$CH_2OH$ |
| $CH_3$—CHOH—CHOH—$CH_2OH$ | $C_6H_5$—CHOH—CHOH—$CH_2OH$ |
| $HOCH_2$—CHOH—$CH_2OH$ | $C_6H_5$—$OCH_2$—CHOH—$CH_2OH$ |
| H—CONH—$CH_3$ | H—CONH—$C_6H_5$ |
| $(C_2H_5)_2N$—$CONH_2$ | $(C_2H_5)_2N \cdots$—$CON(C_6H_5)_2$ |

A change in taste can also be brought about by methylation (FERGUSON and LOWRENCE, 1958), for example:

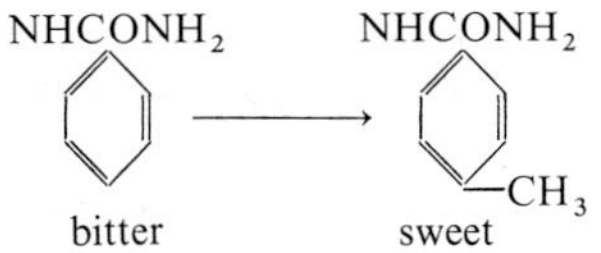

NHCONH$_2$

bitter

$\longrightarrow$

NHCONH$_2$

—CH$_3$

sweet

$H_2N$—$CONH_2$
bitter

$H_2N$—$CON(CH_3)_2$
sweet

As we shall demonstrate below, the interaction between a bitter stimulus and the special bitter-sensitive protein takes place according to the same rules as those govering the reactions of sweet stimuli, which again seems to point to the great importance of hydrogen bonds in this process. There has been shown to be in bitter substances a bifunctional structure, as known for sweet substances, consisting of AH and B components. In this system AH and B are separated by 1.5Å (KUBOTA and KUBO, 1969). The authors postulate that the receptor site contains a similar AH—B system which forms two hydrogen bonds with the AH—B system of the bitter molecules. However, special investigations in this direction are required.

An amount of $10^{15}$ molecules of strychnine is sufficient to induce a bitter stimulus (SKRAMLIK, 1963). Quinine hydrochloride acts as a stimulus in a dilution of 0.00004 $M$, i.e. 0.0016% (PARKER and STABLER, 1913).

# E. Theories of Taste

In what manner do saline, sour, sweet and bitter stimuli make contact with the receptor taste cell? And with what factor do the specific chemical ingredients upon which saline, sour, sweet and bitter stimuli are based react concretely in the taste cell? In other words, what are the primary mechanisms of taste reception which initiate the excitation of the taste cell and the transmission of this excitation through synapses in the form of impulses along the nerve fiber into the central units of the taste analyzer?

Here we should like to recall first the work of LAZAREV (1920) who, starting with the role played by ions in the excitation process, assumed that the taste buds in each tongue papilla of vertebrates contain highly sensitive substances of a protein nature, which were broken down under the effect of an adequate stimulus, while the ionized breakdown products stimulate corresponding nerve terminals. Also of definite historical importance is the theory of RENQUIST (1919), who attributed a special importance to adsorption processes of gustatory substances, which, in his opinion, led to the stimulation of taste buds. The development of histochemistry saw the elaboration of the enzymic theory of taste (KISTIAKOWSKY, 1950; BARADI and BOURNE, 1951a, 1951b, 1953). It was found that when gustatory substances are added to an incubation mixture, they exert a different effect on the activity of the enzymes located in taste buds. Thus, a 2% acetic acid solution inhibits the activity of adenosinetriphosphatase alone, while a 0.5% quinine solution inhibits the activity of almost all phosphatases, but increases the activity of nuclear phosphatase. It was therefore concluded that the initial stage in the interaction of gustatory substances with receptor cells is the activation or inhibition of their enzyme systems. However, it is not possible to state on the basis of the method used by these authors that the changes they detected in enzymic activity are indeed connected with primary processes of taste stimulation. If we wish to understand the primary processes of the reaction between gustatory substances and receptor taste cells, much greater significance must be attributed to BEIDLER's theory (BEIDLER, 1954, 1960, 1961a, 1961b, 1963, 1964, 1965, 1967): he attempted for the first time to trace the primary processes involved in taste reception, starting from the structural characteristics of the plasma membrane of the taste cell. BEIDLER (1954) assumed that gustatory stimuli (molecules or ions) interact with specific sectors of the plasma membrane of a receptor cell; he characterized these sectors as receptor sites. In his opinion, the magnitude (intensity) of a stimulus depends on the number of ions or molecules which interact with the plasma membrane. Starting with the law of mass action and assuming the adsorption of taste molecules or ions with a limited series of equivalent independent receptor sites on the plasma membrane of the receptor cell, BEIDLER derived an equation linking the magnitude of the primary impulse with the concentration of the gustatory substance:

$$K = \frac{Z}{C(N-Z)}, \tag{1}$$

where $C$ is the concentration of the stimulating gustatory substance, $N$ the total number of receptor sites on which taste molecules or ions can be adsorbed,

$Z$ the number of receptor sites which interact with gustatory substances at the stimulus concentration $C$, and $K$ is the equilibrium constant.

Direct measurement of $N$ and $Z$ is impossible. However, since the magnitude of the response of the receptor cell ($R$) is directly proportional to the number of filled receptor sites ($R=Z$), and since a maximum response ($Rm$) is observed at a concentration of the taste stimulus such that all receptor sites are occupied ($Rm=N$), the above equation takes the following form:

$$K = \frac{R}{C(Rm-R)} \tag{2}$$

or

$$\frac{C}{R} = \frac{C}{Rm} + \frac{1}{KRm}. \tag{3}$$

Eq. (3) is the fundamental equation of BEIDLER's taste reception. All parameters in this equation, except for the equilibrium constant $K$, can be measured experimentally. According to this equation, the function, expressed in the coordinates $C/R$ versus $C$, must be a straight line (Fig. 62), and if the linear relationship

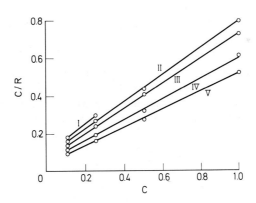

Fig. 62. Summary reaction of gustatory receptors ($C/R$) as a function of the molar concentration of the stimulant ($C$) (BEIDLER, 1964). *I* sodium butyrate; *II* sodium propionate; *III* sodium acetate; *IV* sodium formate; *V* sodium chloride

is established, the equilibrium constant can also be calculated. As long as $K$ does not change, the character of primary reception in the taste cell also does not change.

After determination of $K$ it is also possible to calculate the expended energy of the reaction. The energy consumption or "change of free energy" ($\Delta F$) will be low if $K$ is small. Let us try to perform this calculation by starting, for example, from the premise that the magnitude of the reaction of taste receptor cells to saline stimuli does not change when the temperature varies from 20° to 30°C, and consequently the reaction does not depend on the temperature in the above range (BEIDLER, 1961a). In the equation

$$\Delta F = \Delta H = T \Delta S$$

$\Delta H$ is equal to zero. Since $\Delta F$ can be calculated from the equilibrium constant according to the equation

$$\Delta F = -R T \ln K,$$

we can see that $\Delta F$ (change in the free energy of the reaction) is negative and, therefore, $\Delta S$ (change in entropy) is positive. This means either that the amount of hydration water decreases when ions are adsorbed on the surface of the "receptor", or that the shape of the "receptor" molecule undergoes a slight change when ions are adsorbed on this molecule. Small positive changes in entropy were also found during ion binding of proteins (BEIDLER, 1961a).

The character of the binding of a stimulus to the "receptors" could also be studied by changing the pH of the solution. The magnitude of the reaction to a 0.1 m NaCl solution does not change noticeably over the pH range 3—11. This means that the majority of carboxyl groups in proteins do not take part in the stimulus, although participation of other groups, for example, phosphate groups is possible.

Consequently, the interaction is based not on an enzymic process but rather on a physical adsorption process, including a weak bond between the taste stimulus and the receptor sites of the receptor cell. The complex—stimulus +receptor sites—will be able to dissociate just as readily as it assembles. Thus, taste reception is a multistage process in which the first stages, i.e. the trigger mechanism, correspond to BEIDLER's equation. Later stages are in all probability enzymic, a fact that is confirmed by cytochemical data, and also by tests with sulfhydryl groups (YURIEVA, 1957, 1960a, 1960b; NEJAD, 1961).

What, then, is the nature of the receptor site in the plasma membrane of a receptor cell? BEIDLER (1961a, 1961b) believed that these receptor sites are polyelectrolytes containing a large number of "charged" side chains. The presence of anionic centers, which can adsorb such cations as $Na^+$, $K^+$ or $Ca^{++}$, was also assumed by other authors, and the competitive action of $Na^+$ and $Ca^{++}$ ions was actually demonstrated (NOMURA and SAKADA, 1965). We have already mentioned the data of SHALLENBERGER and ACREE (1967) on the significance of intramolecular hydrogen bonds in the receptor site stimulated by sweet substances. Other receptor sites must be more complex and must be able to recognize the shape of molecules present in certain taste stimuli, for example, L- and D-amino acids. Thus, several different receptor sites must apparently coexist in the membrane of a single receptor cell; this explains why, as established by electrophysiologists, a single receptor cell can react to different taste stimuli.

However, the discovery by DASTOLI and his coauthors of sweet-sensitive and bitter-sensitive proteins in the taste buds of mammals was of decisive importance in understanding the molecular mechanisms of the primary taste reaction (DASTOLI and PRICE, 1966; DASTOLI, LOPIEKES, and DOIG, 1968; DASTOLI,

LOPIEKES, and PRICE, 1968). Similar data on rat taste buds were recently obtained by Japanese researchers (HIJI, KOBAYASHI, and SATO, 1968, 1969) and CAGAN (1971). Thus, specific protein molecules were found to be associated with the receptor sites in Beidler's equation, or, in other words, proteins were found to be the carriers of receptor sites. However, some investigators contest the specificity of "sweet-sensitive" and "bitter-sensitive" proteins in the taste bud cells (KOYAMA and KURIHARA, 1971; NOFRE and SABADIE, 1972).

## 3. Sweet-Sensitive and Bitter-Sensitive Proteins

Starting from the well-established fact that gustatory papillae primarily sensitive to sweet stimuli are found in the front portion of the tongue in cattle and swine, and that bitter-sensitive papillae are found in the back of the tongue (PICK and KARE, 1962; KARE and FICKEN, 1963), DASTOLI and coauthors (DASTOLI and PRICE, 1966; DASTOLI, LOPIEKES, and DOIG, 1968; DASTOLI, LOPIEKES, and PRICE, 1968) have attempted to isolate the proteins present in these papillae. It was found that the protein fraction extracted from taste buds in the front part of cattle and swine tongue was indeed the fraction which

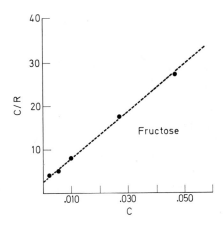

Fig. 63. Plot of the interaction of the sweet-sensitive protein with fructose (DASTOLI and PRICE, 1966). $C$ molar concentration of fructose; $R$ change in refractive index during interaction of the active sweet-sensitive protein fraction with fructose; slope is $1/R_m$, $R_m$ being maximal response; $(1/R_m)(1/K)$ is $y$ intercept where $K$ is the equilibrium constant; $\Delta F = RT \ln K$

reacts with sugar to form a complex. The rate of formation of this complex is not time-dependent and its stability can be correlated with the concentration of a sweet stimulus (Fig. 63). Complexes consisting of a definite solution, containing the protein mentioned above and a sugar of known dilution, were then studied by means of spectrophotometric and mainly refractometric techniques; the latter make it possible to investigate certain specific sweet substances which absorb in the UV region. The results obtained by both methods were the same. Refraction was determined for each extract containing the gustatory substance being tested and for each extract and gustatory substance separately. Data obtained in a test with fructose are shown in Fig. 63. The magnitudes $Rm$ and $K$, i.e. the maximum response and the equilibrium constant, behave according to Beidler's equation. Table 2 shows the relative intensity of a sweet stimulus (sugars) in animals and man.

Table 2. Characteristics of the interaction of sugars with the sweet-sensitive protein from the taste buds of the ox (DASTOLI and PRICE, 1966)

| Sweet substances | $Rm$ | $K$ $(M^{-1})$ | $\Delta F$ (kcal $M^{-1}$) | Relative sweetness, determined in vivo | | | |
|---|---|---|---|---|---|---|---|
| | | | | For man | | | For the dog |
| Fructose | 0.0016 | 1,030 | −4.15 | 1 | 1 | 1 | 1 |
| Saccharose | 0.0008 | 85 | −2.66 | 2 | 2 | 2 | 2−3 |
| Glucose | 0.0017 | 27 | −1.97 | 3 | 3 | 3 | 4 |
| Galactose | 0.0007 | 10 | −1.39 | 4 | − | − | 5 |
| Mannose | 0.0009 | 35 | −0.75 | − | − | − | 2−3 |
| Saccharin | 0.0011 | 226 | −3.25 | − | − | − | − |

Note: $Rm$ is expressed in units of the refractive index.

Thus, Beidler's equation is applicble to the reception of sugars. The free energy $(\Delta F)$, determining the interaction of a protein with sugars can be calculated from the equation $\Delta F = R T \ln K$. The value of the free energy in this case suggests that what takes place is a weak interaction between the protein fraction and sugars rather than a chemical reaction (DASTOLI and PRICE, 1966). The data of SHALLENBERGER and ACREE (1967), according to which perception of a sweet stimulus is based on hydrogen bonds between, for example, a glycol group and the receptor sites of a receptor taste cell, i.e. their sweet-sensitive protein molecules, are in good agreement with the results obtained by DASTOLI and PRICE (1966). It should be mentioned that the interaction between fructose and the protein fraction obtained above did not depend on pH in the range 5.5 to 9.6, but that it dropped sharply at lower pH values.

Thus, from the taste buds of the front portion of cattle and swine tongue it was possible to extract a protein fraction characterized by a clearly expressed trend to form bonds with sweet substances. The relative strength of this bond depends on the sugar concentration and the pH.

The protein fraction obtained from papillae located in the back of the tongue, was found to be bitter-sensitive. It was used to study the interaction between a protein and a bitter substance. As in the investigation of sweet-sensitive proteins, the bitter-sensitive protein never exhibited any dependence upon the reaction time (DASTOLI, LOPIEKES, and PRICE, 1968). For the mathematical expression of the results of their tests, these authors used Beidler's equation. Variations of the refractive index indicating the formation of a complex were used for

$R$, i.e. in determining the magnitude of the response of the receptor cell. The parameters $Rm$ (maximum response) and $K$ (constant) can be easily calculated from a graph. The free energy ($\Delta F$) associated with the interaction of bitter substances with the protein fraction can be calculated as for the interaction of sugars, from the value of $K$ by means of the equation: $\Delta F = RT \ln K$.

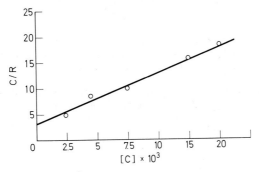

Fig. 64. Plot of the interaction of the bitter-sensitive protein with quinine-HCl (DASTOLI et al., 1968). $R$ change in refractive index during interaction of quinine-HCl with the protein fraction, isolated with 60% ammonium sulfate $C$ molar concentration of quinine-HCl; slope of line is $1/R_m$, $R_m$ being the maximal response; $(1/R_m)(1/K)$ is $y$ intercept, where $K$ is the association constant;
$$\Delta F = RT \ln K$$

Fig. 64 shows the data obtained with quinine hydrochloride, which were found to be typical for all bitter stimuli ($Rm$ and $K$, obtained experimentally, are listed in Table 3 together with corresponding values of $\Delta F$). Linear relations can be clearly observed between the degree of interaction and the concentration, and are consistent with the relative bitterness of the stimulus. The data thus obtained show that the 60% protein fraction from the posterior papillae of the swine tongue is capable of reacting with bitter components to form a complex the stability of which is correlated with the degree of bitterness of the corresponding stimulus.

Table 3. Characteristics of the interaction between bitter compounds and protein extracted from posterior taste buds of swine tongue (DASTOLI, LOPIEKES, and PRICE, 1968)

| Compounds | $Rm$ | $K$ ($M^{-1}$) | $\Delta F$ (kcal $\cdot M^{-1}$) |
|---|---|---|---|
| Guanine—HCl | 0.0014 | 254 | −3.34 |
| Brucine—HCl | 0.0010 | 219 | −3.25 |
| Naringine | 0.0011 | 197 | −3.14 |
| Coffein | 0.0012 | 129 | −2.92 |

Note: $Rm$ is expressed in units of the refraction index. Naringine is a flavoglucoside extracted from the rind of citrus fruits.

The values of $\Delta F$, which are related to complex formation with bitter substances and are slightly higher than the values obtained for sugars, once more confirm the concept that, in all probability, weak physical forces are the principal forces involved in the binding mechanism. The magnitude of free energy, equal to about 5kcal/$M$, is characteristic for hydrogen bonds but not for covalent bonds. These data lead us to believe that the interaction between a bitter-sensitive protein and bitter stimulus is also based on intramolecular hydrogen bonds, the presence of which is due to changes in the conformation of the corresponding stimuli. As was noted earlier, the above authors were unable to identify a time dependence in the variations of the refraction index. Thus, both in sweet-sensitive and bitter-sensitive proteins the function of receptor sites is determined primarily by intramolecular hydrogen bonds.

The authors cited above stress that the protein fraction from papillae located in the front of the tongue do not interact with a bitter stimulus and conversely the protein fraction from papillae in the back of the tongue does not interact with a sweet stimulus. They believe this indicates a substrate specificity on the part of the isolated proteins.

The nature of the sweet-sensitive protein could be studied in greater detail with the aid of modern research methods (DASTOLI, LOPIEKES, and PRICE, 1968). Its molecular weight was found by the molecular sieve method to be 150,000 ± 3,000, and by the ultracentrifuge method 152,000. Ion-exchange chromatography has shown the sweet-sensitive protein to be rather homogeneous

Table 4.  Amino acid composition of sweet-sensitive protein

| Amino Acids | Amino Acid Recov | Amino Acid Residue/100g of Protein (g) | Min Mol Wt (g) | Nearest Integral No. of Amino Acid Residues for 150,000g Protein (g) | Integral Nos. of Residues x Residue Mol Wt (g) |
|---|---|---|---|---|---|
| A | B | C | D | E | F |
| Lysine | 0.212 | 9.05 | 1.414 | 106 | 13.568 |
| Histidine | 0.057 | 2.60 | 5.269 | 28 | 3.836 |
| Amide NH$_3$ | 0.353 | (1.65) | | (177) | (2.478) |
| Arginine | 0.105 | 5.46 | 2.857 | 53 | 8.268 |
| Aspartic acid | 0.261 | 10.00 | 1.150 | 130 | 14.950 |
| Threonine | 0.154 | 5.18 | 1.949 | 77 | 7.777 |
| Serine | 0.175 | 5.07 | 1.716 | 87 | 7.569 |
| Glutamic acid | 0.385 | 16.55 | 779 | 192 | 24.768 |
| Proline | 0.208 | 6.72 | 1.443 | 104 | 10.088 |
| Glycine | 0.207 | 3.93 | 1.450 | 103 | 5.871 |
| Alanine | 0.180 | 4.26 | 1.667 | 90 | 6.390 |
| Cystine ($^1/_2$) | 0.033 | 1.12 | 9.107 | 16 | 1.632 |
| Valine | 0.202 | 6.66 | 1.486 | 101 | 9.999 |
| Methionine | 0.040 | 1.74 | 7.528 | 20 | 2.620 |
| Isoleucine | 0.115 | 4.33 | 2.609 | 57 | 6.441 |
| Leucine | 0.221 | 8.33 | 1.356 | 111 | 12.543 |
| Tirosine | 0.071 | 3.86 | 4.222 | 36 | 5.868 |
| Phenylalanine | 0.090 | 4.41 | 3.333 | 45 | 6.615 |
| Total | | 100.92 | 1.533 | | 148.803 |

Total N is 14.87 %. The values are expressed as moles of acid/0.3 mg of protein. Calculated from the relationship (amino acid residue molecular weight) x 100/per cent of amino acid residue in protein. This number is omitted from the total.

and to contain a large number of cationic groups; data obtained by electrophoresis have shown it to be quite heat resistant, withstanding a temperature increase during its treatment. Titration confirmed the cationic nature of the sweet-sensitive protein. The amino acid composition of the sweet-sensitive protein was also investigated, and this study confirmed the molecular weight of 150,000 obtained by physical methods (Table 4).

Thus, interaction of sweet and bitter stimuli with the receptor cell takes place at the molecular level of cellular organization with the aid of special sweet- and bitter-sensitive proteins. This interaction is not of a chemical nature and appears to be achieved with the aid of hydrogen bonds formed as a result of conformational changes undergone by specific groups found in the stimulating and stimulated substances. Apparently, analogous processes also take place during the interaction of a saline stimulus. Thus, BEIDLER (1954) has shown for mammals and EVANS and MELLON (1962) for flies that the response of saline receptors to a saline stimulus is also effected with the aid of weak (hydrogen?) bonds. Salt-sensitive and acid-sensitive proteins have not been investigated so far. The difficulty here lies in the fact that protein conformation in general is subject to change during complex formation, and this change is reflected in the UV spectrum and contraction index of the complexes. Salts and acids, on the other hand, cause a change in the conformation of any protein.

The task next at hand will involve the investigation of the molecular structure of sweet- and bitter-sensitive proteins. Such an investigation would allow us to trace step by step the way in which conformational shifts induced in these proteins lead to stimulation of the receptor cell and the subsequent transmission of this stimulation in the form of impulses through synapses into the central nervous system.

## 4. Structural Organization of Gustatory Receptor Cells of Vertebrates

Our task here, of course, should consist simply in obtaining an idea, by means of extrapolation, of the location of sweet-sensitive, bitter-sensitive and other receptor proteins in the various structures of receptor taste cells. In fact, if we consider that these proteins, as in photoreceptors, constitute an integral structural part of gustatory receptor cells, it is highly probable that they will be found primarily in the portion of the cellular plasma membrane opposite a taste stimulus. However, as we shall see later, it is not yet possible to give a satisfactory answer to this question. No reliable data are yet available concerning the development or structure of taste cells, not to mention the lack of data on the cytophysiology of such cells. Thus, there are two different concepts concerning the development of taste buds in the tongue of vertebrates. The one concept, based on data obtained by means of light microscopic techniques, holds that taste buds originate in the same way as lateral-line organs (STONE, 1933) from embryonic Schwann cells of growing nerves which penetrate deep into the epithelium from underlying connective tissue (WRIGHT, 1951, 1958, 1964; KURTIEVA, 1953). KURTIEVA's data, obtained in our laboratory, indicate that the development of taste cells forming taste buds takes place in the human embryo as a result of the ingrowing of embryonic Schwann cells connected to peripheral nerve fibers which intrude into the growth layer (Malpighian layer) of the tongue epithelium. The shape of the buds is determined by the pressure of the surrounding epithelium.

The other concept holds that taste cells develop at the embryonic and definitive stages (after gustatory nerves have been cut) as a result of a transformation of the growth layer in the tongue epithelium under the effect of growing gustatory nerve fibers (VON VINTSCHGAU, 1880; TORREY, 1931, 1934; LASHKOV, 1945; GUTH, 1957, 1958, 1963; BEIDLER, 1963; BRADLEY and STERN, 1967). At the present time, this viewpoint seems to be confirmed by electron microscope observations on rat embryos. (Fig. 65) (FARBMAN, 1965a). However, observations in the electron microscope can be interpreted in the light of both the above concepts as regards the genesis of taste bud cells. Whatever the genesis of taste cells in such buds, it is possible that differentiation of the sweet-sensitive protein arises at a sufficiently early stage. It has been shown that 13 to 15-week-old human embryos already exhibit swallowing motions (DAVIS and POTTER, 1946), the intensity of which increases if saccharin is introduced into the allantoic cavity (DE SNOO, 1937; WINDLE, 1940). If a saccharin solution is dyed with methylene blue, it is possible to observe the appearance of saccharin in the urine of the foetus; this fact provides evidence not only of the function of taste cells, but also of the connection between their centers and swallowing muscles. We can assume that differentiation of a bitter-sensitive protein also occurs at the same early stage in the corresponding cells.

What, then, is the structure of taste cells in vertebrates at definitive stages, and how can we obtain an idea of the location site of sweet- and bitter-sensitive proteins in such cells? Taste cells are located in the taste buds. In fish, the latter are present not only in the oral cavity and in the front sections of the gastrointestinal tract, but also, in barbels in the head, in fins and on the outer surface of the body. In amphibians, taste buds are located in the mucous membrane of the oral cavity, in special papillae of the tongue. In reptiles and birds, they are found in the oral cavity and on the tongue. Taste buds of mammals, as we know, are located mainly in the papillae of the tongue: in fungiform papillae on the front two thirds of the tongue, and in circumvallate and foliate papillae at the back of the tongue. The number of taste buds varies greatly and depends on the ecological status of the animal. The taste buds located in the front two thirds of the tongue of mammals are innervated by fibers of the n. facialis and those of the back of the tongue by the glossopharyngeal and vagus nerves. The fibers, upon approaching the base of the taste bud and losing myelin, form the subgemmal plexus and from here a portion of the fibers (intragemmal) enter the taste bud and form synapses with taste cells. Fibers which terminate in the surrounding epithelium are called perigemmal fibers.

Taste buds are oval or "bulbous" in shape, their length is withn the range 30—100 µm and their width 15—70 µm. Taste buds are arranged at right angles to the multilayer epithelial layer of the tongue (Fig. 66). One bud contains 30 to 50 elongated cells, the long axis of which runs parallel to the long axis of the bud. The basal ends of the cells in a taste bud are turned toward the basal membrane which separates the taste bud from the underlying connective

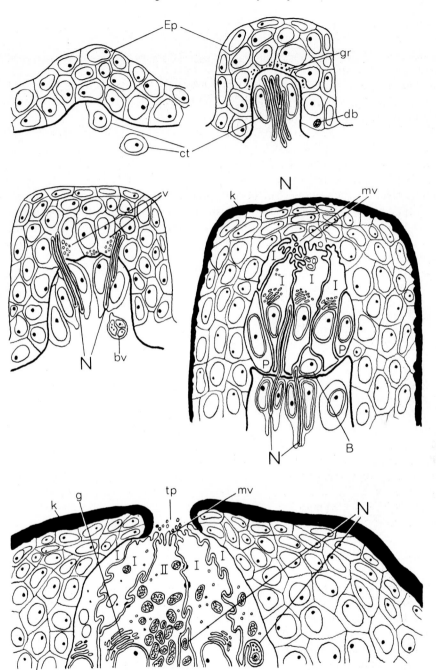

Fig. 65. Diagram showing the major morphological findings in the first five stages of development of the fungiform papilla and its taste bud in the fetal rat (FARBMAN, 1965a). *Ep* epidermis; *N* nerve fibers; *gr* granules; *db* dense body; *ct* connective tissue; *v* vesicles; *bv* blood vessels; *mv* microvilli; *P* peripheral cells; *B* basal cell; *g* Golgi apparatus; *k* keratinized cells; *tp* taste pore; *I, II* type-I and -II cells

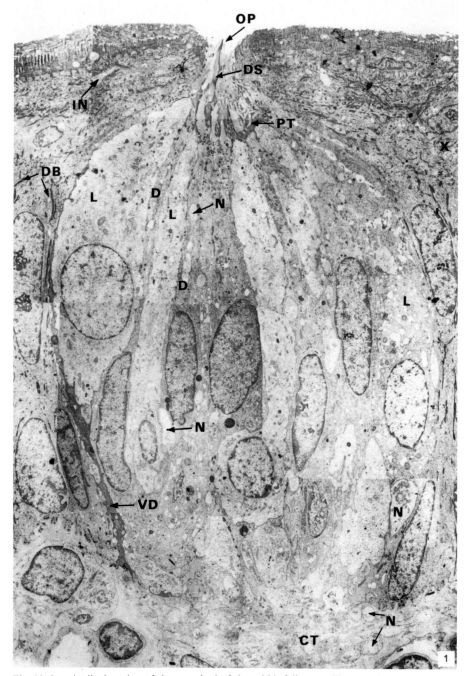

Fig. 66. Longitudinal section of the taste bud of the rabbit foliate papilla (× 8,000) (MURRAY and MURRAY, 1967). *OP* taste pore; *DS* dense matter ("stiff rods"); *PT* taste pit; *L* light cell; *D* dark cell; *N* nerve ending; *CT* connective tissue; *VD* boundary membrane between the taste bud and the connective tissue; *DB* boundary between the tongue epithelium and the taste bud; *IN* epithelium of the papilla

tissue. The apical ends together with the surrounding epithelial cells form a lumen, known as the gustatory canal, which communicates with the oral cavity by means of a narrow gustatory pore. In the light microscope, taste bud cells were clearly distinguished as being of two types: receptor or taste cells, and supporting cells. The first type, the taste cells, was distinguished by a spindle-like shape, a dark cytoplasm and the presence of special dark brads or rods on the apical surface, filling the lumen of the gustatory canal. The terminals of the gustatory nerves are located close to the base of these cells. The second type of cells, the supporting cells, had a similar shape but larger dimensions and a light vacuolated cytoplasm. Other researchers, however, consider such a subdivision as incorrect, since they think the cells in taste buds are continuously degenerating and hence are present at different stages of proliferation and differentiation. For this reason, a subdivision of such cells into taste and supporting cells appears rather artificial. We have already noted that taste buds degenerate after gustatory nerves have been cut and begin to regenerate after nerve regeneration. An intense mitotic activity has been observed in the epithelial cells surrounding the taste bud; in the opinion of some researchers, these cells, as was pointed out above, can be directly transformed into taste cells. According to some data obtained by autoradiography, a taste cell in the taste bud moves towards its center at a rate of about $0.06\,\mu m/h$ or $10\,Å/min$, or $1.4\,\mu m/day$, so that one cell is replaced every 30 hours in the taste buds (DE LORENZO, 1963). According to other data, obtained under the action of colchicine, replacement occurs every 10 hours and the life-span of a taste cell is 10 days (BEIDLER and SMALLMAN, 1965; CONGER and WELLS, 1969). Colchicine blocking of taste buds leads to the disappearance of electrophysiological responses in rats for a period of 4 to 8 hours; these responses appear again during the ingrowing of gustatory nerves (ZOTTERMAN, 1967). If this is the case, then we must assume that there is a change in the connections between taste cells and central neurons and that a "sweet" or "salty" fiber could after regeneration service a "bitter" or "acid" cell, etc. In such a case, in order to avoid confusion, the nearest branches of gustatory nerve fibers probably innervate the newly formed taste cells (BEIDLER, 1963).

The taste buds of lower vertebrates, for example amphibians, are located in the fungiform papillae. In these buds it is possible to distinguish several types of cells, which are in fact present, as we shall see later, also in the taste buds of higher vertebrates. Thus, in the axolotl (FÄHRMANN, HOFFMANN, and SCHUCHARDT, 1965; FÄHRMANN, 1967; FÄHRMANN and SCHUCHARDT, 1967) and in the frog, where the buds are surrounded by ciliated cells according to data obtained in our laboratory by PEVZNER (1970), the upper two thirds of the bud consists of two types of cells (Fig. 67): dark (type-I) cells extending along the entire length of the bud, and light (type-II) cells which are short and wide. Type-I cells are characterized by the greater electron density of their cytoplasm, and their apex consists of narrow finger-like processes. The latter, starting from the upper quarter of the cell, form a compactly built finger-like trunk, which is particularly clearly defined on the side walls; as a result, the central portion of the cell apex has a domelike structure. Both the central dome and the lateral finger-like cell processes are studded with high and frequently ramified microvilli. The plasma membrane coating the finger-like processes has a high electron density; this enables one to trace not only the origin but also the branching character of the processes, which form palisade-like arcades surrounding the central dome of the cell on all sides. The finger-like processes are approximately 6 μm long and 0.5—1 μm wide. It is possible that the bases of adjacent finger-like processes can extend far into the cytoplasm and can even communicate with the cisternae of the endoplasmic reticulum. The nucleus of the cell is generally located in the central portion; it has a segmented character and is characterized by a dense granular content (Fig. 67). A basal body is occasionally found in the upper third of the cell. The mitochondria as a rule have a well-defined rod shape and form prominent clusters in the apical part of the cell; their matrix has a high electron density. A Golgi-apparatus system can be distinguished in the well-defined endoplasmic reticulum, as well as separate sectors of the rough endoplasmic reticulum. Occasional individual secretion granules, lysosome, and multivesicular bodies can be clearly seen in the cells, as well as synaptic vesicles, particularly in the basal portion of the cell, where synaptic contacts with nerve endings can be observed. Nerve endings have a light cytoplasm, and some isolated mitochondria and synaptic vesicles are also found there, they can enter into synaptic contacts both at the base and at higher levels of dark cells.

Light cells are more massive and apparently also extend along the entire length of the taste bud, although it is difficult to observe them in the basal membrane region. Distinct desmosomal structures are visible at the point where light cells come into contact with dark cells in the upper portion of the taste bud (Fig. 67). The apical surface of light cells has an irregular contour and forms a number of irregular swellings, shaped like bulges and depressions or small pits. Individual small and thickened microvilli can be seen on the swellings. The nuclei of light cells are located closer to the base of the taste bud; they have a festoon-like shape and are characterized by the high electron density of the granular chromatin and nucleole. The cytoplasm of the cells contains a large number of vacuoles and granules, concentrated in their apical portion. A centrosome has also been found in the cytoplasm of light cells. Mitochondria look like short, dark rods distributed more or less over the entire body of the cell. Elements of rough endoplasmic reticulum and the Golgi apparatus are clearly visible throughout the cell. Fibrillar structures are present in the cytoplasm of light cells; as in dark cells, individual nerve endings can extend nearly to the base; however, in this case synaptic structures are practically never observed. In regard to the basal cells, which have been described by a number of authors (FÄHRMANN, 1967), it is still difficult to describe them; they are characterized by nuclei of irregular shape and have a granular cytoplasm which apparently forms mesaxonal sheaths around the nerve fibers.

In evaluating the structure of the amphibian taste bud cells described above, we can assume that the dark cells are receptor or taste cells. This assumption is confirmed by the presence of apices and the folded finger-like structure studded with microvilli. The large surface area of the plasma membrane resulting from this folded structure obviously favors contact of the cell with gustatory substances. This portion of the plasma membrane can serve as the location site of both

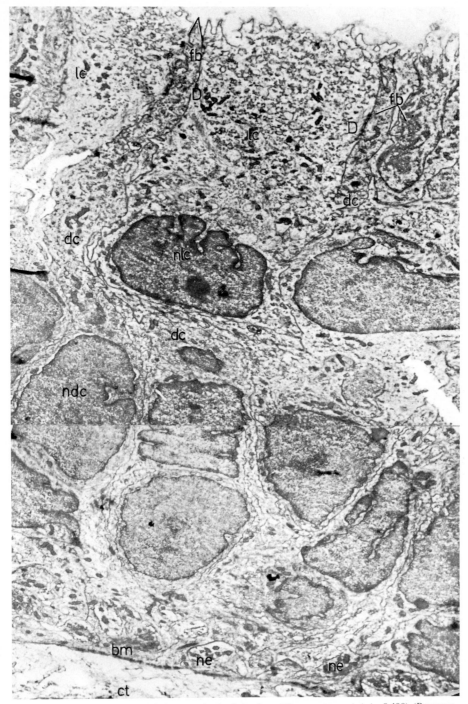

Fig. 67. Longitudinal section of the taste bud of the frog *(Rana temporaria)* (× 8,400) (PEVZNER, 1970). *dc* dark cell; *lc* light cell; *fb* digitiform process; *D* desmosome; *ndc* nucleus of dark cell; *nlc* nucleus of light cell; *bm* basal membrane; *ne* nerve ending; *ct* connective tissue

sweet- and bitter-sensitive proteins, or other special proteins (BEIDLER, 1967). Light cells do not exhibit on their apical surface such a noticeable increase in surface area. The cytoplasm of light cells is completely filled with small and large granules, which indicates their secretory function; it is perhaps more reasonable to classify them as supporting cells. Both dark and light cells are connected by means of desmosomes, which is usually characteristic for the contact of receptor and supporting cells in other sense organs. The basal cells, in view of their indefinite structure, should probably be considered as cambial elements, supplying both dark receptor cells and light supporting cells.

In our opinion, such an assumption can also be derived from the data on the ultrastructural organization of taste buds in mammals (MURRAY and MURRAY, 1960, 1966, 1967; MURRAY, MURRAY, and FUJIMOTO, 1969; NEMETSCHEK-GANSLER and FERNER, 1964; FARBMAN, 1965a, 1965b, 1967; SCALZI, 1967, and others). In the rabbit, both dark and light cells have also been detected in taste buds with the aid of the electron microscope (Fig. 66). However, it is becoming clearer which of these cells should be considered as receptor cells and which supporting cells. Moreover, supporting cells are now being considered as transition stages of receptor cells undergoing differentiation (SCALZI, 1967).

Let us examine briefly the structure of both types of cells. Dark cells have a cytoplasm with higher electron density, are narrow and extend along the entire length of the taste bud from the basal membrane to the gustatory pore.

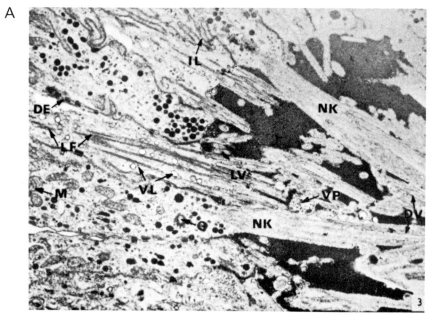

Fig. 68 A and B. Apex of the rabbit taste bud. A. Apical surface of the taste cells, augmented by a system of microvilli, assembled in the form of taste brushes pointing towards the taste pit (× 13,000) (MURRAY and MURRAY, 1967). B. Diagram showing the organization of the brushes (NEMETSCHEK-GANSLER and FERNER, 1964)

B

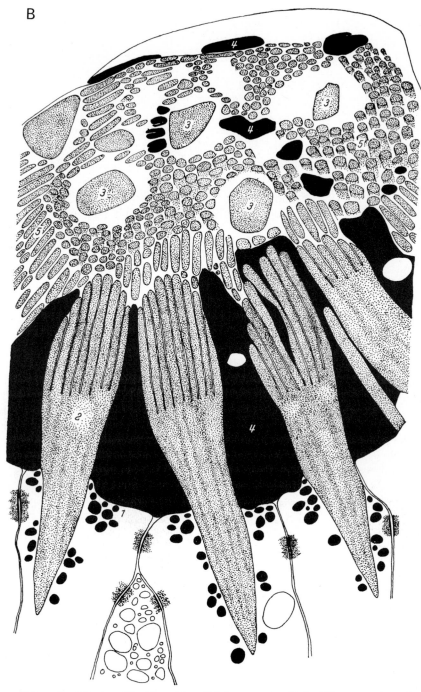

*In A. NK* neck; *DV* microvilli; *VL* vesicles; *DE* desmosomes; *IL* leaf-like connection of cells; *M* mitochondria; *LF* fibril; *LV* base of brush; *VP* substance of "stiff rods". *In B. 1* osmiophilic granules in receptor cells; *2* taste brush covered with microvilli; *3* cross-sections of brush and its microvilli; *4* substance filling the space between brushes ("stiff rods")

In their basal portion, these cells can form lateral processes; their apical surface is narrowed down in the form of a small neck and is studded with a system of microvilli which cover the bottom of the taste pit. The microvilli branch out from the apices of dark cells by means of a small narrow, conical stem, which fans out like a small brush (Fig. 68). The ramifications of this brush consist of 30 to 40 long, narrow digitiform microvilli (NEMETSCHEK-GANSLER and FERNER, 1964). The space between the taste brushes and microvilli is filled with a special electron-dense substance, which apparently corresponds to the "brads" of the light microscope. On the basis of histochemical studies performed in our laboratory (PEVZNER, 1962, 1964a—c, 1966, 1969; VINNIKOV, 1965a, 1965b, 1966a—c), we assumed at one time (VINNIKOV, 1965a, 1965b, 1966a, 1966b) that the substance present in the brads must function like an ion-exchange resin, making it possible for molecules and ions of some gustatory substances to come into contact with the surface of microvilli in the receptor gustatory cell and preventing such contact by other gustatory substances. Microvilli contain thin tubules with a diameter of 130Å. According to up-to-date conceptions, the microvilli are motile and seem to interact actively with the chemical food compounds which are filtered through the brads. In the apical region of the cell a centriole is found, from which a cross-striated root can branch out (MURRAY and MURRAY, 1967). Sometimes it is possible to observe a flagellum, turned towards the gustatory pore and arising from the apex of dark cells. The kinocilium contains $9 \times 2 + 2$ fibrillae (SCALZI, 1967). However, connections of the centrosome with microtubules, rather than with a flagellum, can be observed under the electron microscope (MURRAY and MURRAY, 1967). The presence of fibrillae and microtubules in microvilli makes it possible to compare them with microvilli of other receptor cells. The nucleus of a dark cell has an oval shape and is highly granulated. The cytoplasm contains fine granules, which apparently constitute the prosecretion for the substance present in taste pits. Elongated mitochondria and elements of the Golgi apparatus are more or less uniformly distributed through the entire cell body. Nerve endings filled with mitochondria and synaptic vesicles can enter into synaptic contact with lateral processes of dark cells in the basal portion of the taste bud, thus giving the impression that they penetrate deep into dark cells. The character of synaptic contacts is difficult to trace. Dark cells can combine with each other and with light cells by means of desmosomes.

Light cells have more massive dimensions and contain a large nucleus; their apical surface protrudes into the gustatory pore and is also provided with numerous small microvilli, usually completely enclosed by the substance present in the taste pit. Microvilli of light cells also contain thin fibrillae. The cytoplasm is characterized by uniformly distributed mitochondria, elements of the Golgi apparatus, and smooth and rough endoplasmic reticulum. A centriole can sometimes be observed in light cells. However, it has not yet been possible to establish in a reliable manner the presence of synaptic contacts between light cells and nerve endings (MURRAY and MURRAY, 1967). Since then MURRAY and MURRAY (1969) have demonstrated a third type of cells, characterized by narrow necks or irregular surface at the apical part and the classic chemical synapse at the basal part. The third type of cell is considered to be a receptor cell.

We shall not dwell in detail on the structure of the synapses and nerve endings, which include light endings equipped with a few synaptic vesicles and mitochondria and which appear to be afferent endings, and also dark endings, which are filled with synaptic vesicles and mitochondria and hence must be efferent endings. We shall also not examine here the transitional cell forms,

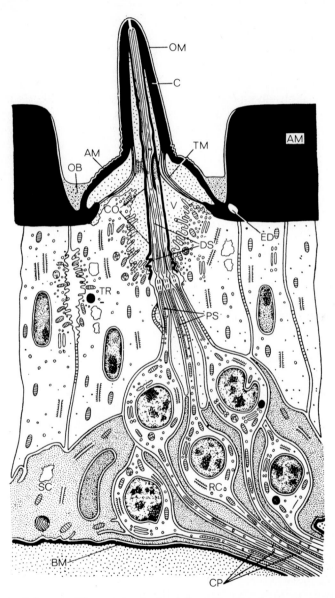

Fig. 69. Structural diagram of the gustatory basiconical sensilla of beetle *(Acilius sulcatus)* (IVANOV, 1969b). *RC* receptor cell; *CP* central process; *BM* basal membrane; *SC* Schwann cell; *TR* trichogen cell; *CO* scolopoid sheat; *V* vacuole; *PS* proximal segment; *DS* distal segment; *TM* thin membrane; *ED* efferent duct; *OB* outer body; *C* cone; *OM* outer membrane; *AM* articular membrane

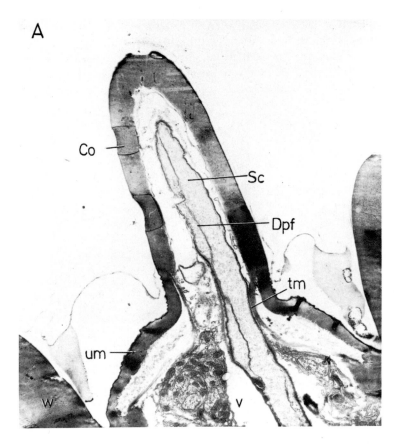

which it is hard to classify as either dark or light cells. Nevertheless, we believe it possible to qualify dark and light cells from a functional standpoint. We also think that in mammals there are sufficiently good reasons to consider dark cells as gustatory receptor cells, and light cells as supporting cells. Such an assumption is supported by the presence in dark cells of mammals of a complex system of motile microvilli, which greatly increases their surface area, as compared to the surface of light cells. As we have seen, a similar large increase in the apical surface with the aid of microvilli was also observed in the dark cells of amphibians. Consequently, if we speak hypothetically about the possible location site of sweet- or bitter-sensitive proteins, it is more logical to associate their location with the larger surface area of the plasma membrane of the motile microvilli in the brushes of dark cells. Regarding the brads, it is hard to state at present what they allow to pass through or what they hold back. However, these brads cover part of the microvilli of dark cells, and apparently completely cover the microvilli of light cells. Thus, whereas in dark cells brads serve in the capacity of a stimulus regulator, in light cells they may simply play a protective role. Of course, we should not ignore the fact that dark cells contain a basal body with a root and a kinocilium. However, the best

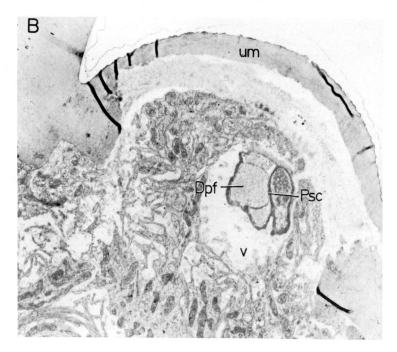

Fig. 70 A and B. Longitudinal (A) and cross-sections (B) of the cuticular section of the basiconical sensilla of the beetle *Acilius sulcatus* (× 20,000) (IVANOV, 1966). *Co* cone; *Sc* scolopoid sheath; *Dpf* distal segment of peripheral process; *tm* thin membrane; *um* articular membrane; *v* vacuole; *Psc* partition of scopoloid sheath; *w* wall of outer skeleton of antennae

argument in favor of a receptor function of dark cells is the presence of synaptic contacts between these cells and nerve endings; such contacts have not established in light cells. Future electrophysiological studies must provide a final solution to the question concerning the nature of dark and light cells. At present, after comparing data obtained with lower and higher vertebrates, we are inclined to consider the dark cells of taste buds as receptor cells and the light cells as supporting cells.

## 5. Structural Organization of Contact Chemoreceptor (Gustatory) Sensillae in Insects

Contact chemoreceptors, i.e., the gustatory organs of insects, are located primarily in oral parts and on distal leg segments, as was established by means of behavioral and electrophysiological tests. They are generally varieties of trichoid and basiconical sensilla (DETHIER, 1963; HODGSON, 1965; WOLBARSHT, 1965; IVANOV, 1969a, 1969b). Under the light microscope they seem to have a similar structure. However, a much more detailed study with the electron microscope has been performed on the sensilla basiconica of dipterous insects (LARSEN, 1963) and in our laboratory on coleoptera (IVANOV, 1966, 1969a, 1969b). According to IVANOV's data (1966, 1969a, 1969b), the cuticular part of thick-walled basiconical sensilla located on the antennae of the beetle *Acilius sulcatus* consists of a cuticular cone connected with the cuticle by a joint membrane. An additional thin membrane, consisting of individual cuticular strands, stretches between the base of the cone and the cuticle canal walls. Each sensilla consists of 4 to 6 bipolar receptor cells, whose bodies lie in the hypoderma lining the cuticle of the antennae. A thin central process, directed toward the central nervous system, extends from the basal pole in the body of each receptor cell (Fig. 69). Lengthwise oriented mitochondria and microtubules can be observed in the cytoplasm of central processes. The opposite, i.e. apical, pole in the body of each receptor cell narrows down into a peripheral process which can be followed up to the apex of the cuticular cone (Fig. 70). Two segments, which differ from a morphological viewpoint, can be distinguished in the peripheral process: a distal and a proximal segment. The distal segment of the peripheral process is a modified cilium; in its cytoplasmic matrix, microtubules and vesicles 200 to 400 Å in diameter can be observed. Distal segments (modified cilia) of receptor cells in the sensilla are located inside a cuticular sheath, attached in the apex region of the cone to its walls. In the cytoplasm of the proximal segment can be seen ribosomes, as well as numerous vesicles and mitochondria extended parallel to the long axis of the segment (Fig. 70).

One of the peripheral processes terminates near the base of the hair and belongs to a mechanoreceptor cell, since it is stimulated by the deflection of the hair. The apex of the mechanoreceptor cell, unlike that of the gustatory cell, is attached to the inner surface of a scolopoid sheath. Thus, in both insects and vertebrates taste sensation is apparently combined with tactile sensation. This assumption is supported not only by morphological but also by electrophysiological data (WOLBARSHT and DETHIER, 1958). The ultrastructural organization of the body of a receptor cell is characterized by the presence of a large nucleus surrounded by a relatively thin layer of cytoplasm (Fig. 71). Mitochondria as well as elements of the Golgi apparatus are uniformly distributed throughout the body of the cell; multivesicular bodies and electron-dense granules are occasionally present. In one of the receptor cells of the organ, a special structure, known as the spherical or onion body was found in the immediate vicinity of the nucleus where the central process branches off from the cell body. This spherical body consists of 10 to 15 concentrically arranged flattened cisterns; the body has a diameter of 10 μm and its functional purpose is not clear.

The peripheral processes of receptor cells and their bodies are surrounded by specialized enveloping cells. The basal parts of receptor cells are surrounded by processes of Schwann cells, which enter into mesaxonal relations with their axons. The nucleus of the Schwann cell is usually located at the level of the receptor cell body. Both the nucleus and cytoplasm of the Schwann cell have very high electron density. Distal to the Schwann cell and surrounding peripheral processes a large trichogen cell is located, extending from the cuticular part of the organ almost all the way to the basal membrane of the hypodermis (SNODGRASS, 1955). The cavity inside this cell, filled with a liquid of unknown composition, is called an extracellular vacuole. The surface of the trichogen cell facing the vacuole is coated with microvilli, filled with vesicles of diameter

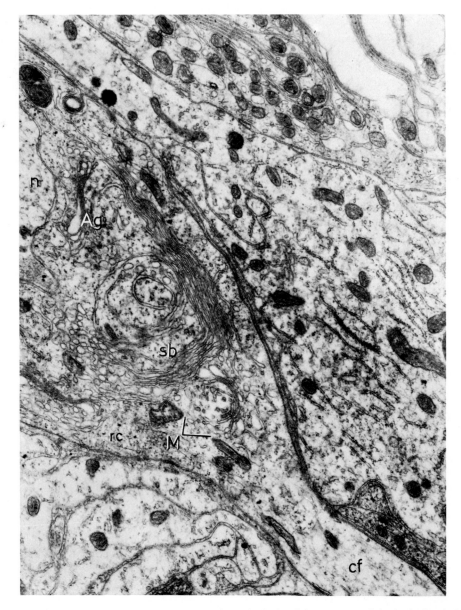

Fig. 71. Branching site of the central process from the body of the receptor cell in the basiconical sensilla of the beetle *Acilius sulcatus* (× 20,000) (IVANOV, 1969b). *n* nucleus; *M* mitochondria; *cf* central process; *sb* spherical body; *Ag* Golgi apparatus; *rc* receptor cell

about 0.1 µm. These cells contain a dark oval nucleus located in their basal portion; they also contain large numbers of elements of the Golgi apparatus and of rough endoplasmic reticulum, as well as multivesicular bodies and various types of granules.

It should be pointed out that supravital observations of receptor cells in basiconical sensilla have not so far discovered any motion of the modified flagella with which the peripheral processes of receptor cells are equipped. Further careful investigations in this direction are needed.

Thus, in insects the receptor surface of gustatory cells is formed at the expense of the plasmic membrane of a modified flagellum, whereas in vertebrates this surface develops at the expense of a complex system of microvilli in brushes. We believe that the sweet- and bitter-sensitive proteins of insects, which have not yet been extracted, are located in the plasma membrane of the modified flagellum. As we shall describe below, many insects respond to a sweet and bitter stimulus in a manner similar to mammals and man.

## 6. Cytochemical Organization of Taste Buds and Function of Taste Cells

We have already stated that the substance present in the "brads", located between brushes and microvilli in the gustatory pit of mammalian taste buds, is considered by us to be an analog of ion-exchange resins, which are capable of "refining" gustatory substances in such a way that their gustatory, stimulating chemical source can interact with the receptor surface, i.e. with the plasma membrane of the microvilli present in gustatory cells. Consequently, this substance must simultaneously play a protective role. The substance present in brads, as was shown by PEVZNER in our laboratory (PEVZNER, 1962, 1964a—c, 1966, 1969), is rich in mucopolysaccharides or mucoproteins, has a high total protein content (three aromatic amino acids), and contains a large number of functional groups of protein molecules (carboxyl and thiol groups). This substance also exhibits a high activity of glycerophosphatase, adenosine triphosphatase, acid and alkaline phosphatases, and 3- and 5-nucleotidases (BOURNE, 1948; ARVY, 1959, 1961; BARADI and BOURNE, 1953, 1959a, 1959b; PEVZNER, 1964c, 1969).

The flagella branching off from the apical end of receptor cells exhibit an adenosine monophosphatase activity (SCALZI, 1966). Microvilli of brushes in dark cells are characterized by a high total protein and a large number of carboxyl and thiol groups, detected here as small granules under the light microscope (PEVZNER, 1962, 1964c). As mentioned earlier, blocking of sulfhydryl groups reduces or completely eliminates sensitivity to a gustatory stimulus in the frog (YUR'EVA, 1957, 1960a, 1960b). Blocking of amino groups also lowers the sensitivity of the gustatory organ (YUR'EVA, 1960b). As shown by studies in our laboratory (PEVZNER, 1962, 1964b, 1964c) and in BOURNE's laboratory (EL-RAKHAWY, 1962a, 1962b), a high activity of succinate dehydrogenase is observed in the apical regions of gustatory cell. The activity of receptor cells is disrupted because of effect on taste buds of malonate, which inhibits the Krebs cycle; however, this activity is restored upon further addition of succinate or fumarate (KOSHTOYANTS and KATALIN-ROZA, 1958). In the same region, as well as in the nucleus-containing portion of receptor cells, high activity of a number of phosphatases is observed, such as glycerophosphatase, adenosine triphosphatase, acid and alkaline phosphatases (BOURNE, 1948; BARADI and BOURNE, 1953, 1959a,

1959b; SIMIDZU, 1957; ARVY, 1959; BARADI, 1963; EL-RAKHAWY, 1963; PEVZNER, 1964c, 1966; ERBENGI and FERNER, 1964; IWAYAMA and NADA, 1967; ZALEWSKI, 1968). We have already pointed out that an enzymic taste theory was formulated on the basis of the fact that gustatory substances act upon enzymes in a different manner, increasing the activity of some enzymes and inhibiting the activity of others (BARADI and BOURNE, 1953).

It has been shown that, in the taste buds of papillae of rats, the activity of adenosine triphosphatase and acid and alkaline phosphatases depends upon the cutting of gustatory nerves, i. e. upon denervation. By qualitative and quantitative methods it was shown that four days after bilateral section, during degeneration of the taste bud, the activity of acid phosphatase increased, while that of adenosine triphosphatase decreased; later both activities vanished. On the other hand, the activity of alkaline phosphatase also gradually decreased and vanished 8 weeks after gustatory nerves were cut (ZALEWSKY, 1968). Further, it was shown that only those taste buds which are innervated by n. glossopharingeus exhibit a change in the activity of alkaline phosphatase (ZALEWSKY, 1969). Unfortunately, the cellular and subcellular processes involving a change in the activity of enzymes were not investigated in this study, which was performed with the light microscope. This would seem to be primarily a matter of degeneration of taste buds and associated changes in the enzymes.

The nucleus-containing part of receptor cells has a high RNA content (PEVZNER, 1962, 1964c, 1969) but a lower total protein content and fewer functional groups of protein molecules than the apical part of the cell. Glycogen is also found in the nucleus-containing portion of the cell (PEVZNER, 1962, 1964c). The synaptic region of taste buds is characterized by a high content of total protein, thiol and carboxyl groups and glycogen (PEVZNER, 1962, 1964c, 1966), and a high activity of succinate dehydrogenase (PEVZNER, 1962, 1964b, 1964c, 1966; EL-RAKHAWY, 1962a, 1962b) and various phosphatases (BOURNE, 1948; BARADI and BOURNE, 1953; ARVY, 1959; PEVZNER, 1962, 1964c; EL-RAKHAWY, 1963; ITOIZ, CARRANZA, and CABRINI, 1966).

A very high level of acetylcholinesterase activity can generally be detected in the synaptic region of taste buds in members of all classes of vertebrates (Fig. 72) (ELLIS, 1959; BARADI and BOURNE, 1959a; GEREBTZOFF, 1959; ARVY, 1961; EL-RAKHAWY and BOURNE, 1961; PEVZNER, 1962, 1964a, 1964c, 1966, 1969; HODOSH and MONTAGNA, 1963; SCALZI, 1966). A comparatively high monoamine oxidase activity has also been observed in this region; monoamine oxidase is an enzyme involved in the metabolism of catecholamine (GOLDSMITH and ELLIS, 1961). In view of these facts, we can assume that transmission of the nervous impulse arising in the receptor cell takes place mainly by means of a cholinergic mechanism, although, of course, we cannot definitely exclude the possibility that catecholamines, i. e. an adrenergic mechanism, are involved in this process. The above assumption is supported by biochemical data showing that the acetylcholine content is considerably greater in the region of gustatory papillae than in the surrounding epithelium. Further, the cutting of gustatory nerves, leading to the degeneration of taste buds is accompanied by a fall in acetylcholine content down to one eighth of the original level (BRÜCKE, HELLAUER, and UMRATH, 1948). The application of specific concentrations of acetyl-

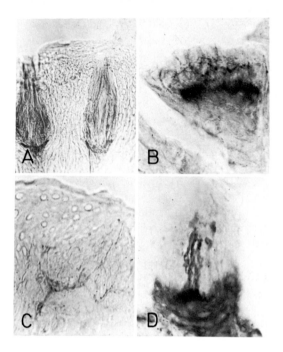

Fig. 72A—D. Acetylcholinesterase activity in the synapse region of taste buds of (A) the carp,
(B) the grass frog, (C) the steppe turtle, and (D) the pigeon (PEVZNER, 1964b)

choline and acetylcholinesterase-inhibiting compounds considerably increases
the response of gustatory cells in frog tongue to gustatory substances (LANDGREN,
LILJESTRAND, and ZOTTERMAN, 1954; SKOUBY, ZILSTORFF-PEDERSEN, 1955;
KIMURA, 1961).

We shall not dwell here on the strictly chemical characteristic of the light
cells that we believe to be supporting cells of taste buds. These cells appear
to contain much the same biologically active chemical compounds as dark
receptor cells, but the amount of such compounds is less and enzyme activity
is considerably lower. We consider this further proof of their functional nonequiva-
lence. Thus, the ultrastructural picture of the organization of receptor and supporting cells in taste buds coincides with their histochemical characteristics. The
structural and cytochemical organization of gustatory cells suggests that, although
the primary processes in the stimulation of receptor cells are associated with
the interaction between a specific protein and a definite gustatory stimulus
and are not enzymic processes, they still lead to a stimulation of the gustatory
cell. This stimulation is based on multistage activation of numerous enzymes
and associated substrates, as well as of other biologically active chemical compounds located in the ultracellular structures of gustatory receptor cells. All
of these factors culminate in the release of acetylcholine onto the postsynaptic
membrane where it is bound to a special cholinoreceptive protein. This process,
in turn, is regulated by the hydrolyzing action of cholinesterase. It is possible
that catecholamines are also involved in this process. As a result, ionic processes

arise on the surface of synaptic membranes, accompanied by the formation of biopotentials, which are transmitted from the gustatory cell along nerve fibers as impulses to the central nervous system. We shall not consider here the possible role that efferent innervation may play in the excitation of gustatory cells, since electrophysiological data concerned with this aspect are not at present available.

The cytochemical organization of gustatory cells described above applies only to vertebrates; no data are available for insects.

## 7. Electrophysiological Investigations

We have already mentioned that electrical stimulation of papillae in the human tongue can induce four types of taste sensation (BÉKÉSY, 1964, 1965). When a current generator supplies vibrations at a frequency of 30 to 40 cps, both saline and acid papillae are stimulated, while sweet papillae are stimulated at 70 cps and bitter papillae at 100 cps. Chemical stimulation of the same papillae in man induced similar sensations at whatever concentration of solutions (BÉKÉSY, 1966). BÉKÉSY, therefore, concluded that the quality of taste is the same for each individual papilla stimulated by either electrical or chemical means. The papillae are characterized by their strictly localized sites on the surface of the tongue according to whether they are saline, acid sweet or bitter papillae.

Anatomical differences have been found between acid-saline and bitter-sweet papillae, and these differences are expressed in their shape and blood supply (BÉKÉSY, 1964, 1965).

Investigations of taste papillae of rats and hamsters with the aid of microelectrodes introduced into single gustatory receptor cells (KIMURA and BEIDLER, 1956, 1961; TATEDA and BEIDLER, 1964; BEIDLER, 1966) have shown that these papillae constitute a live battery, the source of their electrical energy being the nonuniform distribution of $Na^+$ and $K^+$ on the surface of the cell membrane. The contents of the cell have an electronegative charge in contrast to the surface. The membrane potential is 30 to 50 mV. A taste stimulus acts upon the cell to produce a slowly changing potential, the receptor potential. The receptor potential varies for the same stimulus from 15 to 45 mV. The researchers found that no single receptor cell responds only to an acid, only to a saline, or only to a sweet stimulus. The majority of individual receptor cells respond to all taste stimuli, but the sensitivity of the cell varies. Thus, every taste cell can respond to more than one stimulus, and sometimes responds to all four taste stimuli (BEIDLER, 1966). Unlike gustatory papillae, taste receptors therefore are practically nonspecific. We must assume that the composition of the cytoplasmic membrane of microvilli of one and the same cell includes, along with complex sweet- or bitter-sensitive proteins, some sort of compounds (are these also proteins?) which interact with the various cations and anions present in salty substances and the $H^+$ of acid substances.

How is the depolarization of the plasma membrane transmitted in the synapse region to the endings of the gustatory nerves? Here there is a definite disagreement between the data obtained by cytochemistry and by electrophysiology. ESAKOV (1966) was able to demonstrate that blocking acetylcholine or cholinesterase does not affect the spontaneous activity of gustatory nerve fibers but significantly modifies their response to adequate stimuli. On this basis, ESAKOV concludes that a cholinergic system modifies to a considerable extent the polarization properties of impulses travelling along the nerve fiber. Under the effect of a stimulus, the discharge of a single nerve fiber is characterized first by a high-frequency pulsation of 1 to 2 sec duration, followed by a stable discharge during, the entire time of action of the stimulus.

A study of the action currents recorded from single fibers of the frog gustatory nerve has made it possible to distinguish four types of fibers: D fibers, responding primarily to divalent salts, saccharose and water; M fibers, responding mainly to monovalent salts; Q fibers, responding to quinine; and A fibers, responding to acids (SATO and KUSANO, 1960). Continuing these studies, KUSANO (1960) investigated the responses of 108 single fibers in the gustatory nerve of the frog and found that 51 fibers were of type M, Q, or A, and that 11 fibers responded to only one stimulus. The remaining 46 fibers responded to a wide variety of compounds, although different stimuli induced different responses. Thus, the nerve fibers of the frog do not apparently possess absolute specificity.

In tests performed by KONISHI and ZOTTERMAN (1963), where biopotentials were recorded from a small branch of the gustatory (IX) nerve of the carp, about half of the fibers investigated exhibited a differential sensitivity, and only a quarter had absolute specificity. The remaining 28 % of the fibers were relatively non-specific and responded to one or two stimuli. Finally, 18 % of the fibers responded to all stimuli, with the exception of common salt (NaCl) and quinine hydrochloride.

In man, bioelectrical responses were obtained from chorda tympani during surgical operations (DIAMANT et al., 1963, 1965). At the temperature of the tongue surface, water does not cause an increase in nervous activity. However, the action of NaCl at a concentration of 0.01 $M$ or higher coincides with the average threshold of this salt in man (PFAFFMANN, 1955). Sugars, saccharin and alcohol were quite effective, in particular saccharose, which had a threshold of about 0.02 $M$.

To summarize, we can say that in vertebrates a sweet stimulus can be recognized by the most sensitive fibers, saline and bitter stimuli by the least sensitive, and an acid stimulus by any kind of fiber. By recording action currents from the n. glossopharyngeus (IX) of rats, cats, and rabbits, it has been possible to show topographically that the response to quinine predominates in the posterior one-third of the tongue, which is less sensitive to NaCl than the front two thirds of the tongue (YAMADA, 1967).

Thus, the number of strictly specific gustatory fibers, and also of gustatory cells, is smaller in vertebrates than that of nonspecific fibers. Specific fibers are still present in vertebrates, but their number varies in different animals, the largest number being found in apes and, of course, in man (ZOTTERMAN, 1967).

In insects, biopotentials can be recorded from contact (gustatory) sensilla (MORITA and YAMASHITA, 1959; EVANS and MELLON, 1962; ELIZAROV, 1965;

ELIZAROV and SINITSINA, 1969). Several types of impulses could be distinguished according to the magnitude of their amplitude. A volley of impulses with the same amplitude corresponds to the activity of one of the receptor cells in a sensillum. On this basis, if the sensilla of the fly *Formia* are stimulated with a 0.5—1.0 *M* solution of NaCl or other salt, it is possible to isolate a special cell, which is specific with respect to salts and is called the L-receptor. Another cell of the sensilla is stimulated by solutions of glucose, sugar, etc., and is called the S-receptor. The third type of cell is an aqueous or W receptor; it is stimulated when pure water acts upon the sensilla. If the hair is bent at the same time as gustatory impulses are registered, it is possible to record mechanical or M-impulses, arising in the sensilla due to the presence of a mechanoreceptor cell.

Careful bioelectric tests carried out on receptor sensilla have shown that the impulses of a sugar receptor cell have a positive polarity, while those of a saline cell have a negative polarity (DETHIER and HANSON, 1965; ELIZAROV and SINITSINA, 1969). The generator potential of a gustatory chemoreceptor cell in insects is a slow negative oscillation with an amplitude of several millivolts; this potential increases rapidly the instant the stimulus starts to act and is maintained at a constant level throughout the duration of the stimulus action. Against the background of this oscillation, impulses can be observed that have a positive polarity and a frequency that remains constant as long as the stimulus exerts its effect (ELIZAROV and SINITSINA, 1969). When the gustatory cell is stimulated with calcium chloride and guanine, the generator potential assumes the opposite sign, the receptor membrane is hyperpolarized, and the impulses vanish (MORITA and YAMASHITA, 1959). The total generator potential can be recorded when sensilla are stimulated by a mixture of compounds which excite several receptor cells (HODGSON, 1964, 1965). Inhibition processes have been observed in W-cells when octolamine or stimulants for other cells (saccharose, NaCl) are added to distilled water. The inhibiting action of a mixture of sugar and salt solutions on chemoreceptor cells is observed at any given concentration of these compounds within the range 0.01 to 1 *M* (ELIZAROV and SINITSINA, 1969). It is assumed that inhibitory effects are associated with the presence in plasma membranes of selective molecular sectors that react with molecules of the stimulus. Therefore, the interaction of an excitatory stimulus with membrane molecules would induce depolarization of the membrane, whereas the interaction of an inhibitory stimulus with membrane molecules would induce hyperpolarization (HODGSON, 1965). However, more direct confirmation of the correctness of BEIDLER's theory (1964) is available. There has been shown to be a connection between the concentration of NaCl in a solution and the frequency of the action potentials obtained from chemoreceptor contact sensilla in the fly. The frequency of the response to 0.05 *M* NaCl does not change at pH 3 to 8, and the magnitude of the free energy is also insignificant. Thus, the primary interaction of a taste stimulus with the plasma membrane of the modified flagellum in the receptor cell of insects (and of the receptor cell in vertebrates) is not an enzymic process (DETHIER, 1963).

In insects, electrophysiological studies have disclosed in practically all cases that receptor cells in contact (gustatory) sensilla have a specific structural and functional character. In vertebrates in which the presence of special sweet- and bitter-sensitive proteins can be established, this specialization, as we have seen, is rather more relative.

# 8. Conclusion

A study of the chemical structure of taste stimuli shows, in general, that the taste of salts depends on both anion and cation, that an acid stimulus is determined by hydrogen, and that a sweet stimulus is apparently associated with intramolecular shifts taking place between the hydrogen bonds of the active centers of the sweet-sensitive protein and those of the gustatory substances; a bitter stimulus is determined both by the structure of the molecule (intramolecular hydrogen bonds as in the system sweet-sensitive protein—sweet substance) and the presence of certain functional groups, e.g. phenyl groups. Insignificant structural changes may be accompanied by considerable changes in the character of the gustatory stimulus. With what does the stimulus interact in the receptor cell? In this respect, we have to give credit to BEIDLER, who in 1954 proposed his famous "taste equation", which reflects in a reasonably correct way the course of the mechanism that triggers taste reception. His conclusion, that the interaction of a taste stimulus with receptor sites in the plasma membrane of the receptor cell is based on physical processes of the adsorption type and not on enzymic processes, has been confirmed by the most recent biochemical investigations. In this respect, it is difficult to overestimate the discovery in mammals of a sweet-sensitive protein located in taste buds in the front portion of the tongue, and of a bitter-sensitive protein located in taste buds in the rear portion of the tongue (DASTOLI and PRICE, 1966; DASTOLI, LOPIEKES, and DOIG, 1968; DASTOLI, LOPIEKES, and PRICE, 1968; HIJI, KOBAJASHI, and SATO, 1968, 1969). Both proteins form with sweet and bitter stimuli complexes that are not time-dependent and exhibit a linear dependence upon the molar concentration of the stimulus. Apparently, these proteins contain "active" centers; their interaction with sweet and bitter stimuli is based on London-type hydrogen bonds.

Thus, the taste reception of sweet and bitter stimuli and also, as we believe, of acid and saline stimuli, takes place at the molecular level of organization of these stimuli proper and of gustatory receptor cells. At present, it still difficult to determine in a direct way the location site of gustatory proteins in the plasma membrane of receptor cells. However, we can assume that in human embryo development these proteins—at least sweet-sensitive ones—are synthesized at a fairly early stage. This assumption is supported by the fact that a 13-week-old human fetus can swallow amniotic fluid sweetened with saccharin. The protein opsin in visual cells and the sweet- and bitter-sensitive proteins in gustatory cells can be considered as protein mutations that determine the specific character of the structure and function of receptor gustatory cells. Unfortunately, it is still not clear, at least in the case of vertebrates, which of the cells in taste buds are receptor cells, and which are supporting cells. The gustatory cell of vertebrates, in our opinion a dark cell, performs its function mainly with the aid of a system of brush-like microvilli. We must assume that gustatory proteins are located in the plasma membrane of their microvilli.

In vertebrates, electrophysiological studies have shown that the same gustatory cell, as well as adjacent sensory nerve fibers, is able to respond to a number of gustatory stimuli, and not only to a sweet or only to a bitter stimulus. Consequently, different protein molecules, sensitive not only to sweet but also to other gustatory stimuli, must be located in the same gustatory cells. Thus, in vertebrates, molecular differences in taste reception have not yet found their structural reflection at the cellular organization level, in the same way as in color vision. In insects, the situation is different; their contact gustatory sensilla contain receptor cells whose peripheral processes are modified flagella. With the aid of electrophysiological methods it is possible to distinguish several types of strictly specialized receptor cells, namely a saline or L-cell, a sugar or S-cell, and an aqueous or W-cell. Thus, in these ancient phyla, taste reception, like visual reception, is already reflected not only at the molecular but also at the cellular level of organization. There can be no doubt that in insects these types of reception are based on the same molecular principle as in vertebrates. Molecular processes start in the plasma membrane of microvilli or of a modified flagellum during interaction with a corresponding taste stimulus, for example, with molecules of sweet-sensitive and bitter-sensitive proteins, during which they change their conformation (this represents the primary conversion of energy or its encoding). These processes trigger a whole series of ionic and enzymic shifts in the subcellular structures of the receptor cell. Attesting to this fact is the complex cytochemical organization and high enzyme content of the receptor cell. As a result of the ionic and enzymic shifts that characterize the stimulation of a gustatory cell, a nervous impulse is initiated by means of which the gustatory cell transmits encoded information through synapses and along gustatory nerve fibers to the central nervous system. Naturally, the picture thus outlined still contains a number of blank spots, showing how much still remains to be done in order to achieve a deeper understanding of the mechanism of taste reception.

# Chapter VI

# Smell

## 1. Introduction

The remote character of the functioning of the olfactory organ is based on a simple phenomenon: molecules of an odorant are separated from the main bulk and, being volatile, are wafted around by air currents. They are thus capable of interacting with olfactory cells. In this particular case we are concerned with the interaction of molecules of an odorant with the receptor cells of the olfactory organ, hence the problem of function posed by this sense organ was always a problem of molecular biology. Up to the present, despite an abundance of theories of olfaction, the nature of the interaction of odorant molecules with an olfactory receptor cell has not yet been elucidated. Until recently, researchers have been primarily concerned with the chemical structure and shape of odorant molecules, and considerable progress has been made in this direction. However, we still do not know what substances are present in receptor olfactory cells, the molecules of which react with odorant molecules.

No one doubts that it is such a mechanism that triggers stimulation of the olfactory cell and its transmission as an impulse through synapses to the central nervous system. However, the molecular mechanism underlying the primary interaction between the olfactory receptor cell and the odorant molecule that leads to the first energy conversion is still not clear. In this respect, the only encouraging prospect seems to be to compare the mechanisms of olfactory and gustatory reception. We shall first consider briefly the characteristics of the molecular structure of odorant and of certain recent olfaction theories, also the evolution of the structural, cytochemical and functional organization of receptor cells present in the olfactory organs of vertebrates and certain invertebrates (insects), in order to gain a clear idea, not only of what has already been accomplished, but also of what remains to be done on the problem of olfaction.

## 2. Structure of Odorant Molecules. The Problem of Their Interaction with Olfactory Cells. Theories of Smell

The chemical properties of compounds are known to be associated with their structure; however, molecules of different structure may have a similar smell, and vice versa. Let us compare a number of substances having a "roselike" smell (WRIGHT, 1964, 1966):

Rosetone

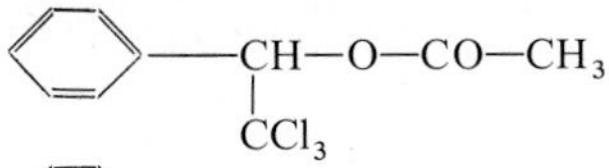

$$CH-O-CO-CH_3$$
$$|$$
$$CCl_3$$

Phenylethanol

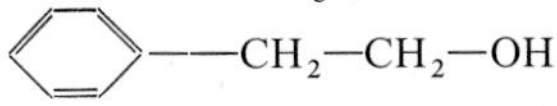

$$CH_2-CH_2-OH$$

Geraniol

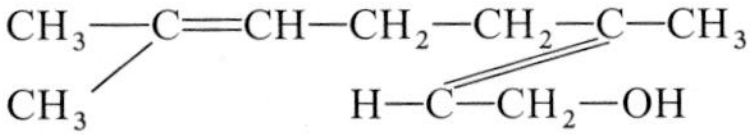

$$CH_3-C=CH-CH_2-CH_2-C-CH_3$$
$$CH_3 \qquad\qquad H-C-CH_2-OH$$

Pelargol

$$CH_3$$
$$\;\;\;\;\;CH-CH_2-CH_2-CH_2-CH-CH_3$$
$$CH_3 \qquad\qquad\qquad CH_2-CH_2-OH$$

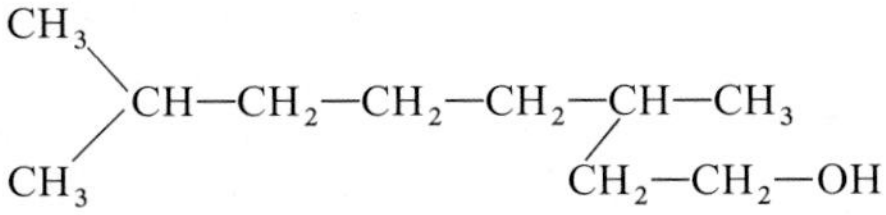

Here is another example of compounds with a camphor smell:

Camphor

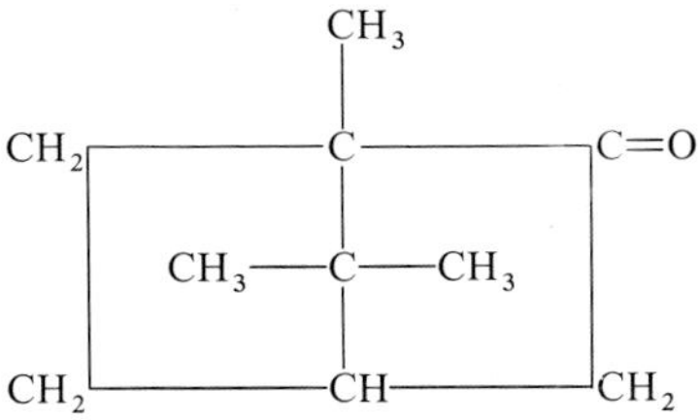

$$CH_3$$
$$CH_2 \qquad\qquad C \qquad\qquad C=O$$
$$CH_3-C-CH_3$$
$$CH_2 \qquad\qquad CH \qquad\qquad CH_2$$

Chloroethane

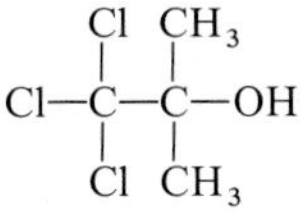

$$Cl\;\;CH_3$$
$$|\;\;\;\;|$$
$$Cl-C-C-OH$$
$$|\;\;\;\;|$$
$$Cl\;\;CH_3$$

Ethyl-tret-butyl ether

$$CH_3$$
$$|$$
$$CH_3-CH_2-O-C-CH_3$$
$$|$$
$$CH_3$$

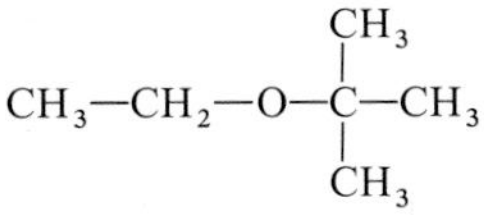

Now let us take an example of odorants which have molecules of similar structure but different odors (BRAUN, KRÖPER, and WEINHAUS, 1929):

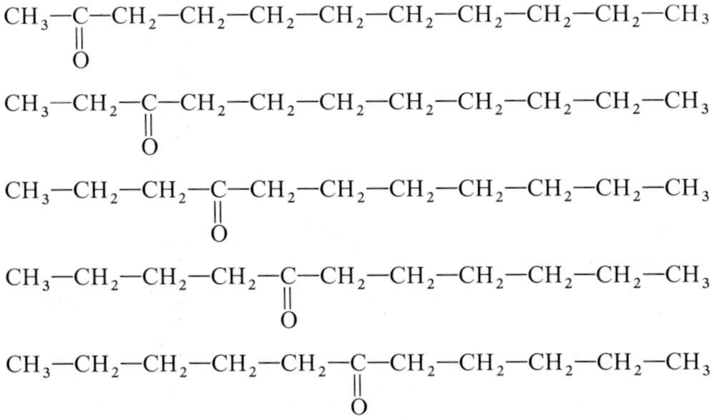

$$CH_3-C-CH_2-CH_2-CH_2-CH_2-CH_2-CH_2-CH_2-CH_2-CH_3$$
$$\;\;\;\;\;\;\|$$
$$\;\;\;\;\;\;O$$

$$CH_3-CH_2-C-CH_2-CH_2-CH_2-CH_2-CH_2-CH_2-CH_2-CH_3$$
$$\;\;\;\;\;\;\;\;\;\;\;\;\|$$
$$\;\;\;\;\;\;\;\;\;\;\;\;O$$

$$CH_3-CH_2-CH_2-C-CH_2-CH_2-CH_2-CH_2-CH_2-CH_2-CH_3$$
$$\;\;\;\;\;\;\;\;\;\;\;\;\;\;\;\;\;\;\|$$
$$\;\;\;\;\;\;\;\;\;\;\;\;\;\;\;\;\;\;O$$

$$CH_3-CH_2-CH_2-CH_2-C-CH_2-CH_2-CH_2-CH_2-CH_2-CH_3$$
$$\;\;\;\;\;\;\;\;\;\;\;\;\;\;\;\;\;\;\;\;\;\;\;\;\|$$
$$\;\;\;\;\;\;\;\;\;\;\;\;\;\;\;\;\;\;\;\;\;\;\;\;O$$

$$CH_3-CH_2-CH_2-CH_2-CH_2-C-CH_2-CH_2-CH_2-CH_2-CH_3$$
$$\;\;\;\;\;\;\;\;\;\;\;\;\;\;\;\;\;\;\;\;\;\;\;\;\;\;\;\;\|$$
$$\;\;\;\;\;\;\;\;\;\;\;\;\;\;\;\;\;\;\;\;\;\;\;\;\;\;\;\;O$$

All these compounds have an odor resembling that of rue, but with the shifting of the carbonyl group (—CO—) towards the middle of the chain the rue odor becomes weaker and gradually shades into a fruity odor.

Another example (WINTER and GAUTSCHI, 1962) refers to two synthetic isomeric compounds:

$$CH_3—CH_2—CH \atop \underset{\displaystyle CH—CH_2—CHO}{\|}$$
trans

$$HC—CH_2—CH_3 \atop \underset{\displaystyle HC—CH_2—CHO}{\|}$$
cis

The compound with the *cis* configuration had an odor of fresh greens, while the *trans* compound had nothing in common with it.

In the synthesis of the attractant of the Mediterranean fruit fly *Ceratitis capitata* (WRIGHT, 1964), called siglure, it was found that if this compound has the *cis* configuration

it has no biological activity and does not attract males, whereas the *trans* form can be used as a lure for males.

WRIGHT (1964), in addition, devotes special attention to optical isomerism, which occurs when a molecule contains a carbon atom bound to four atoms or atomic groups. The four valences of the carbon atom are directed in space so as to form equal angles with each other; such a molecule can exist in both right-handed and left-handed forms. Compounds of this type, for example, the right- and left-handed forms of methanol, have identical odor (DOLL and BOURNOT, 1949). There are no known cases where one of the isomers has an odor and the other has none (WRIGHT, 1964). WRIGHT concludes from this that, since enzymes are stereospecific, enzymes of the receptor cell cannot take part in the interaction of this cell with odorant molecules, otherwise the right- and left-handed forms of the odorant would be perceived in a different manner. For this reason WRIGHT rejects KISTIAKOWSKY's theory of the perception of odorants (KISTIAKOWSKY, 1950), which was based on data obtained by BARADI and BOURNE (1951a, 1951b, 1953). This theory postulated that enzymes located in olfactory cells, particularly the supporting cells, are inhibited by odorant molecules.

Thus, we have to agree with the conclusion reached 40 years ago by DYSON (1926, 1928a, 1928b, 1929, 1931, 1938), that it is impossible at present to explain rationally the phenomenon of odor from the standpoint of the chemical structure of odorant molecules, neither qualitatively, nor quantitatively.

A great deal of attention has been directed lately, not so much to the structure as to the geometry of the molecule. Thus, AMOORE (1962a, 1962b, 1970) starting from the assumption made by MONCRIEFF (1951) that the odor of a compound depends on the shape of its molecules and on how accurately this molecule can be "inscribed" into a "specific site" on the surface of a receptor cell, formulated his stereochemical theory of olfaction. This theory postulates that compounds of similar odor must also have a similar molecular geometry. If the conformation of a molecule of the compound corresponds specifically to only one site on the surface of the receptor cell, such a compound will possess a "primary" odor. If only part of the odorant molecule fits into a site of appropriate shape, then such a compound will possess a complex odor. Since the number of different shapes of site is assumed to be small, the number of "primary" odors will accordingly also be small. Starting from the theory of probability and using as a basis the frequency of a given odor and molecular models, AMOORE (1962a, 1962b) distinguished seven "primary" odors among the abundance of organic odorants: 1. camphoraceous, 2. pungent, 3. ethereal, 4. floral, 5. minty, 6. musky, and 7. putrid[1]. The remaining complex or mixed odors are made up of two or more primary odors. Thus, the seven primary odors resemble the three primary colors: red, green and yellow.

From the molecular size and shape of the compounds endowed with primary odors, AMOORE calculated the approximate dimensions of the molecules and corresponding specific sites on the surface of receptor cells. The ethereal molecule has a rod-like shape, therefore, it must have an elongated site; its length is 18Å, its width 5Å, and its depth 4Å. The camphoraceous molecule is rounded, with a diameter of 7Å, and its site is shaped like an elliptical cup, 4Å deep, 9Å long, and 7.5Å wide. The musky odor molecule is also rounded, being 7Å in circumference, and its receptor site is slightly larger, having a width of 9Å and a length of 11.5Å. The receptor site for a molecule of floral odorant consists accordingly of a circular depression with 9Å in diameter with a deeper outlet 4Å wide, starting at the center and extending 7.5Å from the edge of the circular portion, etc. Minty odor molecules are a "wedge-shaped" shape and contain an electrically polarized group of atoms, capable of forming a hydrogen bond in the vicinity of the "wedge peak".

Pungent and putrid odors do not fit into this scheme. The molecules responsible for these odors have indefinite shape and size. The pungent odor group is

---

[1] AMOORE later (1965) modified his seven primary odors to seven or more classes.

associated with compounds whose molecules have a positive charge and a high affinity for electrons. Putrid odors, on the other hand, are emitted by molecules having an excess number of electrons, known as nucleophilic molecules.

Thus, every site "traps" an odorant molecule having the corresponding conformation. A complex molecule occupying two different sites belonging to the same receptor cell has a complex odor.

AMOORE's theory was supported by the fact that it is sometimes possible to predict the odor of a compound from the shape of its molecule. For example, the probable odor of molecules of the following three compounds was predicted (RUBIN, APOTHEKER, and LUTMER, 1962):

1.
$$CO\text{——————}O$$
$$HC\underset{\diagdown CH_2-CH_2 \diagup}{\overset{\diagup CH_2-CH_2 \diagdown}{\phantom{x}}}C-CH_2-CH_3;$$

2.
$$CO\text{——————}O$$
$$HC\underset{\diagdown CH_2-CH_2 \diagup}{\overset{\diagup CH_2-CH_2 \diagdown}{\phantom{x}}}C-CH_2-CH_2-CH_2-CH_3;$$

3.
$$CO\text{——————}O$$
$$HC-CH_2-CH_2-\underset{\diagdown CH_2-CH_2 \diagup}{\overset{\diagup CH_2-CH_2 \diagdown}{\phantom{x}}}C-CH_2-CH_2-CH_2-CH_2-CH_2-CH_2-CH_2-CH_3$$

The molecule of the first compound is a rather compact sphere and fits in the best possible manner into the "camphoraceous" site. The molecule of the third compound has a very long "tail" and, therefore, fits a "floral" site best. The second compound corresponds, in molecular shape and size, to both types of site mentioned above and hence would be expected to yield a combination of both odors. These predications were confirmed in practice (JOHNSTON and SANDOVAL, 1962). In addition to the above compounds, several analogous compounds were synthesized and found to have the predicted quality and intensity of odor (JOHNSTON and SANDOVAL, 1962). Thus, the stereochemical theory of olfaction has a number of achievements to its credit, a fact which should be taken into account.

However, this theory completely ignores the question of what happens after the molecule has entered the specific site on the surface of the plasma membrane of the receptor cell? What does the molecule react with after entering the site? The theory does not touch on the reasons why the molecule stays in the hole, nor does it explain how potentials arise in response to the occupying of the site by the molecule, nor how the intensity of the odor is perceived. Consequently, the theory based on the stereochemical shape of odorant molecules proved incapable of solving the problem of how such molecules interact with specific but still unidentified molecules of some biologically active chemical substances present in the plasma membrane of the receptor cell, i.e. the problem of the primary processes basic to olfaction. The situation was not improved by attempts to modify this theory by proposing, instead of occupation of sites, silhouette photographs of molecular models of odorants, the profiles of which can be correlated with functional groups in the molecules.

In this respect, the "quantum" theory of olfaction deserves special attention. This theory starts from the premise that intramolecular vibrations, which are subject to quantization rules, constitute an inherent property of odorant molecules. In other words, the physical basis of an odor is not connected with the size, shape or reactivity of the molecules present in odorants, but rather with their intramolecular vibration (DYSON, 1938; WRIGHT, 1966). The same molecular vibration frequency can be found in odorants with the most varied chemical structures and chemical properties. As a result of the vibrations of atoms, and also of their atomic components and the molecules as a whole, there arise electromagnetic waves, and it is these that are responsible for the Landsberg-Mandelshtam-Raman effect (effect of combination light scattering) and also for the absorption of infrared rays by a compound. DYSON (1938) assumed that osmetic frequencies, i.e. those to which the nose is sensitive, correspond to wave numbers in the range 1,400 to 3,500 cm$^{-1}$. According to WRIGHT (1964), however, only wave numbers below 500 are of importance. This author cites data to show that molecules of compounds of similar odor must be characterized by similar low-frequency vibrations. For example, odorants with an almond odor have the following vibration frequencies (in cm$^{-1}$):

| Nitro-benzene | Benzo-nitrile | α-Nitro-thiophene | Butyro-nitrile | Benzal-dehyde |
|---|---|---|---|---|
| 176 | 172 | 169 | 179 | 130 |
| 252 | – | – | – | 225, 237 |
| 397 | 320, 381 | 376 | 370 | – |
| 435 | 405, 460 | 442 | – | 439 |
| 532 | 549 | – | 524 | – |

WRIGHT maintains that this shows rather convincingly the connection between the almond odor and the low-frequency vibrations of molecules of all these compounds.

According to WRIGHT (1964), the vibrations of the odorant molecule must have a low-frequency character, must encompass the entire molecule or its major portion, and must contain components normal to the surface of the plasma membrane of the receptor cell. WRIGHT believes that there are 95 primary odors and that each has a corresponding type of olfactory receptor cell, which can be stimulated by molecular vibrations of a frequency of 3—30 cm$^{-1}$. Most odors consist of a combination of primary odors[2].

---

[2] According to more recent data, the frequency of molecular vibrations in odorant molecules can apparently be correlated with the frequency of their bioelectric coding in olfactory bulbs (WRIGHT, HUGHES, and HENDRIX, 1967). However, this correlation does not depend on the chemical identification of the stimulating molecule. Moreover, not all molecular vibrations possess osmotic activity.

According to WRIGHT's theory (1964), for odorant molecules to cause stimulation of olfactory cells, they should not only come into intimate contact with such cells but must also act at the same time on the "olfactory pigment" present in these cells. Molecules of "olfactory pigment" absorb low-frequency vibrations emitted by molecules of odorants; this is followed by a series of energy conversions, culminating in nerve impulses transmitted to the central nervous system. Thus, the primary trigger mechanism that determines odor reception is the interaction of the quantum energy of molecules present in odorants with the pigment found in olfactory receptor cells.

What is the nature of this "olfactory pigment"? Up to the present, neither the chemical nature of the pigment in olfactory cells nor its location has been clearly determined. According to some data the pigment extracted from the olfactory mucosa consists of phosphatids (GEREBTZOFF and PHILIPPOT, 1957; PHILIPPOT and GEREBTZOFF, 1958), while according to other data this pigment consists of light-resistant, free and protein-bound carotenoids and vitamin A (BRIGGS and DUNCAN, 1961, 1962; DUNCAN and BRIGGS, 1962). An olfactory pigment has been isolated from the olfactory mucosa of cattle (KURIHARA, 1967), and the following three fractions were obtained: 1. a fraction soluble in organic compounds, 2. a water-soluble fraction, and 3. pigment granules. The third fraction was found to be the heaviest and bound to a protein. The chromoprotein isolated from the pigment granules exhibited an absorption peak near 260 nm, and three pigments could be extracted from it. A similar chromoprotein was extracted from the water-soluble pigment fraction. Finally, apart from these pigments, $\beta$-carotene and cholesterol could be extracted from the olfactory mucosa.

The exact location of carotenoid and vitamin A pigments in structures of the olfactory mucosa has not yet been determined, much less their location in olfactory cells. Some researchers even deny that such pigments are present at all in the olfactory mucosa of a number of animals (JACKSON, 1960). However, ROSENBERG and co-workers have been able to establish in vitro the formation of a weak bond or "complex" between an adsorbed gas molecule and some crystals of carotenoid pigments ($\beta$-carotene) (ROSENBERG, MISRA, and SWITZER, 1968). At the same time, the conductivity of such carotenoids, which are semiconductors, exhibits sharp changes. The surface conductivity of $\beta$-carotene increases by up to 103 and is proportional to the partial pressure of oxygen in the surrounding atmosphere; this effect completely disappears when pure nitrogen is substituted for oxygen. However, in gases possessing an odor, e.g. carbon dioxide, nitrous oxide, butanol, hexanol and particularly ammonia and methanol, nitrogen induced an increase in conductivity. The conductivity of carotenoids varies according to a definite law under the effect of various alcohols and ethers. It is possible to detect a fatigue and regeneration effect in the semiconductor $\beta$-carotene when it is subjected to frequent and repeated action of an odorant compound. Therefore, the $\beta$-carotene of the olfactory mucosa may also change its physical properties in the presence of odoriferous gases. Where are carotenoid pigments located? In the opinion of ROSENBERG, MISRA, and SWITZER (1968) presumably in the plasma membranes of olfactory cells, where precisely the weakly bound (donor—acceptor) complex between the carotenoid and the odorant molecule is formed. As a result, the conductivity of the semiconductors (carotenoids) increases, thus causing depolarization of the plasma membrane of the olfactory cell.

Unfortunately, these concepts turn out to be highly speculative when we attempt to apply them to an olfactory cell. As we have already mentioned, carotenoids and vitamin A are found in any cell possessing a flagellum or cilia, and their concrete molecular location site in membranes, with the exception of the visual cell, has not yet been clarified. The loss of smell in cases of vitamin A deficiency and its restoration in anosmetic patients after administration of vitamin A can be explained on the basis of its general, nonspecific action.

THOMPSON stated (1957) that molecules containing the isotope deuterium instead of hydrogen, for example $H_2S$ and $D_2S$, have a similar odor, although in this case there is a significant change in the frequency of fundamental molecular vibrations.

When some of the hydrogen atoms in the molecule of the sex attractant of the melon fly *Dacus cucurbitae* are replaced by deuterium, a noticeable shift of absorption peaks in the infrared region is observed, yet no changes were noted in the attractive properties. Moreover, some compounds having a similar structure and analogous infrared spectra failed to attract insects (DOOLITTLE *et al.*, 1968).

Optical isomers have identical molecular vibration frequencies although they differ in the character of their odors. Molecules with almost identical vibration frequencies have dissimilar odors. Conversely, compounds with similar odors have different vibration frequencies. Thus, we are confronted with the paradoxical status of the theory: two of its original postulates are subject to criticism, namely both the quantum properties of odoriferous molecules and the assumed presence in the olfactory cell of receptive chemical compounds, such as carotenoids and pigments. Nevertheless, there can be no doubt whatsoever that work should continue in both directions.

Theoretical attempts are being made to clarify the processes involving the interaction between odorant molecules and the plasma membrane of olfactory cells. Thus, DAVIES and TAYLOR (1957, 1959) assume that it is possible to effect a quantitative determination of the stimulation of olfactory cells, based on adsorption phenomena. When odorant molecules are adsorbed by cell membranes, a change in permeability to $Na^+$ ions and a depolarization of membranes occur, accompanied by the appearance of an action potential. Threshold stimulation can be achieved, provided a definite number of odorant molecules is adsorbed on the surface of the olfactory cell. To calculate the magnitude of this adsorption, we can use Langmuir's equations:

$$\frac{X}{Cd} = K\frac{L}{A},$$

where $X$ is the mean concentration of odorant molecules per $cm^2$, $C$ is the mean concentration of odoriferous molecules per $cm^3$ over the adsorptive surface, $d$ is the membrane thickness (about 10 Å), and $K (L/A)$ is the adsorption constant of odorant molecules supplied from the air into a lipidaqueous medium. The number of pits (N) in a given olfactory cell containing P odorant molecules is given by Poisson's equation:

$$N = \frac{ne^{-Jx}(Jx)p}{P!},$$

where p! is the minimum number of odorant molecules adsorbed by the receptor pit at the threshold excitation, n is the number of receptor pits of each receptor cell (cell surface divided by J), and J is the area of the pit. From these two equations we can derive the stimulation threshold of the olfactory cell (O T), described by the equation:

$$\log O T = \frac{\log p!}{P} - \log \alpha d - \frac{\log n}{P} - \log K \frac{L}{A}.$$

Unfortunately, none of these parameters can be determined experimentally, except for the stimulation threshold. K (L/A) can be determined, assuming that the plasma membrane of the olfactory cell resembles a mixture of gasoline, ether and water, whose partial coefficient can be determined experimentally. The value p arbitrarily designates the unit of the strongest odor (β-ionone), the magnitude of which is four times greater for the hypothetical very weak acids. If we substitute these values in the theoretical equation, and if we assume that the surface has a thickness of 10Å, we obtain an area of 64Å for the receptor pit J and a number of 45,000 such receptor sectors approximately for each olfactory cell.

With the above parameters, one can calculate the stimulation threshold (O T), if the constant of adsorption between air and the lipid-water phase and the value of p are known. The value of p can be found once the size and shape of the odoriferous molecules are known. However, in determining the olfactory threshold it was found that the number and size of the receptor sectors do not depend on the quality of the odor (MOULTON and BEIDLER, 1967).

DAVIES (1965) explains the well-known phenomenon of fatigue of the olfactory receptor as follows: adsorption of odorant molecules causes depolarization of the plasma membrane of the olfactory cell but, since the subsequent supply of odorant molecules with inhaled air is retarded, the ionic concentration necessary for the subsequent depolarization is not maintained. The above author also assumes that the membrane of a receptor cell has a varying degree of resistance to the penetration of odorant molecules. In his opinion, this assumption is basic to odor differentiation; it is difficult, however, to agree with this conclusion. The most serious objection to this theory is that the plasma membrane of the receptor cell lacks a substrate that can code an olfactory stimulus.

BEETS (1957) assumes that the character of an odor is determined by specific functional groups, and also by the conformation, shape and size of the odorant molecule. In his opinion, the different intensity of musk odors is due to the nature of the functional groups.

In seeking to understand the mechanism of olfactory reception, significance must also be attributed to data showing that different odorant molecules are adsorbed in different ways by olfactory cells according to the duration and degree of adsorption. Such data were obtained by MONCRIEFF (1961) on the basis of tests in which he determined the lag time of the response reaction on the part of a tested subject. The subject assessed the quality of the odor after the passage of air containing a definite concentration of an odorant through small pulverized pieces of the olfactory mucosa of nasal cavity of freshly slaughtered cows. On the basis of such tests, MONCRIEFF (1961) built a model of the olfactory organ, which can react immediately to the presence of odorants. This model is based on a recording of temperature changes during adsorption on an organic film of the odorant molecules. In the same way as in the olfactory organ, a concentration and selective accumulation of odorant molecules takes place in the model as a result of adsorption. Differentiation of odors is connected with the different degree and rate of adsorption.

Thus, in closing this section, we have to admit that some important information on the nature of odorant molecules is still lacking. Apparently, both the structure and shape of these molecules as well as their quantum activity play an important role. However, these molecules must also possess some sort of additional and still unknown physical or chemical properties, which are specifically responsible for their odor. In fact, the perception of odors in man is practically unlimited, although the evolution of the human olfactory organ has remained at the same level for centuries.

The situation is equally unsatisfactory in regard to answers to the following questions: With what does an odorant molecule interact in the receptor portion of the plasma membrane of the olfactory cell, and what is the subsequent fate of this molecule? What kind of biologically active compounds are represented by the molecules present in this membrane? Are they carotenoids, including vitamin A? Or are they chromoproteids? At present, it is hard to say. However, we can state, by analogy with the visual and gustatory cells, that some sort of universal protein molecules are involved, located with a strict dimensional orientation in the plasma membrane of the olfactory cell, which interact with an odor molecule and, depending upon the quality of the latter, undergo a gradual change in conformation. It is, in fact, the conformation that in the final analysis determines the character of the odor perceived. This interaction process is also the trigger mechanism responsible for the stimulation of an olfactory cell.

In this respect, the attempts made by ASH (1968, 1969), ASH and SKOGEN (1970) to investigate the molecular mechanisms of olfactory reception appear very encouraging. Conformational changes in the molecule, which can be detected by differential spectroscopy, are induced by subjecting preparations of rabbit olfactory mucosa to the action of aqueous solutions of odoriferous compounds, such as linalool or linalyl isobutyrate and other odoriferous compounds, used either separately or together. [Thus, the above author has followed the scheme of tests performed by DASTOLI and PRICE (1966) on taste buds.] The preparation tested by ASH was obtained by curettage of the rabbit olfactory mucosa and consists of receptor cells with antennae, supporting cells, and the mucus which covers the olfactory epithelium.

According to ASH and SKOGEN (1970), the interaction between the stimulus and the preparation was always followed by a spectral change with a maximum at 267 nm. On the basis of these data, ASH (1968) advanced the hypothesis that the activity of the olfactory preparation in the 267 nm region is due to the formation of a complex, including a molecule of the stimulus and of a specific ingredient (proteins or lipoproteins) in the olfactory mucosa. The change in configuration is associated with complex formation and is accompanied by a rearrangement of the electron field around the chromophore group; ASH thinks this is what is responsible for the absorption in the 267 nm region. Similar conformational changes may act as the trigger mechanism effecting a change in the permeability of membranes which ensure the chemical sensitivity of biological systems. Thus, the assumption is made that formation of protein complexes occurs in the process of olfactory reception at the moment when an odorant molecule interacts with the olfactory receptor cell. Similar assumptions are also made by DRAVNIEKS (1962) and by ROSENBERG et al. (ROSENBERG, MISRA, and SWITZER, 1968). ASH (1968) believes that we are not dealing here with an enzymic activity. This belief is supported by the fact that at low concentrations of the olfactory preparation a higher activity could be observed than at high concentrations of the same preparation. The plateau of the curve depends on the concentration of the preparation. When the fresh preparation is allowed to stand at room temperature for more than 4 hours, its activity decreases to an insignificant extent, whereas all preparations are rapidly inactivated when the temperature is raised to 68 °C. Denaturation at 68 °C disrupts the activity of the nonstimulated preparation, and also modifies the absorption ability of preparations which were heated after the activation period. Low temperatures and freezing did not exert a noticeable effect on the activity of the olfactory preparation.

ASH assumes that the characteristic feature of olfactory reception can be linked to the structure of olfactory cells, whose olfactory knobs come into direct contact with odorant molecules. He considers the fact that other cells are sensitive to these molecules as indication that common mechanisms of molecular interaction are involved. Thus, the above study outlines biochemical perspectives for investigating the primary processes of olfactory reception. It is still too early to predict the final results of studies in this direction, but already we can hope that these studies will be extended to include a greater number of odorants and also the careful isolation of one, perhaps even several specific olfactory proteins, with simultaneous determination of their location site in olfactory cells. As has been shown, the olfactory protein, when stimulated, requires ascorbic acid as a cofactor. In this respect, there is a striking analogy with the processes occuring during stimulation of rhodopsin, which takes place with the participation of retinal as an "intermediary". Similar molecular processes testify to the presence of olfactory proteins in insects (RIDDIFORD, 1970). Thus, in the male silkworm *Antheraea pernii* and other insects the response to sex pheromone is inhibited by formaldehyde applied to the sex sensilla, which are known to bind the imidazole and sulfhydryl groups of the protein and the $\beta$-amino groups of lysine and arginine. Indeed, a protein that showed two basic bands ($\alpha$ and $\beta$) on the electrophoretogram was isolated from the sex sensilla of males. The $\alpha$ band seems to correspond to the receptive protein of males toward the female pheromone. When the female was labeled with tritiated hydrogen, in two of 20 cases the $\alpha$ band showed some radioactivity. The similar molecular mechanism of olfaction and gustation has recently been shown to present in American cockroach (ROZENTAL and NORRIS, 1973). Thus, in insects olfactory reception does involve molecular processes.

The question of the magnitude of the absolute olfactory threshold, i. e., the minimum concentration of an odorant capable of inducing an olfactory sensation, was being tackled until recently on the basis of different methods. For this reason, quantitative data on threshold concentrations of odorant had merely an orientational significance, as was correctly pointed out by BRONSHTEIN (1950). For example, in man, the threshold, expressed in terms of the number of molecules entering the nasal cavity, depends upon the duration of action and concentration of the odorant, and also upon the velocity of the current of air or gas. The influence exerted by the velocity of the air flow on the magnitude of the threshold can be linked with its effect on the adsorption of the odorant by the mucous epithelium of the nose. It was found that the threshold is almost constant for short-acting stimuli, while for longer-acting stimuli it is proportional to the duration of the stimulus. Thus, the molecular concentration of the odorant becomes the controlling factor. For very short-acting stimuli the threshold has a tendency to rise because the volume of aspired air is very small. Consequently, according to DE VRIES and STUIVER (1961), great significance must be attributed to the volume of the nasal cavity that must be filled before the odorant reaches the olfactory mucosa. On the basis of an analys of data relating to the threshold of olfactory sensation, DE VRIES and STUIVER (1961) have established that the threshold of a single human olfactory cell does not exceed eight molecules for corresponding odorants with very low threshold. However, for an olfactory sensation to arise, the participation of at least 40 olfactory cells is required, each of these cells react toward one or several odorant molecules.

The sensitivity of insects to odors is quite comparable with human data. Thus, one-millionth of a picogram ($10^{-18}$ g) of the sex attractant extracted from the glands of female silkworm moths causes excitation in males of the species *Bombyx mori* (WRIGHT, 1964).

To sum up, despite the large number of research studies and olfaction theories available to us, we are still only at the beginning of research on the molecular mechanism of the initial stage in the process of perception of odorant molecules.

# 3. Structural and Cytochemical Organization of the Olfactory Cells of Vertebrates

The olfactory organ of vertebrates consists of the olfactory mucosa of the nasal cavity in higher vertebrates and olfactory sacs in lower vertebrates. The development and structure of the olfactory organ in vertebrates has been very fully studied, although some functional correlations still cause difficulties. Under the light microscope it has been definitely established that the olfactory mucosa of the nasal cavity, as well as of Jacobson's organ, where olfactory cells are also present, is laid down and develops in the same way as the eye cup during the early embryonic stages in the front portion of the embryonic neural plate

(GAWRILENKO, 1910; SHMAL'GAUZEN, 1950; VINNIKOV and TITOVA, 1957a). In the course of its further development the eye cup does not sever its connection with the brain at any stage, whereas the future olfactory mucosa becomes separated from the central nervous system primordium at certain stages of its embryonic growth and later is again attached to it. Further, in contrast to the rudiment of the eye and neural plate, which are converted into the neural tube and bathed in the internal medium of the fetus, the rudiment of the olfactory, as well as the definitive organ, remains in contact with the external environment (for further details see Ya. A. VINNIKOV and L. K. TITOVA: *Morphology of the Olfactory Organ*, 1957a). Unfortunately, the development of the olfactory mucosa, including its receptor layer, has been studied so far only under the light microscope. HIS in 1889 had already established that in human embryos there are originally no traces whatsoever in the mesenchyme of an olfactory nerve between the olfactory bulbs in the brain and the olfactory pit, where the epithelium of the future olfactory mucosa is located. Later, the epithelium of the pit begins to undergo intensive karyokinetic division. Pearshaped elements resembling neuroblasts are the products of cell division. The neuroblasts move towards the "mesodermal" surface of the epithelium and form prominences, which are gradually transformed into the olfactory nerve. These data were later confirmed by GROTH (1939) and PEARSON (1941).

The cytological characteristics of the differentiation of olfactory cells were traced under the light microscope by VINNIKOV and TITOVA (1957a) in different members of all classes of vertebrates. In fish, it was possible to show the development of olfactory cells whose processes may be threadlike, rod-shaped or cone-shaped. In amphibians, the development of special bulges, known as olfactory knobs, can be clearly observed on the distal ends of peripheral processes of olfactory cells. In the classic histological literature the tips of the peripheral processes of the olfactory cells were called "olfactory vesicles". The term "olfactory knobs" was proposed in 1949 by VINNIKOV and TITOVA.

Hairs develop both on the surface of the peripheral processes of embryonic olfactory cells, as well as on the surface of the surrounding supporting cells. In birds (chicken embryos) regressive processes, observed on the 15th day of incubation, lead to reduction of the total area of the olfactory mucosa. In human embryos, it is possible to observe an ingrowth of the ciliated epithelium into the olfactory receptor layer. Bowman's glands apparently develop at the expense of such displaced sectors of the respiratory epithelium.

In human embryos at 13 cm length some characteristic features are observed in the distribution of cellular elements in the receptor layer of the olfactory mucosa. The upper portion of the receptor layer consists of peripheral processes of rod- and cone-shaped olfactory cells, terminating in olfactory bulbs in the formative stage; nucleus-containing parts of olfactory cells are located below the upper portion. Supporting elements, characterized by light, spherical nuclei, are located between olfactory cells in the upper, middle and lower portions of the mucosa. In human embryos at 18 to 29 cm length the appearance of longitudinal striation can be observed in the peripheral processes of rod-shaped cells. The peripheral processes of olfactory cells terminate in olfactory knobs on the apex of which two to three hairs can be observed.

A few words now about the development of the olfactory bulbs in which the central processes of the olfactory cells terminate, and where synapses with mitral and bristle neurons are formed. In human embryos 5.5 to 6.5 cm long the olfactory bulbs still have a well-expressed cavity (which later disappears) lined with an ependyma that communicates with the cavity of cerebral ventricles. The central processes of the olfactory cells, accompanied by glial cells and running in the fila olfactoria of the olfactory nerve, extend up to the front end of the olfactory bulbs. Fibers entwine from all sides the front portion of olfactory bulbs and fit tightly against them. At the same time, the terminals of olfactory fibers, gathering in large bundles, penetrate the tissue of the olfactory bulbs and form the rudiment of olfactory glomerules, where synaptic contacts are established with dendrites of mitral and bristle cells in the process of development. Electron microscopic studies (OCHI, 1967) have shown that there is intense differentiation of mitral cells and formation of synapses with olfactory fibers in rats during the postnatal period. Simultaneously, the first appearance of synaptic vesicles in olfactory presynaptic endings can be observed, followed by a thickening of synaptic membranes, which occurs in rats between the 12th and 17th day of postnatal life; a cytochemical differentiation of olfactory bulbs, associated with the development of mediators, also takes place during the same period. A similar investigation is planned on the development of the olfactory cell in vertebrates from the viewpoint of its ultrastructural and molecular organization.

Studies performed by VINNIKOV and TITOVA (1949, 1957a) still with the light microscope, allow us to conclude that there is a considerable similarity between olfactory and visual cells. From the basic principles governing ontogenesis and phylogenesis, these authors derived the premise that ocular and olfactory rudiments not only have a common origin in the embryonic tissue of the neural plate and that both olfactory cells and photoreceptors of vertebrates are primary sensory cells, but also that a number of their structural and physiological characteristics coincide. The olfactory cells of a number of members of all classes of vertebrates have been studied with the aid of the electron microscope in the author's laboratory (BRONSHTEIN and IVANOV, 1965; BRONSHTEIN, 1966; BRONSHTEIN and PYATKINA, 1966, 1968, 1969a, 1969b). These data will be presented later in this book.

According to the data of MOULTON and BEIDLER (1967), a lamprey has 800,000 olfactory cells, an adult man $10^7$, a rabbit $10^8$, and an Alsatian dog $2.24 \times 10^9$. The corresponding area of the olfactory receptor epithelium in man is $10 \, cm^2$, in the rabbit $9.3 \, cm^2$, and in the Alsatian dog $196.46 \, cm^2$. Thus, the rabbit has 120,000 olfactory cells per $cm^2$ of olfactory epithelium, and man 10,000 cells. In all probability, the number of cells present in the olfactory receptor layer determines whether an animal is classified as macrosmatic, having a well developed sense of smell, or as microsmatic, having a poorly developed sense of smell.

Olfactory cells in all types of vertebrates have a strikingly similar structure which testifies to a unique mechanism of function (Fig. 73). These cells have an elongated, bipolar shape. A peripheral and axonlike process extends from the nuclear cytoplasmic body. Central processes form fibers of the olfactory

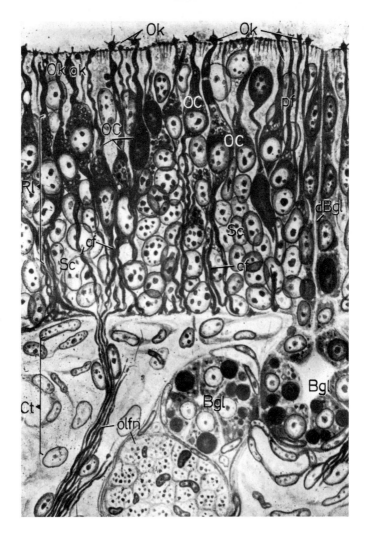

Fig. 73. Olfactory lining of the rabbit. Immersion, objective 90, eyepiece 10 (VINNIKOV and TITOVA, 1957a). *Rl* receptor layer; *OC* olfactory cells; *pf* peripheral process; *Ok* olfactory knob; *Okok* olfactory knobs drawn into the receptor layer (olfactomotor phenomena); *cf* central processes of olfactory cells; *olfn* olfactory nerve bundle, cut lengthwise and crosswise; *Bgl* efferent duct of Bowman's gland; *Sc* supporting cells; *Ct* connective tissue

nerve. As in photoreceptors, two or three types of cells with rod- and cone-shaped peripheral processes can be distinguished under the light microscope among the olfactory cells of vertebrates (DOGIEL, 1886; VINNIKOV and TITOVA, 1957a); these processes terminate at the distal end in specialized bulges, known as mobile olfactory knobs (VINNIKOV, 1956a, 1956b; VINNIKOV and TITOVA, 1957a). Olfactomotor phenomena, i.e. movements of the olfactory knobs, were first detected by VINNIKOV and TITOVA (1949, 1957a). These movements consist in the protrusion of the olfactory knobs into the lumen of the olfactory organ or their retraction deep into the olfactory receptor layer, depending upon the functional state. It is assumed that olfactomotor phenomena are associated with adaptation processes, which are well known to occur in the olfactory organ.

The surface of the olfactory knobs is covered with sensitive hairs, or antennae in our terminology (Fig. 74); some vertebrates have several antennae (15—20 in the dog, squirrel and rabbit) and others only one (some species of fish), which is accordingly thicker. The average length of these antennae is 15—30 µm, and their diameter at the base is 0.25—0.3 µm. In our laboratory KOSTANYAN (1971) has shown that the length of the antennae in *Triturus vulgaris* (amphibia) can increase during their seasonal migration from water to land. As a rule, short microvilli are located between the antennae; the latter are submerged in a liquid medium, which in land vertebrates is secreted by Bowman's glands. We must assume that processes involving the interaction of odorant molecules with the olfactory cell take place in the plasma membrane of the antennae.

In insects, as we shall demonstrate later, anatomic relations are such that only the ramified apex of the antenna in an olfactory receptor cell, located close to pores in the chitin, can come into contact with molecules of odoriferous compounds. The presence of a large number of mobile antennae in vertebrates greatly increases the chances that a given molecule will land on the receptor membrane of an olfactory cell. According to calculations performed by BEIDLER (1964), if every olfactory cell in a mammal is equipped with 13 antenne and each antenna is 100 µm long and 0.15 µm wide, and if there are $10^8$ receptor cells, then the entire surface area of these antennae will amount to 600 cm², or approximately the same as the surface of the animal's entire body. The general outline of the antennae and their position at the apex of the receptor cell have recently been studied by the scanning electron microscope (BARBER and BOYDE, 1968).

As was shown by BRONSHTEIN (1964) in our laboratory, antennae in the olfactory cells of vertebrates are characterized by a continuous automatic motion, quite different in character and amplitude from the pulsation of ciliated cells. This motion is asynchronous and has a pendulum-like character, bending and funnel-shaped. As a result, the apices of antennae move through a complex trajectory that encompasses a wide zone above the free surface of the receptor cell, and so increases the possibility of contact between the antenna and odorant molecules. Addition of ATP leads to barely noticeable changes in the character of the motion of olfactory antennae. However, addition of ATP to glycerinized cells with immobile antennae was accompanied by restoration of their motion. When olfactory cells were placed in an incubation medium containing nitroblue tetrazolium, used for the detection of oxidative enzymes, the motion of the antennae ceased because the oxidative function of the mitochondria was blocked by formasan deposits on their cristae. Subsequent addition of an ATP solution restored the automatic motion of the antennae. These experiments show once more that the factor responsible for the motion of antennae is the energy of the ATP generated by mitochondria of the olfactory knobs.

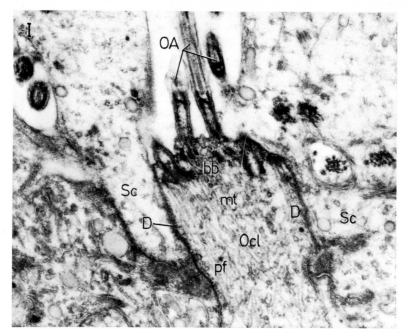

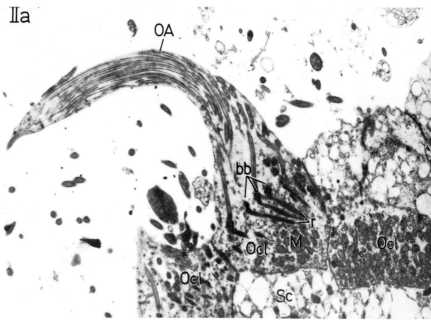

Fig. 74 I—V. Apex of olfactory cells (I) of the river lamprey *(Lampetra fluviatilis)* (× 20,000); (II) of the catfish *(Silvius glanis)*. a longitudinal section (× 9,500), b cross-section (× 57,000); (III) of the grass frog *(Rana temporaria)* (× 30,000); (IV) of the turtle *(Testudo horsfieldi)* (× 24,000); (V) of the monkey *(Cercopithecus)* (× 47,000) (BRONSHTEIN and IVANOV, 1965; BRONSHTEIN and PYATKINA, 1966, 1968, 1969a, b). *Ocl* olfactory knob; *OA* olfactory antennae (for II—complex antenna, seen in longitudinal section (a) and cross-section (b); *bb* basal bodies (for III and V—with pedicles); *mt* microtubules; *D* desmosomes; *Sc* supporting cells (for III—with secretion granules and microvilli); *Sg* secretory granules; *pf* peripheral process (for IV—with microtubules); *mv* microvillum; *M* mitochondria; *r* rootlets

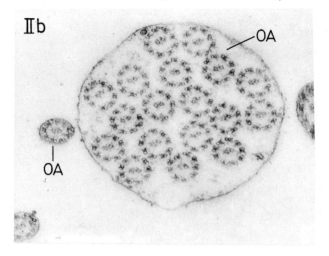

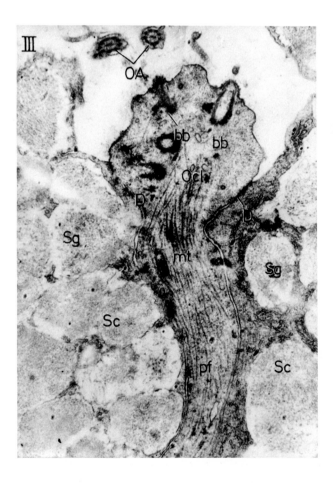

Electron microscopic studies have shown that antennae contain 9 pairs of peripheral and 2 central fibrils (Fig. 74), coated by an extension of the cellular plasma membrane. Some fish, amphibians, reptiles and birds contain a complex consisting of 2—3—10—12 sets of 9 pairs of peripheral and 2 central fibrils located under single plasma membrane, as BRONSHTEIN and PYATKINA (1966, 1968, 1969a) observed for the first time. In this case, the antenna has the character of a complex flagellum, or macrocilium (Fig. 74, II). In other cases, the antenna contains a normal set of fibrils and thins out in the proximal section with a constant loss of a large number of fibrils (REESE, 1965); it may also contain moniliform bulges along its course (REESE, 1965).

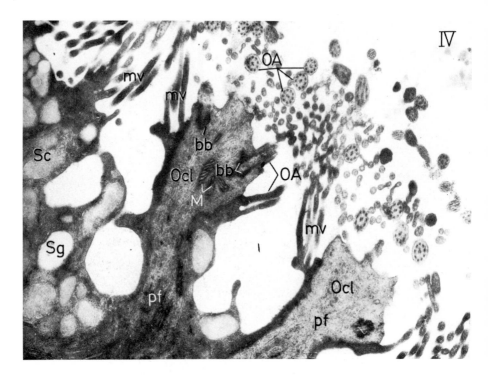

As histochemical studies have shown, the composition of olfactory antennae includes lipids, proteins containing a large number of sulfhydryl groups, and phosphatases. They do not contain any nucleic acids, oxidative enzymes or acetylcholinesterase (BRONSHTEIN, 1965).

In the cytochemical reaction for ATPase it is possible to detect under the electron microscope the extensive localization of the enzyme in the plasma membrane of antennae, which therefore possess, like fibrils, high ATPase activity (Fig. 75). The apex of an olfactory hair is usually filled with a homogeneous or granular osmiophilic substance of still unknown chemical composition (BRONSHTEIN and PYATKINA, 1969a).

Electron histochemistry has also revealed products of the histochemical reaction for $Na^+$, in the form of small spherical crystals with a diameter of 250Å and without any apparent order in the matrix of frog antennae, between fibrils, or more frequently in the vicinity of the plasma membrane. Individual reaction products also remain outside the antennae and in residues of the mucus coating the olfactory mucosa (BRONSHTEIN and PYATKINA, 1969a). Recently the potassium and sodium content was determined in the mucus covering the olfactory

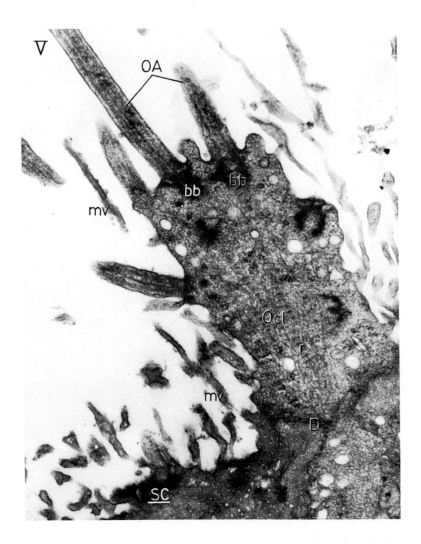

epithelium of the frog *Rana temporaria* and the guinea pig *Cavia cobaya* by means of flame spectrophotometry (BRONSHTEIN and LEONT'EV, 1972). Samples of the olfactory mucus of the frog contain $104.6 \pm 10$ meq $Na^+$ and $69.6 \pm 7$ meq $K^+$ per kg wet weight. The corresponding values for the guinea pig are $75.8 \pm 6$ and $77.4 \pm 7$ meq/kg.

So far it has not been possible, by either cytochemical or electronmicroscopic methods, to detect any carotenoids (including vitamin A) or olfactory pigments in the plasma membrane of antennae, in their matrix, in olfactory bulbs, or in the cellular cytoplasm. However, ascorbic acid was revealed biochemically in the olfactory epithelium (KURIHARA, 1967).

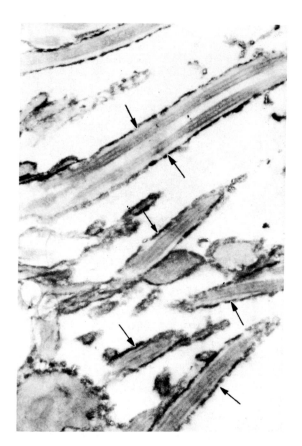

Fig. 75. Activity of ATPase localized in the plasma membrane of olfactory antennae of the grass frog (× 40,000) (BRONSHTEIN and PYATKINA, 1969a). *Arrows* indicate the localization site of ATPase; determination of ATPase was by the method of WACHSTEIN and MEISSEL

The proximal end of antennae, which joins the cytoplasm of the olfactory knob with a diameter of from 1 to 2 μm runs on into the basal bodies; the latter have the usual structure and are equipped with feet directed toward the center of the olfactory knob. Numerous microtubules 180—200Å in diameter, or cross-striated rootlets radiate from the basal bodies (Fig. 74). In some animals, for example in the dog (OKAHO, WEBER, and FROMMES, 1967), these tubules and rootlets may be responsible not only for regulating the motion of the antenna but also for olfactomotor phenomena.

The olfactory knob also contains vacuoles and mitochondria. The number of mitochondria increases at the spot where the olfactory knob joins the peripheral process. The olfactory, as pointed out by BRONSHTEIN (1966), is one of the important cytochemical centers of the olfactory receptor cell; it contains a high concentration of protein sulfhydryl and carboxyl groups and lipids, and the activity of phosphomonoesterases is well expressed in the knob, while the activity of oxidative enzymes is clearly apparent in the mitochondria. Cytochemical data, obtained in our laboratory by BRONSHTEIN (1965), have recently been confirmed with by biochemical methods (KOCH, 1969). Differential centrifugation of the olfactory mucosa gives a fraction consisting of olfactory knob, including their membranes, antennae, basal bodies and vesicles; 56 % of the total enzymic acitivity in such a fraction must be attributed to $K^+$- and $Na^+$-ATPase acitivity. There is also high activity of cytochromoxidase, which increases in a particularly significant way following treatment with desoxycholate, while the activity of ADN-cytochromoxidase decreases. Treatment with desoxycholate also reduces the acitivity of $Mg^{++}$-, $Na^+$- and $K^+$-ATPase.

The peripheral process connecting the olfactory knob with the body of the receptor cell has a length of the order of $20—90\,\mu m$. From a cytochemical standpoint, this sector is poor; it contains, as noted above, microtubules or rootlets connected to basal bodies (Fig. 74). These microtubules, which appear cross-striated under the light microscope, led VINNIKOV and TITOVA (1949, 1957a) to conclude that a contractile substance, designated myoide, is present in the peripheral process; this substance is responsible for olfactomotor phenomena. The body of the olfactory cell does not contain any specific structures; a nucleus, mitochondria, granules, lysosomes, elements of the Golgi apparatus, membranes of the rough-surface endoplasmic reticulum, and sometimes a centrosome are all found here. The presence of a centrosome was reported by MULVANEY and HEIST (1967), and in studies performed in our laboratory (KOSTANYAN, 1971). The nucleus-containing portion of the olfactory cell contains RNA and various proteins, including enzymes. We must assume that it is this portion of cell that synthesizes the protein indispensable for the normal vital activity and functioning of the cell.

A central process extends from the lower pole of the olfactory cell; its diameter at the branching-off point may vary from $0.2$ to $0.5\,\mu m$ in different animals. The central processes of receptor cells, while still being part of the receptor layer, are arranged in clusters, which later, after being coated with Schwann cells, continue into the appropriate connective tissue and form the clusters, stems and fila olfactoria of the olfactory nerve. Schwann cells usually form a mesaxon around a large number of fibers, often exceeding several hundred, which reach the olfactory bulbs of the brain, where they form synaptic contacts with dendrites of mitral neurons and cells with spikes in what are called the olfactory glomerules. As electron microscopic studies have shown, the diameter of individual fibers in the area of olfactory bulbs may vary from $80—90$ to $200—300\,\mu m$ or more (ANDRES, 1965). By examining longitudinal sections one can see that this difference in diameter is associated with the fact that each fiber can form along its entire length spindle-like thickenings which seem to correspond to the varicosal thickenings seen under the light microscope. Nerve fibers are characterized by the fact that they contain a large number of "neurotubules", the diameter of which may be as large as 200Å, and "neurofilaments" of diameter up to 40Å. The number of tubules may range from 1 to 10. Occasionally, membranes are found, i.e. elements of the endoplasmic reticulum.

Telodendrons of olfactory fibers, having an average diameter of 250Å and adhering tightly to each other, are found in the area where the olfactory glomerules are located. From 10,000 to 25,000 fibers can be found in the glomerules of the white rat. The cytoplasm of olfactory fibers becomes thicker, and the neurotubules terminate in a thin, agranular network. The neuroplasm is poorly discernible and has a large number of micropinocytosic invaginations and "acicular" vesicles. Mitochondria and synaptic vesicles are located in even more distal segments of telodendrons found in the fibers of olfactory cells; these mitochondria and synaptic vesicles have a diameter within the range 350 to 750Å. Orbicular synaptic membraneous complexes, 200 to 250Å thick, are located between filled synaptic vesicles telodendrons, and the light ramifications of dendrites found in mitral cells and cells with a rosette (ANDRES, 1965). In the cytoplasm of dendrites can be found elements of a loose agranular endoplasmic reticulum and individual vesicles 300—600Å in diameter, assembled in groups, can break off from this reticulum. The intercellular clefts of a glomerule are distinguished by some sort of contrasting content. The activity of oxidative enzymes and acetylcholinesterase can be detected cytochemically in the region where glomerules are present.

A few words now about supporting cells; these are regularly found between receptor cells, frequently surrounding separate fields or groups of olfactory cells, particularly in lower vertebrates. These cells are connected to receptor cells by means of regularly positioned desmosomes. In cyclostomes and in fish supporting cells are equipped with flame cilia (BRONSHTEIN and IVANOV, 1965; BRONSHTEIN and PYATKINA, 1966). In other animals, and particularly in higher vertebrates, these cells are coated with microvilli. Supporting basal cells are frequently located only at the base of the receptor layer; these supporting cells contain a very large number of ultracellular structures and also numerous biologically active chemical compounds. These cells are also capable of secretion; there is no doubt whatsoever that supporting cells perform a significant trophic function with respect to olfactory receptor cells.

In land vertebrates the surface of the olfactory mucosa, as already mentioned, is coated with an aqueous secretion, secreted primarily by Bowman's glands; the latter are not found in fish, in which the secretory activity is performed by supporting cells (VINNIKOV and TITOVA, 1957a). The substance secreted by these glands forms a monolayer on the surface of the cellular receptor layer and constitutes a direct medium for the free diffusion of odorant molecules which are poorly soluble in water. It is possible that this secretion also takes part in the removal of odorant molecules from receptor cells after their stimulation. The chemical composition of the mucus which covers the olfactory mucosa and the significance of this mucus for both the movement of antennae and the interaction between antennae and odorant molecules are being very intensively studied in our laboratory. Histochemically, Bowman's glands can be colored by PAS reagent. Since these glands are mixed, the substance secreted by them is both serous and mucous; in some animal species it may contain acid mucopoly-saccharides, while in other species it may contain mucoproteins, glycoproteins, neutral polysaccharides, etc. The nasal mucus of man contains 2—3 % mucin, and its pH lies in the range 6.6 to 7.0. BRONSHTEIN and PYATKINA (1969a), using Komnic's electron-cytochemical method (KOMNIC, 1962), have detected voluminous $Na^+$ reaction products in Bowman's glands. Such reaction products, e. g. crystals of Na pyroantimonate, may reach dimensions of up to 500—700 Å in the cells Bowman's glands, indicating the presence of a considerable concentration of $Na^+$. These products are also found in large amounts in the composition of the total secretion in Bowman's glands, which is secreted onto the surface of the olfactory mucosa. Excretion of $Na^+$ by nasal glands is known to take place in certain birds in connection with their marine habitat (FÄNGE, SCHMIDT-NILSEN, and ROBINSON, 1958). As we shall see later, in the organ of olfaction the function of Bowman's glands in supplying $Na^+$ to the surface of the olfactory mucosa may help to provide a complete gradient between the internal and external environment of the antennae in olfactory cells.

## 4. Functional Shifts of the Structural and Cytochemical Organization of Olfactory Cells in Vertebrates

What happens to the olfactory cell when it is stimulated by odorant molecules? At present, very little information is available to us in this respect. Apparently technical difficulties have prevented urgently needed *in vitro* studies of the effect of odorant molecules on the movement of antennae of olfactory cells. Also not clarified is the content of carotenoids and other pigments in antennae, to which some researchers, as we have seen, ascribe the role of "receptors" of odorant molecules. While we assume that the first encoding transformation, i. e. interaction with odorant molecules, takes place in the plasma membrane of motile antennae of olfactory cells, we still know nothing about the nature of the structural and cytochemical changes which take place at the same time in the membrane or matrix of the antennae. Most of the available information concerns the body of the receptor olfactory cell and reflects later stages in the perception of odorant molecules.

Thus, the studies of BOURNE and BARADI (BOURNE, 1948; BARADI and BOURNE, 1951a, 1951b, 1953, 1959a) dealt with the distribution in the receptor layer of the olfactory mucosa of a number of enzymes capable of hydrolyzing phosphoric acid esters, such as glycerophosphate, hexose diphosphate, adenosine triphosphate, and also yeast and muscle adenylic acids and non-specific lipases. Moreover, whereas the presence of enzymes in antennae had appeared doubtful under the light microscope, esterase and acid phosphatase activity was detected in the body of olfactory cells. Supporting cells were found to contain the largest number of enzymes. In some cases, it was possible to detect cholinesterase activity in single olfactory cells of the rabbit; this activity was localized in peripheral and central processes (BARADI and BOURNE, 1959a). When small amounts of vanillin, mint, anise oil, bush red pepper extract, tea, coffee and acetic acid were added to the incubation medium, different changes in the enzymic (phosphatase) activity were noted. For example, acetic acid inhibited the reactions of all enzymes. Mint and anise oil inhibited only the 5-nucleotidase activity, pepper suppressed the ATPase, esterase, lipase activities and the activity of acid phosphatase, etc.

Thus, according to BARADI and BOURNE (1953), odoriferous molecules inhibit enzymic reactions in the cytoplasm of olfactory cells, thereby causing shifts in the concentration of a number of compounds, and this finally leads to the appearance of an olfactory stimulus. Different compounds inhibit different enzymic reactions and at the same time act simultaneously upon several such reactions. On this basis, as already discussed, KISTIAKOWSKY (1950) proposed his enzymic theory of olfaction, a critique of which was given above. There has also been some criticism of the methodology used in the study of BARADI and BOURNE (VINNIKOV and TITOVA, 1957a).

BRONSHTEIN (1965) noted that, when odoriferous compounds (thymol, camphor, clove oil) were allowed to act upon the isolated olfactory mucosa *in vitro*, an olfactomotor reaction and a redistribution of RNA, proteins and sulfhydryl groups were observed in olfactory cells. Simultaneously, he noted increased secretion of the substance secreted by Bowman's glands. GOMAZKOVA (1963), using biochemical methods, found that the phosphatase activity of olfactory mucosa homogenates decreases when odorants are added to the incubation medium. These few investigations show that specific stimulation of olfactory cells causes a number of shifts on the part of the basic biologically active chemical compounds present in their cytoplasm. It is obvious that these cytochemical changes are the consequence of a primary transformation that takes place in the antennae when molecules of odorants act upon their plasma membrane. However, we do not at present understand the cytochemical picture of the second transformation, i. e. the transmission of a nervous impulse to the central nervous system, which takes place in the synapses, i. e. in the olfactory glomerules.

## 5. Structural Organization of Olfactory Cells of Insects

Behavioral and electrophysiological studies have shown that placoid and certain varieties of trichoid, basiconical and coeloconical sensilla act as olfactory receptors in insects (Fig. 76). These sensilla may be located on antennae, palpi and ovipositors. For example, bees carry approximately 3,000 sensilla on each antenna (DETHIER, 1963).

The structural organization of insect sensilla has been studied under the light microscope. The number of receptor cells making up a sensillum may vary (4–6–12–18–20–50) according to the character of the sensillum. Electron-microscopic studies by IVANOV on antennae of the bee and the beetle *Acilius sulcatus* (IVANOV, 1966, 1968, 1969a, 1969b) and by ERNST (1969) on the carrion beetle *Necrophorus* (Coleoptera) have shown that the receptor cells of sensilla have a bipolar shape (Fig. 77); they consist of a nuclear-cytoplasmic body and a central and peripheral processes. The cellular cytoplasm has an extraordinary wealth of organoids: endoplasmic reticulum, elements of the Golgi apparatus, mitochondria, etc. (Fig. 78). The central process runs in the direction of the

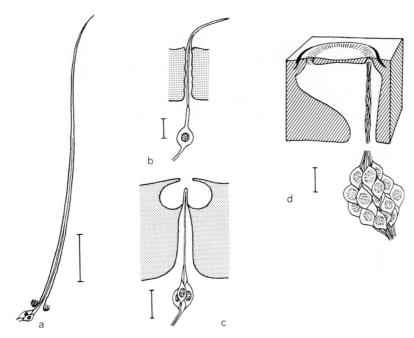

Fig. 76a—d. Examples of four types of olfactory sensilla in insects (ERNST, 1969). a Trichoid sensillum
(*Antherea pernii*); b basiconical sensillum (*Necrophorus vespilio*); c coeloconical sensillum (*Locusta
migratoria*); d placoid sensillum (*Apis mellifiera*). Receptor cells in sensilla are adjacent to cuticular
portions. Peripheral processes of receptor cells penetrate into the interior of hairs (a—c) or into
the groove of the cuticular plate. Scale: for a and b — 50 μm, for c and d — 5 μm

central ganglions; this process, as well as the cellular body, is located in a
mesaxon formed by Schwann cells. The peripheral process has a complex structure;
at a certain distance from the nuclear-cytoplasmic body it forms a narrow
bridge or snare node, which divides it into an inner and outer segment (Fig.
79). At the snare point lies the basal body, from which 9 pairs of peripheral
fibrils (the 2 central fibrils are absent) extend over a short distance, while cross-
striated rootlets with a striation period of 650—700 Å branch off into the inner
segment. Thus, the outer segment of the peripheral process can be considered
as a modified flagellum or cilium, quite similar to the antennae of olfactory
cells in vertebrates. Flagellate structures were detected for the first time in
sensillum cells by SLIFER with the electron microscope (SLIFER, 1961; SLIFER
and SEKHON, 1961). The structure of the outer segment is rather complex;
it is a large elongated cylinder of uniform thickness with a ramified apex from
which extend a number of digitiform processes arranged at right angles (Fig.
77). Various indefinite structures, including vesicles, can be observed in the
light matrix of the digitiform processes. The plasma membrane of these ramifications, which greatly increase the total surface area of peripheral processes, lies
directly next to the pores of the cuticular part of the sensillum. Up to 180—360
pores are found on the surface of the cuticular cone of the basiconical sensillum
in the fly *Phormia regina* Mg; these pores make up 7—14 % of the cone area

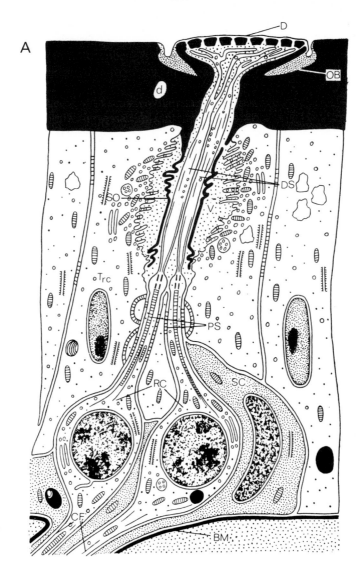

Fig. 77 A and B. Structure of insect sensilla. A. Structural diagram of the placoid sensillum of the beetle *(Acilius sulcatus)*, based on electron microscopic data (IVANOV, 1969a). *RC* receptor cells; *CF* central process; *Trc* trichogen cell; *SC* Schwann cell; *v* vacuole; *SO* scolopoid sheath; *DS* distal segment; *d* efferent duct of gland; *PS* proximal segment; *OB* outer body; *D* cuticular disk-shaped plate with pores; *BM* basal membrane. B. Reconstruction of the basiconical sensilla of the carrion beetle *(Necrophorus)* (ERNST, 1969). This diagram shows one third of the length of the olfactory hair *Ri*; the cuticle adjacent to the hair is shown in a size equal to 17—20 μm, as well as a portion of the adjacent epithelial layer *C* and *C*[1]; *A* axon; *Ad* outer segment of peripheral process; *ID* inner segment of peripheral process; *B* basal membrane; *CK* canals of the cuticle; *DS* sheats of the peripheral process; *PKa* pores; *PKe* pore chambers; *PTr* pore tubes; *PT* pore recesses; *Si* receptor cell; *SL₁* fluid in vacuole No. 1; *SL₂* fluid in vacuole No. 2; *trZ* trichogen cell; *Flp* finger-like processes; *NT* neurotubulus; *DZ* bifurcations of the peripheral process; *tZ* tormogen cell

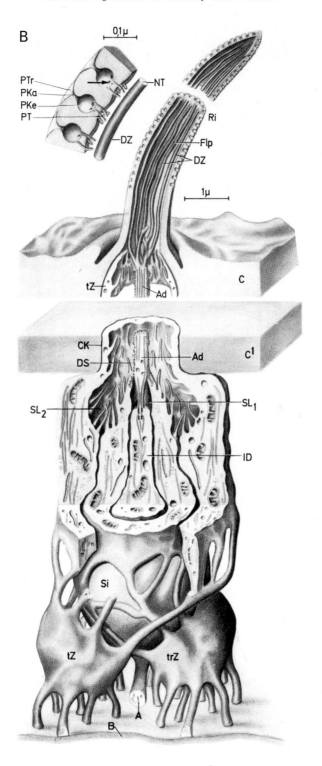

(DETHIER, LARSEN, and ADAMS, 1963). The diameter of these pores is 0.088 μm on the inside and 0.075 μm on the outer surface. The walls of the cuticular cone of distant chemoreceptors in the silkworm are perforated with 3,000 pores. The carrion beetle *Necrophorus* has 13,000—17,000 pores (Fig. 77 B). Each pore, with a diameter of 50—60 Å, leads into an extended chamber from which several small tubules 100—200 Å in diameter extend in the direction of digitiform pro-

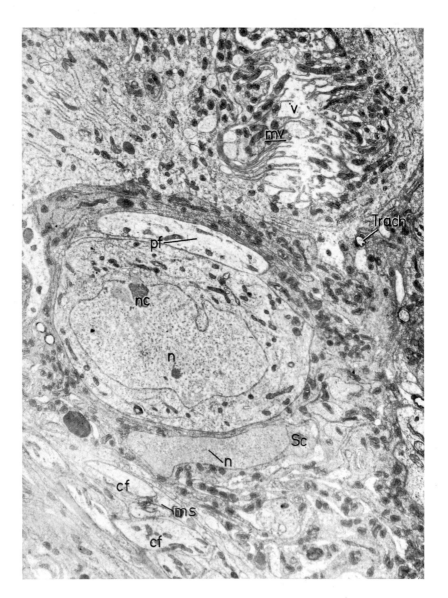

Fig. 78. Longitudinal section of the hypoderm lining the cuticle of the antenna in the beetle *Acilius sulcatus* ( × 20,000) (IVANOV, 1969b). *ms* mesaxon; *n* nucleus; *nc* nucleolus; *Trach* tracheole; *cf* central process; *pf* peripheral process; *Sc* Schwann cell; *mv* microvilli; *v* vacuole

cesses. Tangential sections of the placoid sensillum of *Acilius sulcatus* and *Necrophorus* clearly show that each pore is surrounded by six adjacent pores (IVANOV, 1969a, 1969c; ERNST, 1969). Such a hexagonal arrangement is obviously the most economical and effective way of utilizing the area occupied by the pores (Fig. 80). The pores are characterized by a rather complex shape and have the form of a funnel the mouth of which opens into the disk cavity. In *Acilius sulcatus* the diameter of the pore is 0.04 μm at its widest section and 200Å at the narrowest section.

It is obvious that in insects interaction between molecules of odorants and the olfactory cell can take place only in the pore area of the sensillum; lying close to this area are the distal sections of the peripheral process in the receptor cell, this process being a modified flagellum. Hence, an inverse extrapolation is possible, as was performed above with respect to vertebrates, where we believe such interrelationships are also found in the antenna region. Incidentally, insects have, in addition to olfactory antennae, unicellular glands that are apparently homologous to Bowman's glands in vertebrates. Special tests with colloid silver have shown that the liquid bathing the digitiform processes of the peripheral segment in the olfactory cell communicates with the external orifice of the pore through which molecules of odorants enter (ERNST, 1969). Consequently, in both insects and vertebrates, before such molecules can act upon the receptor cell, they must be dissolved in this liquid. The liquid on the outside apparently originates from the substance secreted by special glands and that inside from the liquid in the vacuole, which will be described later in this chapter.

IVANOV (1969a, 1969b) pointed out that the presence of pores and their number and diameter constitute the most important morphological features of olfactory organs in insects. From the number and diameter of pores we can calculate the effective surface area that interacts with molecules of odorants; from this figure we can then calculate the reaction threshold in terms of the number of molecules present in a unit area of the receptor cell.

At the present time, no cytophysiological (other than electrophysiological), cytochemical or electron microscopic studies are available, concerning shifts in the structural organization of insect olfactory cells during stimulation by odorant molecules. It is therefore not possible to give more than a hypothetical functional interpretation of the structure of sensilla. In this connection, we should discuss briefly the enveloping cells of sensilla surrounding the peripheral process of receptor cells. The distal processes of receptor cells are located inside the scolopoid sheath, which apparently protects these cells from mechanical shock (SLIFER, PRESTAGE, and BEAMS, 1959) and simultaneously acts as an effective insulator (DETHIER and WOLBARSHT, 1956). The portion of the trichogen cell that borders on a special liquid reservoir or vacuole (Fig. 77 A, B) is covered with numerous microvilli and folds of the cytoplasmic membrane and under these are located large numbers of vesicles 400Å in diameter. The cytoplasm of the trichogen cell contains numerous mitochondria, smooth and rough endoplasmic reticulum membranes, Golgi apparatus complexes, and multivesicular and dense bodies. The function of the vacuole in the trichogen cell, the contents of which are replenished by secretion, has been assumed to be to prevent the peripheral process from drying up (SNODGRASS, 1926; SLIFER, 1961). As we have seen, it is possible that molecules of odorants are dissolved in the liquid that fills the vacuole in the pore area (ERNST, 1969). However, in the trichoid mechanoreceptor sensillum of the bee, for example, there are no pores connecting the outer and inner medium, yet a vacuole is present. Undoubtedly, intensive metabolic exchanges take place between the trichogen cell and the vacuole. The chemical composition of the vacuole and the contents of vesicles, an accumulation of which is observed in microvilli, are unknown; after osmium tetroxide fixation they appear to be electron-transparent. Apparently, trichogen cells not only secrete the liquid contents of the vacuole, but also maintain its salt composition constant. The vacuole contents of the trichogen cell fill up the cavity inside the cuticular parts of sensilla; these contents are also in contact with distal sections of the peripheral processes in receptor cells. Similar structural relationships are observed in Corti's organ of vertebrates, where receptor hair cells are also surrounded on nearly all sides by an endolymph with a particular salt composition. This liquid plays a definite role in the depolarization of membranes of the stereocilia and plasma membrane found in a hair receptor cells during stimulation, when biopotentials of Corti's organ arise.

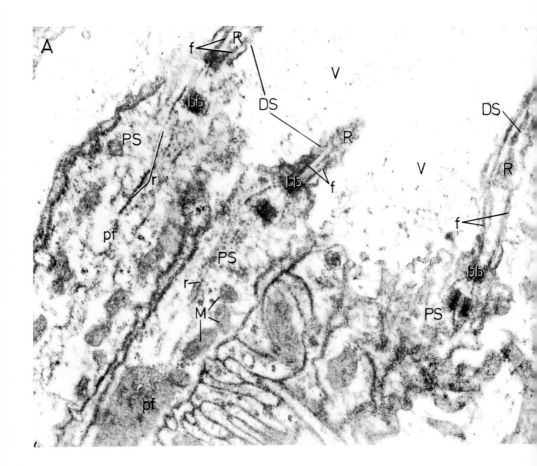

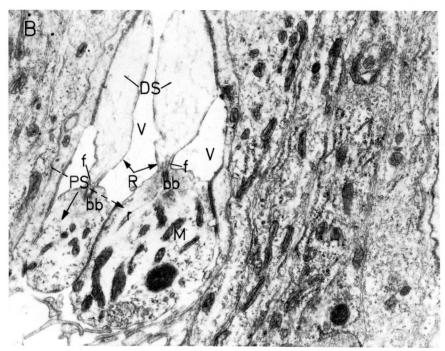

Fig. 79 A and B. Peripheral processes of receptor cells (IVANOV, 1969b). A. Peripheral process (*pf*) of a receptor cell in placoid olfactory sensillum of the bee *Apis mellifera* (×45,000); B. Site at which the proximal segment of the peripheral process of the receptor cell in the laminated organ of *Acilius sulcatus* is converted into a modified cilium (*R*) (×10,300). *PS* proximal segment of the peripheral process; *DS* distal segment of the peripheral process; *bb* basal body; *f* peripheral fibrils of the distal segment; *M* mitochondria; *r* rootlet; *V* vacuole

Although vertebrates and insects exhibit a basic similarity in the structural and functional organization of their receptor olfactory cells, a number of clearcut differences can be noted; these do not, of course, prevent the cells from performing a similar function, i.e. the reception of odorants. For example, as we have pointed out, the molecular concentration thresholds of odorants generally coincide in vertebrates and insects; a definite relationship can also be noted in vertebrates and insects-between the number of receptor cells and the acuity of odor perception, which, in turn, is determined by the ecology of the species. The same applies to the "agreeable" and "disagreeable" character of an odor for different species among both vertebrates and insects. Thus, the evolution of the olfactory organ in vertebrates and insects is characterized by both parallel and divergent features.

## 6. Electrophysiological Investigations

If a microelectrode is placed on the surface of the olfactory mucosa of a frog and an air stream carrying odorants is directed to that spot, a slow multiphase negative potential is recorded. This is called an electro-olfactogram by analogy with the retinogram (OTTOSON, 1956). This potential is characterized

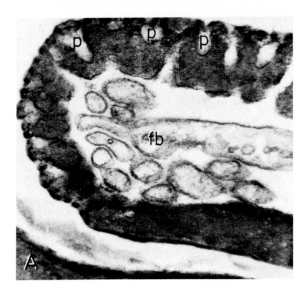

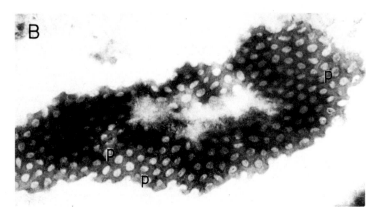

Fig. 80 A and B. Apex of the disk of the placoid sensillum in *Acilius sulcatus* (IVANOV, 1969 b).
A. Sector of the placoid sensillum: disk with pores (*p*) and digitiform processes (*fb*) (× 58,000);
B. Pores (*p*) arranged according to a hexagonal packing type (× 45,000)

by a rapid growth phase and a relatively slow decline; it varies with the concentration of the stimulus and the animal species. According to some investigators,
different olfactograms correspond to different odors (OTTOSON, 1956); others
have observed no such difference (TAKAGI and SHIBUYA, 1960a, 1960b). OTTOSON
(1963) believes that the electro-olfactogram is a homolog of the generator potentials of other sense organs, since during stimulation by odorants there occurs
a variation and summation of the discharge of olfactory cells and of the neuronal
activity of the olfactory bulbs. However, other investigators deny that a correlation
exists between the electro-olfactogram and the bulb potentials (TAKAGI and

OMURA, 1960; MOZELL, 1964a, 1964b; SHIBUYA, 1964). It has been shown that, when the olfactory nerve is cut, the amplitude of the electro-olfactogram decreases as the number of olfactory cells diminishes as a result of degeneration (TAKAGI and YAJIMA, 1965). The electro-olfactogram seems to represent a complex potential connected with Bowman's glands, supporting cells, etc., and including the generator potential arising in receptor cells (MOULTON and BEIDLER, 1967). Thus, the electro-olfactogram includes numerous components connected with the passage of molecules of odorants along the olfactory mucosa.

When a microelectrode is introduced into an isolated olfactory cell, its response can assume different forms. Most olfactory cells have their own "rate of discharge" or phase activity in the absence of any odorant activity. It has been established that cells which do not discharge spontaneously respond to an odor by responses such as "on", "on-off", and "off". Some spontaneously discharging cells can respond by a reaction of "on" inhibition, i.e. stimulation follows inhibition, and inhibition follows stimulation. The remaining spontaneously discharging olfactory cells do not react to odors (TAKAGI and OMURA, 1960).

We have already stated that in the olfactory mucosa of the frog it has been possible to obtain responses from eight types of olfactory cells, which correspond to the primary odors expressed in the shape of the odor molecules (LETTVIN and GESTELAND, 1965). In the olfactory bulbs of the rabbit it is possible to record slow potentials, connected with individual olfactory glomerules, when one of the eight above-mentioned classes of odoriferous molecules is allowed to act on the olfactory mucosa (LEVETEAU and MACLEOD, 1966). Only 3 pairs among the 35 glomerules isolated exhibited the same activity spectrum. ADRIAN (1951a, 1951b) has established that certain odors can be distinguished according to their relative effectiveness in the rear and front portions of olfactory bulbs. In confirmation of these data, it was possible to demonstrate the existence of a latero-medial differentiation in the responses to a given group of odors (MOZELL, 1964a, 1964b).

Of considerable interest are the attempts of TAKAGI and coworkers to analyze the role of $Na^+$ and $K^+$ in the generation of an electro-olfactogram (TAKAGI et al., 1968). We believe these attempts should be correlated with the data quoted above on the localization of $Na^+$ in the slime of olfactory receptor epithelium, obtained in our laboratory by BRONSHTEIN and PYATKINA (1969a).

In order to find out whether electronegative potentials (i.e. the electro-olfactogram of the olfactory mucosa) constitute a generator potential, a study was made of the changes in the ionic composition of the surrounding medium. When saccharose, lithium, choline or tetraethylammonium ions, or hydrazine were substituted for $Na^+$ in the Ringer's solution bathing an isolated olfactory mucosa, the amplitude of the electro-olfactogram first decreased and then vanished. In a potassium-free Ringer's solution, the amplitude of a negative olfactogram first increased and then decreased. When the $K^+$ concentration in the medium was increased parallel to the decrease of $Na^+$ in the medium, the amplitude of the negative electro-olfactogram first decreased, then vanished, and finally exhibited a reversal of polarity. When the $K^+$ ions in the medium were replaced by an equimolar amount of saccharose, lithium, choline or tetraethylammonium ions, hydrazine or sodium, the previous polarity of the electro-olfactogram was restored. However, this restoration was complete only in the presence of Na⁺. Thus, it was possible to demonstrate the essential role played by $Na^+$ and $K^+$ in the generation of a negative electro-olfactogram. On this basis, TAKAGI and his colleagues (TAKAGI et al., 1968) concluded that a negative electro-olfactogram consists of both a generator and a positive potential.

Data obtained by BRONSHTEIN and PYATKINA (1969a) suggest that Bowman's glands supply $Na^+$, which is distributed over the surface of the olfactory mucosa. This makes it possible for us to unravel the mechanism of depolarization of the plasma membrane in antennae of vertebrate olfactory cells during interaction with odorant molecules. If, as the above authors propose, we assume there is a change in the $Na^+$ permeability of the antenna membranes during this interaction, then as a result of this change $Na^+$ ions from the surrounding medium are able to reach the cytoplasm and cause a depolarization of the plasma membrane, expressed in the form of a generator potential. The significance of $Na^+$ in this process was also noted by OTTOSON (1963). Sufficient energy for these exchange processes is supplied by the high ATPase activity of the plasma membrane. However, no biopotentials could be recorded from antennae of olfactory cells, nor from outer segments or rhabdomers of photoreceptors. Nevertheless, recording of biopotentials from the olfactory cell body and its axon is stopped when antennae are exposed to the action of ether and chloroform vapors. If the action of these narcotics is of short duration, potentials again arise when the olfactory mucosa is stimulated by odorants (AI and TAKAGI, 1963).

In insects, two potentials, a negative (depolarizing) and a positive (hyperpolarizing) potential, have been recorded in a single olfactory cell. It was established that the role of the negative potential is excitation (generator potential), while that of the positive one is inhibition of the receptor (SCHNEIDER, 1957a, 1957b, 1957c; BOECKH, 1962; SCHNEIDER, LACHER, and KAISSLING, 1964; KAISSLING and RENNER, 1968).

Thus, data obtained with insects reinforce the viewpoint that two types of potentials of opposite polarity interact in the electro-olfactogram. Thus, if electrodes are applied to the distal and proximal antenna terminals of *Bombyx mori*, which is then stimulated by a stream of odorants, a potential or electro-olfactogram is recorded; its amplitude is determined by the concentration of the odorant and its shape by the type of odorant. Under the action of a narcotic, the response vanishes. A sex attractant induces an electro-olfactogram only in males of *Bombyx mori* (SCHNEIDER, 1962). In members of the subfamily Saturniidae, attractants from females belonging to different species do not exhibit species-specificity, although the attractant of the female *Bombyx* does not exert any effect on male moths of the family Saturniidae.

Certain olfactory sensilla on the antennae of the beetle *Necrophorus* consist of a single receptor cell. By recording the bioelectric activity when these sensilla were subjected to the action of odorants, it was possible to detect a slow generator potential; a volley of impulses could be observed against the background of this potential, with the maximum impulse frequency corresponding to the ascending phase of the slow potential. Responses to stimulation with several odors differed in the amplitude and growth steepness of the slow potential; this was accompanied by a change in the frequency of the impulse spectrum (BOECKH, 1962). It was found that the stimulating or inhibiting effect of a number of fatty acids depends upon the number of carbon atoms in the chain (see Table 5). The negative generator potential and the frequency of afferent impulses in

Table 5. Responses of the olfactory sensillum of the carrion beetle *(Necrophorus vespiblio)* as a function of the carbon chain length in a fatty acid series (BOECKH, 1962)

| Compound | Formula | Number of carbon atoms | Reaction |
|----------|---------|------------------------|----------|
| Cycloheptanone | $CH_2(CH_2)_5CO$ | 7 | − |
| Propionic acid | $CH_3CH_2COOH$ | 3 | − |
| Butyric acid | $CH_3CH_2CH_2COOH$ | 4 | + |
| Caproic acid | $CH_3(CH_2)_3CH_2COOH$ | 6 | + |
| Heptanoic acid | $CH_3(CH_2)_4CH_2COOH$ | 7 | + |
| Caprylic acid | $CH_3(CH_2)_5CH_2COOH$ | 8 | + |
| Pelargonic acid | $CH_3(CH_2)_6CH_2COOH$ | 9 | + |
| Capric acid | $CH_3(CH_2)_7CH_2COOH$ | 10 | 0 |
| Stearic acid | $CH_3(CH_2)_{15}CH_2COOH$ | 18 | 0 |
| Oleic acid | $CH_3(CH_2)_7CH—CH(CH_2)_7COOH$ | 18 | + |

Note: (−) hyperpolarization of the cellular membrane, inhibition; (+) depolarization of the cellular membrane, stimulation; (0) no response.

a volley reached its minimum value under the action of vapors of an acid with four carbon atoms in the chain, and its maximum value when the acid had seven or eight carbon atoms in the chain. Any further increase in the number of carbon atoms caused a decline in the response, and it vanished under the action of capric acid, which has 10 carbon atoms in its molecule. In *Necrophorus*, a similar effect is caused by molecules of fatty acids having less than six carbon atoms in the molecule. Tests carried out by ELIZAROV and SINITSYNA (1969) have shown that the same odorants used in large concentrations repel mosquitos, whereas in small concentrations they exert an attracting effect. The above authors point out that similar properties are exhibited by certain repellents although their attractive effect is insignificant at low concentrations. On the other hand, many attractants act as repellents at high concentrations. However, compounds that act as repellents at very low concentrations show no change in this effect when the concentration is increased.

Recordings of biopotentials from the olfactory sensilla of the moth *Antheraea pernyi*, which has three receptor cells, have shown that this moth possesses specific reception only for molecules of certain odorants (SCHNEIDER, LACHER, and KAISSLING, 1964). Thus two cells in the sensillum respond to stimulation by phenyl acetate, terpineol, isosafrole, geraniol, etc., by generating volleys of impulses of different intensity. The third cell, which generates high-amplitude impulses, is excited only by molecules of sex attractant and does not respond to other odorants. Collating the electrophysiological and biochemical data (RIDDI-

FORD, 1970), we can assume that recognition of the quality of odoriferous molecules in insects takes place at the molecular level of the organization of the receptor cell, namely of its outer segment which, as we have seen, is a modified cilium. The plasma membrane of this cilium must contain molecules of the olfactive proteins that interact with odorant molecules. Thus, in insects molecular olfactory specificity has found its expression in the course of evolution in the form of morphologically and functionally differentiated separate types of receptor olfactory cells.

# 7. Conclusion

The problem of olfaction, like that of gustation, is a problem of molecular biology. All contemporary olfaction theories are designed to lead to an understanding both of the structure, shape and physical nature of odorant molecules, and of the organization of the olfactory cell and the plasma membrane of its motile antennae, which must contain molecules of olfactive proteins capable of interacting with odorant molecules. On the basis of a careful study of the chemical structure of a number of odorant molecules, we cannot affirm that chemical structure alone determines the character of the odor emitted by these molecules (DYSON, 1926, 1938). The results of investigation of the stereochemical conformation of odorant molecules were somewhat more encouraging (AMOORE, 1962a, 1962b). The synthesis of certain odorant molecules having a definite conformation has made it possible to predict their odor. However, it is not at all clear in what way the conformation of a molecule determines the nature of its odor, nor is it clear what substance this molecule interacts with in the hypothetical corresponding "specific site" of the plasma membrane, nor what is the exact nature of this interaction. Attempts have been made to associate the properties of an odorant molecule with its quantum intramolecular vibrations, which act in a specific manner upon carotenoids or other pigments present in cells of the olfactory mucosa (WRIGHT, 1964). However, this theory is also beset by a number of difficulties; these concern not only the nature of the vibration of odoriferous molecules, but also primarily the location site of the carotenoids or pigments upon which the quantum energy of odorant molecules appears to act. There are other possible concepts regarding the nature of both odorant molecules and the compounds with which they interact. Thus, we are only in the initial guesswork stages concerning the chemical and physical nature of odorant molecules, the number and variety of which is constantly being added to. Their novelty, however, does not prevent such molecules from supplying information to our olfactory cells, although the evolution of these cells in primates was apparently completed long ago, and in any case prior to the appearance in the environment of man and animals of modern synthetic odorants. We can assume that all odorant molecules, despite their great variety, possess some common chemical and physical properties, still unknown to us, that give them their odorant character. Perhaps there are some kinds of universal chemical groups present in all odorant molecules and gustatory substances.

A study of the ultrastructural organization of olfactory cells in vertebrates and insects shows that the interaction of odorants with these cells takes place at the molecular level in the plasma membrane of motile antennae. The evolution of olfactory cells in vertebrates and insects, based on a cell equipped with flagella, has led to the elaboration of similar molecular mechanisms under the effect of the similar physical and chemical properties of odorant molecules. The specific reactions of receptor cells always arise in the plasma membrane; this is the first energy conversion and constitutes the trigger mechanism that induces depolarization of the receptor cell membrane and the appearance of bioelectric activity, which is transmitted via the synapses to the central nervous system. With what does an odorant molecule interact in the plasma membrane? This question still presents certain difficulties, although we assume that the reaction involves carotenoids, including vitamin A or some other olfactory pigment. In the first place, it has not yet proved possible to identify an ordered or somehow organized localization of such compounds in the membranes of olfactory cell antennae. Moreover, it is equally probable that such compounds are located in the supporting cells of the olfactory mucosa, or even in the appropriate connective tissue. We therefore believe the correct course is to initiate [as has been done by ASH (1968, 1969), ASH and SKOGEN (1970), and RIDDIFORD (1970)] a search in the plasma membrane of antennae for some specific proteins and accompanying cofactors possessing specific sensitivity for certain odorant molecules as at present classified. As discussed above (Chapter V) such "sweet-sensitive" and "bitter-sensitive" proteins have already been isolated from cells of taste buds. Using analogous methods, workers have begun studies to isolate olfactive receptive proteins in vertebrates and insects, whose olfactory cells are known to have a similar structural and functional organization. In theory, the cellular and molecular mechanisms of olfactory reception in vertebrates and insects ought to be universal. However, further intensive investigations will be neccesary for the complete decoding of olfactory mechanisms.

Chapter VII

# Hearing

## 1. Introduction

Among all sense organs, the most complex transformations occurring during reception of a stimulus are those observed in the organ of hearing, found only in the most highly organized animals, namely vertebrates and insects. Sound reception must be considered as mechanoreception that has attained the highest stage of development. With the aid of such a system of mechanoreceptors an animal can determine the character of the substrate with which it comes into contact, the velocity of a stream of water or air, the depth of immersion, the pressure of a liquid in its own vessels and cavities, the movement and position of its own muscles and joints (proprioception), changes in the Earth's gravitational field and angular accelerations, vibrations, and finally, sounds of specific frequency and intensity. In vertebrates, mechanoreception takes place with the aid of special encapsulated and nonencapsulated corpuscles, as well as by means of specialized secondary sensory cells that have no central process of their own and transmit information directly to synapses, but are equipped with a cluster of stereocilia polarly opposed by a single kinocilium containing $9 \times 2 + 2$ fibrils. In insects, mechanoreception is achieved by means of sensilla. The peripheral process of receptor cells in sensilla is a modified flagellum containing $9 \times 2 + 0$ fibrils, which is attached to the cuticular elements of sensilla.

In vertebrates, the secondary sensory receptor cells of Corti's organ, the hair cells, constitute what is called the acoustic-lateral system in which lateral-line organs, semicircular canals, sacculus and utriculus are onto- and phylogenetically combined. The sacculus and utriculus come into direct contact with a stimulus, or, as we shall see in the next chapter, receive it by means of a small number of transformations, for example cupula deviation or the action of a standard mass of otolith. In Corti's organ, under the action of the energy of sonic frequencies, a series of complex mechanical (in the middle ear) and hydrodynamic (in the inner ear) transformations take place. These transformations lead to the appearance in the region of the antennae-stereocilia of hair cells of shearing forces that develop because of the motion of basilar and tectorial membranes. This sets off a complex mechanochemical process, which is associated with the triggering of substrates and enzymes of the cholinergic system located in the region of stereocilia of hair cells. It follows that the plasma membrane of the stereocilia of hair cells is the final site of application of all the energy conversions which a sound stimulus undergoes in the middle and inner ear.

In the plasma membrane of the stereocilia the energy of molecules that take part in wave transmission is converted in an equivalent manner into molecular processes of the kind associated with nerve conduction in the synaptic region.

The two contemporary theories of hearing, namely the mechanoelectrical theory (DAVIS, 1957, 1958, 1960, 1961) and the cytochemical theory (VINNIKOV and TITOVA, 1961, 1962a, 1962b, 1963, 1964; VINNIKOV, 1966a, 1966b, 1969) attempt to explain, each in its own way, the primary stimulation processes, i.e. the trigger mechanism of a hair cell in Corti's organ. However, as we shall show in our further presentation, these theories do not contradict so much as supplement each other.

Unfortunately, there is still a shortage of data concerning the character of the mechanochemical processes occurring during the auditory stimulation of hearing organs (chordotonal and tympanal organs) in insects. Judging from the similarity of their structural and functional organization to those of vertebrates, we can assume *a priori* that an analogy is present here.

Last but not least important in connection with the transformations of an auditory stimulus, is the problem of what constitutes an adequate stimulus. Indeed, how does a receptor auditory cell respond adequately, by means of its mechanochemical molecular mechanism, to the action of the energy of molecules that take part in wave transmission and are present in a sound wave, in spite of the many highly complex transformations which this wave undergoes on its way from the tympanic membrane to the stereocilia of hair cells? What does the general effect of sound on any cell really consist in, and what must this cell, which has been converted into a receptor cell during the course of evolution, transmit to the central nervous system in the form of encoded information?

We believe that quantitative cytochemical data on the general effect exerted by sound waves upon living tissue are rather revealing in this respect; such data were obtained some time ago by CHAMBERS and FLOSDORF (1936), NASONOV and RAVDONIK (1947) and for the cochlea by VINNIKOV and TITOVA (1961, 1964) and VINNIKOV and SOKOLOVA (1961).

The nonspecific effect of an auditory stimulus has recently been investigated on embryonic tissues by VOINO-YASENETSKII (1965), SVIDERSKAYA (1967, 1968a, 1968b) and by SVIDERSKAYA and GRIGOR'EVA (1969).

New data on the ultrastructural level of organization of hair cells in vertebrates (birds and mammals) and insects, as well as their cytochemical characteristics both when these cells are in a state of relative rest and when they are subjected to shifts under the effect of an auditory stimulus, convey a clearer idea of the structural and functional organization of hair cells and enable us to compare them with other receptor cells. These are the problems confronting us in the present chapter.

## 2. Auditory Stimulus, its Nonspecific and Specific Effect, and the Evolution of Auditory Receptor Mechanisms

Molecules of air or a liquid are in constant motion (thermal or Brownian), hence reception of the energy of their thermal vibrations is of no use to the organism. Sound, that is, the synchronous, nonrandom oscillation of molecules of gas or liquid, is, however, perceived by the hearing organ as useful information. The action of a single molecule is not perceived by the organism, but it does perceive well-defined or synchronous vibrations of a group of molecules, i.e. a sound wave.

Thus, an auditory stimulus is an aggregate of sinusoidal mechanical waves, where each wave can be characterized by frequency and amplitude. The motion of a sound wave causes the particles of the medium in which the sound is propagated to be mixed. The propagation velocity of sound and its attenuation with distance depend upon the properties of the medium. Thus, the velocity of sound in air at 20 °C is equal to 343 m/sec, while in water it is 4.7 times greater. The intensity of sound is usually expressed as the density of sound energy and is measured in dynes/cm². The faintest sound that can be heard by man has an intensity of about 0.0001 dyne/cm². The threshold of optimum audibility for man, at an oscillation frequency of 1,000 cps (cycles per second) is approximately equal to 0.0002 dyne/cm². The intensity of sound, measured in dynes/cm², is usually expressed in relative units known as decibels (10 times the logarithm of the ratio of two values of sound intensity). The standard usually adopted in constructing the scale of sound intensity (decibels) is the audibility threshold for man. At the low-frequency end of the sound range (below 50 cps) acoustic reception overlaps with vibroreception. Some animals are able to perceive only low frequencies, so that for these animals vibration and sound are essentially the same thing. However, in most animals sound and vibration are perceived by different organs (see Chapter VIII).

Under normal conditions the cells and tissues of the internal organs are protected from the mechanical action of a sound wave by skin (in vertebrates) or chitin (in insects). Why is such protection necessary? What is the essence of the nonspecific effect of an auditory stimulus upon the cell? What mechanisms enable such a stimulus to be converted into a specific stimulus and perceived in the form of the corresponding information?

CHAMBERS and FLOSDORF (1936) have shown that sounds of high frequency and intensity in the audible range are capable of causing denaturation (i.e. damage) of native proteins *in vitro*. Thus, a direct sound effect could damage the proteins in a living cell.

NASONOV and RAVDONIK (1947) stained isolated frog sartorius muscles with Neutral Red and Cyanol and subjected them to the action of sound frequencies ranging from 200 to 10,000 cps and having the same intensity (95 db). They found that muscles subjected to the action of sound absorb larger amounts of dye than do controls. Maximum dye absorption was observed in the frequency range 2,500 to 3,000 cps. In this range muscles also respond to the action of sound by prolonged contraction. It was further found that, at the same frequency, the intensity of frog muscle staining with Neutral Red depends upon the intensity of sound. When the epithelium of frog renal tubules was subjected to the action of sound, maximum dye (Phenol Red) binding was also observed at a frequency of 2,500 to 3,000 cps (NASONOV and ROZENTAL, 1950). Analogous data were obtained with Neutral Red staining of neurons in spinal ganglions of the rat (NASONOV and RAVDONIK, 1950; ROMANOV, 1954). We should mention the fact, noted for the first time by NASONOV, that the vital sorption of a dye by living tissues of vertebrates subjected to the action of sound falls within the range of the human audiogram.

There was obviously a problem in applying the same method to measure the effect of a sound stimulus on Corti's organ isolated *in vitro* and on the same organ when it formed part of the whole organism. It proved possible to set up such tests in connection with the elaboration of the method comprising the vital isolation of the cochlea (VINNIKOV and TITOVA, 1959, 1961, 1963, 1964).

Under the action of sound of varying duration (15 and 30 min, 2,4 and 6 hours) and frequency, hair cells located on the upper coils of the cochlea exhibited changes at low frequencies, and those located on the lower coils of the cochlea at high frequencies. There was a change in cell shape, a rounding off, swelling or contraction of the nucleus, and vacuolation of the cytoplasm. Vital staining with Neutral Red was accompanied by a decrease in the number of deposited granules, as against controls, or by complete disappearance of the granules. A striking fact was that the dye absorption curve under the action of sound exhibited, both in the cochlea isolated *in vitro* and in the cochlea forming part of the whole organism, increased sorption in the region of 2,000 to 2,500 cps and resembeld that observed in the tests of NASONOV and RAVDONIK (1947) (Fig. 81). This shows that sound energy is perceived in a similar manner by the cytoplasm of hair cells in Corti's organ, which are specialized with respect to sound, and by the cells of other tissues, which are not specialized in this respect. Thus, all tissues, including Corti's organ, respond to sound by means of a similar, nonspecific reaction. However, hair cells, though they

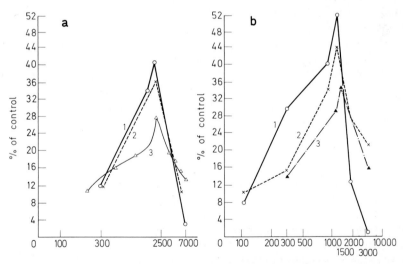

Fig. 81a and b. Staining of the cochlea with Neutral Red under the effect of sound of differing frequency and identical intensity (95 db) during 30 min (a) and 1 hour (b) (VINNIKOV and SOKOLOVA, 1961). Sound frequencies in cps are plotted along the abscissa, and dye sorption (in % with respect to the control) is plotted along the ordinate. *1* cochlea *in vivo*; *2* cochlea *in vitro*; *3* frog sartorius muscle

respond to sound by means of a general and essentially nonspecific reaction, are able to utilize this reaction as a specific response to the sound stimulus. This reaction is probably determined by the character of the acoustic "resonance", i.e. by the change in the conformation of the protein molecules in the protoplasm of animal cells. Corti's organ, when it is part of the whole organism, does not come into direct contact with sound, therefore this original tissue reaction is preserved; if this were not so, sound perception would not be able to reflect concrete reality.

Such an adequate reflection of acoustic energy became possible thanks to the mechanical process of resonance (which arose during evolution) induced by acoustic frequencies in the auxiliary structures present in the middle and inner ear. These structures carry to the hair cells mechanical vibrations, strictly identical to sounds, in the form of wave movements with amplitudes of up to 1% of the diameter of a hydrogen atom (FATT and KATZ, 1950, 1951) of the endolymph, perilymph, the basilar and tectorial membranes.

How, then, is the hair cell able to preserve this original reaction to a sound stimulus, while differentiating its frequency and intensity and repeating and recalling it an infinite number of times? In other words, what are the molecular mechanisms that arose in the course of the evolution of an auditory receptor cell and how do they enable this cell to encode the information supplied by a sound stimulus, i.e. to act as transducer of this information and of its intensity and frequency, and to convert the sound stimulus and transmit it in the form of nerve impulses through synapses to the central nervous system? We shall now attempt to answer these questions.

In hearing organs, i.e. Corti's organ of vertebrates, and the chordotonal or tympanic organ of insects, sound waves received from the surrounding air or water are transmitted through a system of solid or liquid structures and thereby undergo a number of energy conversions. Thus, the hair cells do not come into direct contact with a sound wave, but are stimulated only by an energy equivalent of this wave.

Corti's organ in mammals is located on the basilar membrane (Fig. 82 A). This membrane consists of several layers: an upper fibrous layer on which Corti's organ is located, an upper homogeneous layer, a lower fibrous layer, and a lower homogeneous layer on which the endothelium lining the tympanic surface is located (ENGSTRÖM, 1955; IURATO, 1962a, 1962b). Corti's organ includes two systems of receptor cells: three rows of outer hair cells and one row of inner hair cells. Corti's organ in birds does not exhibit differentiation into outer and inner hair cells. Nevertheless, birds can perceive sounds in the range 10 to 20,000 cps. According to some authors (SCHWARTZKOPFF, 1963), the cochlea and the organ of Corti in birds have some differencies. Each receptor cell is crowned with a bundle of stereocilia, to which in mammals a basal body is polarly opposed (Fig. 82 B), and in birds one kinocilium. The stereocilia are apparently attached by their crowns to the lower surface of the tectorial membrane (VINNIKOV et al., 1965; KIMURA, 1966; KOICHEV, 1969a, 1969b). This kind of attachment, which is common for mechanoreceptors, makes possible the direct transmission of shearing forces to the stereocilia plasma membrane. The tectorial membrane is a noncellular fibrous formation consisting of glycoproteins (BAIRATI, JURATO, and PERNIS, 1957). Two nerve plexuses—an inner and an outer one—approach the base of the hair cells in the cochlea; their fiber terminals form synaptic contacts with the hair cells (VINNIKOV and TITOVA, 1961). Fibers of the spiral plexuses are formed by dendrites of neurons in the

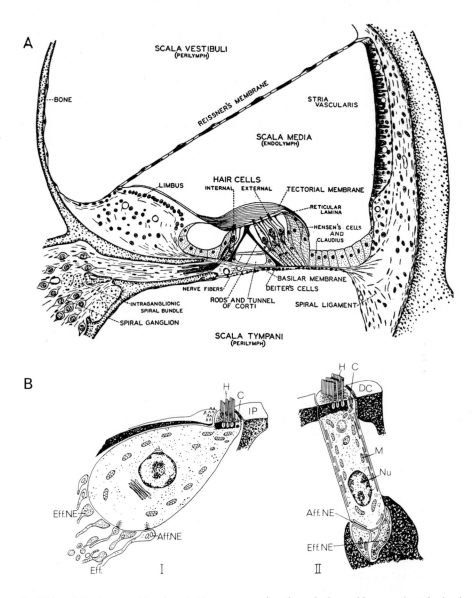

Fig. 82 A and B. Organs of hearing. A. Transverse section through the cochlear canal at the level of the second (lower) turn of the cochlea of a guinea pig (DAVIS, 1957). B. Semischematic diagram of the inner (*I*) and outer (*II*) hair cells of the organ of Corti in mammals (WERSÄLL *et al.*, 1965). *H* stereocilia; *C* centriole (basalbody); *M* mitochondria; *Nu* nucleus; *Aff. NE* afferent nerve endings; *Eff.NE* efferent nerve endings; *DC* Deithers' cells; *IP* inner pillars; *Eff.* efferent nerve

spiral ganglion, and also by efferent fibers of Rasmussen's olivo-cochlear bundle (RASMUSSEN, 1960).

The physical transformations caused by the action of a sound wave in the inner ear, i.e. in the cochlea, were analyzed for the first time by BÉKÉSY (VON BÉKÉSY, 1947, 1948, 1949a, 1949b, 1951a—1951c, 1952a—1952c, 1953a, 1953b, 1954, 1956, 1957a, 1958b, 1959, 1960a, 1960b). This author observed directly under the microscope the vibrations occurring in various areas of the cochlea when the latter was subjected to sinusoidal oscillations of the stapes. The localization in the cochlea of regions of maximum amplitude depends upon the frequency of the vibrations. The amplitude maximum shifts in a wave-like manner along the cochlear wall in a direction away from the stapes. The magnitude of the shift of the maximum oscillation region, at a given change in frequency $\Delta n/n$ (where $n$ is the frequency), represents the mechanical resolving power. In the basal portion of the cochlea are located receptor cells that perceive both high and low frequencies, whereas in the upper part of the cochlea only low frequencies are perceived.

What is the position during acoustic stimulation of the receptor cells in Corti's organ, which are located on the highly mobile basilar membrane facing the less mobile tectorial membrane?

It is assumed that under the effect of acoustic stimulations the cochlea can bend in both a lateral (radial) and a longitudinal (helical) direction. This must cause the appearance of shearing forces (DAVIS, 1958) between the surface of the hair cells and the tectorial membrane on the one hand, and the basilar membrane on the other hand. These shearing forces must bend the stereocilia of receptor cells, resulting in the appearance of biocurrents or a microphonic potential, i.e. stimulation of the receptor cell (DAVIS, 1958). The outer hair cells in the organ of Corti, judging by the orientation of the basal body, will be depolarized when the stimulus bends the cochlear in a radial direction; the inner hair cells in the organ of Corti will be depolarized when the direction of the stimulus along the axis of the cochlear canal is helical (WERSÄLL, FLOCK, and LUNDQUIST, 1965). In this connection, it is generally believed that the bending of the stereocilia and their subsequent polarization are associated with deformation of the plasma membrane, and this is quite sufficient to produce a mechanical stimulation of the cell, in the same way as in other mechanoreceptors, for example in the Pacinian corpuscles (GOLDMAN, 1965; IL'INSKII, 1966; MIRKIN, 1966a, 1966c; CHEREPNOV, 1968). Thus, according to DAVIS (1953, 1954, 1958, 1961, 1965), if the deformation by bending stereocilia causes a change in the resistance of the plasma membrane, then the potential difference in the system: hair cell-endolymph-perilimph amounts to 70—80 mV, respectively. Thus, a voltage of 150 mV is applied to the membrane of the stereocilia.

However, we believe that this explanation overlooks one more primary molecular structure which is located in the stereocilia and whose function precedes the appearance of biopotentials. What we have in mind here is that acetylcholine has been detected in the endo- and perilymph of birds, mammals and fishes (DACHA and MARTINI, 1942; GISSELSON, 1950). According to most recent data, the concentration of acetylcholine in the perilymph and endolymph of the cat is on average $459.5 \times 10\,\gamma/ml$ (the concentration was measured by the method of Cersten). Brief stimulation of the cochlea with sound (2,000 cps at 120 db for 10 min) results in the concentration of acetylcholine increasing to 988 $\gamma$/ml, i.e. a 20,000 times increase. When the olivo-cochlear bundle is cut, the content of acetylcholine is only half as much. Thus, there is an acetylcholine efferent which disappears after cutting of the nerve, and an acetylcholine afferent which persists under the same conditions (PLUZHNIKOV and YANTAREVA, 1971; KIBYAKOV et al., 1973).

Thus, the presence of a cholinergic mechanism in the cochlea has been confirmed. Moreover, histochemical methods have established that there is acetylcholinesterase activity in the synaptic region of Corti's organ (CHURCHILL, SCHUKNECHT, and DORAN, 1956; VINNIKOV and TITOVA, 1958b, 1961, 1964; ANICHIN, 1968; KANEKO and DALY, 1969). Under the action of high-frequency sound, the enzymic activity of acetylcholinesterase was found to increase in the region of synapses and the spiral plexus at the base of the cochlea, and to increase under the action of low-frequency sound mainly at the apex of the cochlea (VINNIKOV and TITOVA, 1958b, 1961, 1964; ANICHIN, 1964, 1965, 1968). From these facts we are entitled to draw the conclusion that synaptic transmission by receptor cells in Corti's organ takes place with the aid of a cholinergic mechanism. It is true that some authors consider this mechanism to apply to both afferent and efferent synapses (VINNIKOV and TITOVA, 1961, 1964), while others consider its function to be restricted to afferent synapses (ROSSI and CORTESINA, 1962a, 1962b, 1963; ROSSI et al., 1964). The enzymic activity of acetylcholinesterase has been observed in synaptic structures of lateral-line organs in fish (TITOVA and ARONOVA, 1964), in synapses of labyrinth cristae and maculae of cyclostomes, fishes, amphibians, reptiles, birds and mammals, and also in synapses of Corti's organ in birds and mammals (TITOVA and VINNIKOV, 1964; VINNIKOV, TITOVA, and ARONOVA, 1965). Transmission in afferent synapses is possibly realized by GABA (FLOCK and LAM, 1974). However, it was found that in Corti's organ this enzyme is present not only in the synaptic region, but also in the cytoplasm and in stereocilia of hair cells (VINNIKOV and TITOVA, 1961, 1964; KANEKO and DALY, 1969). The activity of the enzyme in stereocilia varies according to the acoustic stimulus (VINNIKOV and TITOVA, 1961, 1964; ANICHIN, 1968).

Thus, not only the transmission but also the perception of a stimulus by hair cells in Corti's organ, in contrast to other organs of the acoustico-lateral system, probably takes place by means of a cholinergic mediator system, which includes the acetylcholine of the endolymph, and, according to modern concepts, a cholinoreceptive protein and acetylcholinesterase, localized in stereocilia of receptor cells in Corti's organ. Consequently, the final transformation, in the case of sound stimulation, takes place as a result of the action of shearing forces in the region of bending stereocilia and is primarily associated with the triggering of the cholinergic system, followed by depolarization of the plasma membrane. The cholinoreceptive protein is apparently localized in the plasma membrane of stereocilia, and interacts with the acetylcholine of the endolymph and with acetylcholinesterase. The enzyme was detected by us histochemically under the light microscope (VINNIKOV and TITOVA, 1961) and has also been observed with the electron microscope by KANEKO and DALY (1969). The data of IURATO (1971), who considers the localization of acetylcholinesterase in the region of stereocilia of hair cells to be an artefact, do not seem to me to be convincing. There will be a more detailed discussion of this molecular mechanism in the following section.

The differentiation of hair cells is accompanied by a restructuring of their cellular and molecular organization which finds expression in their ability to synthesize the cholinoreceptive protein and acetylcholinesterase and to supply these compounds not only to the synaptic region, but also to another structure, the stereocilia. We believe that this novel localization of these two proteins was the result of a change in the genetic code. This change would have been associated in the course of evolution with certain peculiarities in the perception of an acoustic stimulus, or more precisely with its equivalent energy conversions in the outer, middle and inner ear.

The above presentation indicates how complex is the path by which a nonspecific cellular reaction to an acoustic stimulus is finally converted into a specific reaction, and what complex structural and molecular mechanisms were selected in this case during the course of evolution. It is interesting to note how the complex chain of energy conversions of a sound stimulus has finally led to the mechanochemical utilization of a specific synaptic cholinergic mediator system.

All the above information refers to the evolution of the molecular organization of the auditory receptor cell in vertebrates. In regard to insects, such data are practically nonexistent. In insects, there are a number of structural characteristics associated with the transformation, in the course of evolution, of the universal mechanoreceptor cell into an auditory cell. The location of chordotonal and tympanic organs in different parts of the insect body indicates that these organs have formed independently of each other in the course of evolution, although it is possible that the proprioceptor organs of arthropods, located in the region of limb articulation, should be considered the structural precursors of chordotonal organs (HOFFMAN, 1964). As we know, the hearing organ of insects is represented either by chordotonal sensilla or by the tympanic organ. These can be located on the first abdominal segment *(Acrididae)*, in the lower part of the front legs (grasshoppers and *Kryllidae*), and also in the hind body and other sections of the body (some *Papilionaceae* and butterflies, cicads, and crickets). Although the anatomical structure of the tympanic organ of insects differs considerably from that of the hearing organ of vertebrates, the nature of the transformation of an auditory stimulus is nevertheless in many respects identical in both insects and vertebrates. For example the tympanic organ of the locust is located in a special depression along the side of the first abdominal segment. This organ consists of a tympanic membrane, lying at an angle of 45° and partially concealed by the anterior and posterior folds of the integuments. On the inside, closely adhering to the tympanic membrane, is a large air sac and several other smaller sacs, which communicate with the external environment by means of a stigma, comparable with the Eustachian tube of vertebrates. The connection of the tympanic membrane with the tracheal system maintains the former in a stretched state. In addition, muscles also seem to be involved in the stretching of this membrane (SHVANVICH, 1949). Several thickenings are found on the inner surface of the tympanic membrane: the plicate corpuscle (Rinnenförmiges Körperchen), the palisade corpuscle (Stilförmiges Körperchen), the conical process (Zapfenförmiges Körperchen), and the pear-shaped vesicle (Birnförmiges Körperchen). It is here that the receptor cells making up the sensilla are located and from them extend branchlets of the dorsal nerve of the third thoracic segment. The membrane on which these structures are located is essentially an invaginated cuticle coated on the outside with hypodermal epithelium. The membrane is 2—3 μm thick, becoming thicker at the posterior edge, and its elasticity is accordingly greater at this spot. On the inside, the tympanic membrane is coated with the epidermis of the tracheal sacs. Thus, the tympanic membrane is coated with epithelium on both sides and is located in an air medium. It is quite obvious that, in its anatomical and physiological position, the tympanic membrane of insects combines the role of the tympanic membrane, the oval foramen membrane, the basilar membrane and the tectorial membrane found in vertebrates. Thus, in insects, an auditory stimulus is converted in a similar way to what occurs in vertebrates, although these conversions in insects are effected more economically and involve a smaller number of structures.

In the same way as in other insect sensilla, the receptor cells of chordotonal and tympanic organs are equipped with two processes: a central process, which

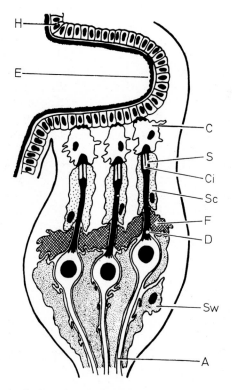

Fig. 83. Diagram of longitudinal section through the receptor region of the tympanic organ of the locust *(Locusta)* (GRAY, 1960). *H* hypoderma; *E* base of process; *C* cap cell; *S* fibril; *Ci* flagelliform process; *Sc* scolopoid cell; *F* fibrous covering cell; *D* peripheral process; *Sw* Schwann cell; *A* axon

is an axonlike fiber, and a peripheral process, which is a modified flagellum containing 9 pairs of peripheral fibrils (Fig. 83). The peripheral process consists of a proximal and a distal segment; the apex of this process adjoins a cap cell, by means of which the entire receptor system is attached to the tympanic membrane. Thus, as occurs in Corti's organ, the receptor cells are stimulated by shearing forces which arise during the movement of a tympanic organ. Such stimulation is due to the attachment of the apex of a distal segment of the

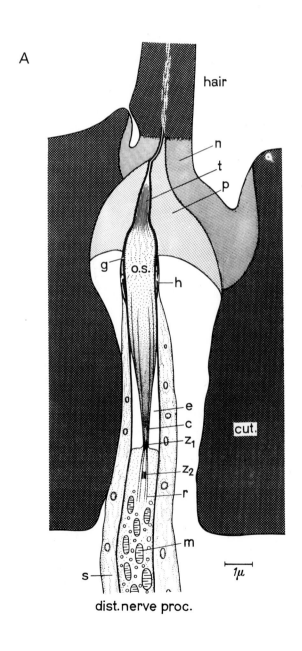

**B**

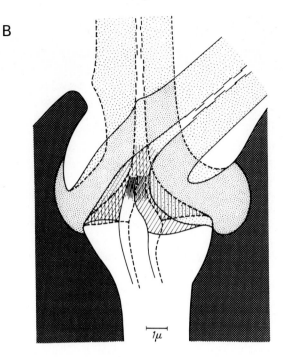

Fig. 84 A and B. A. Diagram of a mechanoreceptor hair-plate sensillum of the bee (THURM, 1965a, b). In A: *c* ciliary structure; *cut* cuticle; *e* extracellular space; *g* granules; *h* cuticular sheath; *m* mitochondria; *n* joint (hair) membrane; *o.s.* peripheral segment; *p* cap; *r* root fibers (cross-striated root); *s* Schwann or trichogenic cell; *t* tubular body; $Z_1 Z_2$ centriole. B. The distortions of the hair base with bending of the hair: resting position—dashed lines; maximally bent position—solid lines. From photomicrographs of a section *in vitro*

peripheral process of the receptor cell to the base of a cap cell. As in other mechanoreceptor cells, a structure analogous to the tubular body of other mechanoreceptor sensilla can be observed in the apical area of the flagellum of chordotonal and tympanic organs. This structure is probably the receptive sector of the receptor cell, where the primary processes of reception of a mechanical stimulus take place.

Indeed, data obtained by a number of authors (GOLDMAN, 1965; GÖRNER, 1965; THURM, 1965a, 1965b), as well as by IVANOV in our laboratory (1968, 1969a, 1969b) show that the structural organization of receptor cells in the mechanoreceptor hair organs of certain insects (*Acilius sulcatus, Apis mellifera, Culex pipiens,* etc.) hardly differs at all from that of the tympanic organ of the locust, as investigated by GRAY (1960). The only differences are those found in the cuticular section of mechanoreceptors, a short, needlelike hair connected to the upper edge of the hair canal by a thin connective membrane. The base of the hair protrudes slightly into the canal cavity and is connected, in turn, to the canal walls by means of an accessory hair membrane (Fig. 84). The peripheral process extended by the receptor cell toward the base of the hair attaches in the area of a notch located on the surface of the hair.

It is assumed (THURM, 1965a, 1965b) that bending of the hair, which in this case acts as a rigid bar (this fact is readily confirmed by direct observations), leads to the appearance of mechanical stresses in the region of the hair base, which is connected to the canal walls by means of the accessory hair membrane. It is natural to assume that the latter has the properties of a flat spring, i.e. it is capable of bending under the action of applied forces but cannot stretch or contract (IVANOV, 1969a, 1969b). Deformation of the hair in the region of its base in turn causes a stretching of the scolopoid membrane connected to the walls of the notch. Running inside the scolopoid membrane is the peripheral process of the receptor cell: this process contains a special structure—the tubular body—in the region subjected to deformation as a result of the events described above, and this leads in the final account to the appearance of the generator potential in the receptor cell.

According to THURM (1965a, 1965b), the compression of the peripheral process of the receptor cell at the level of the tubular body is an adequate stimulus for this mechanoreceptor. The threshold is approximately equal to a 2% bending of the cuticular hair, corresponding to a variation of 30Å in the diameter of the nerve ending, or 0.5% if the diameter is of the order of 0.6 μm. THURM (1965a, 1965b) points out that the latent period of the receptor potential in hair plates, Vater-Pacini corpuscles, and muscle spindles is more or less identical and equal to 0.2 msec. The similarity of the receptor potential in muscle spindle and in hair plates is remarkable. The relationship between the receptor reaction and oxygen supply is also similar. Thus, 2 minutes after the start of oxygen deprivation (anoxia), generation of the receptor potential decreases in hair plates, and after 10 minutes it is almost completely blocked. We think this fact suggests that during the deformation of the membranes, some kind of active biochemical processes occur and that these precede the disruption of the ionic equilibrium and depolarization.

Thus, the problem of the stimulation of the plasma membrane at the moment of its deformation by a mechanical stimulus is a very complex one. In a special analysis of this problem, GOLDMAN (1965) considers several possibilities: 1. the membrane possesses piezoelectric properties, i.e. electric discharges can be generated directly at the expense of a mechanical shift; 2. pressure may exert a direct effect on the structure of the membrane; 3. mechanical forces may filter water through the membrane, thus creating a "streaming potential"; 4. there may be formation or dissociation of some kind of substance that exerts an effect on the properties of the membrane; 5. the permeability of the membrane undergoes a change under the action of a mechanical force. The last assumption is the most generally accepted, since it results from tests in which the stimulus and the electric reaction are recorded simultaneously. Thus, 10% compression from both sides of a circular peripheral ending (terminal) will cause a 0.5% change in the surface area of its membrane, provided the volume is constant, yielding a depolarization of 10 mV. A similar depolarization can be induced by a doubling of the $Na^+$ permeability of the membrane. If the molecules in the membrane have hexagonal packing, a free space equal to about 10% remains between the molecules. In the case of square packing, this free space would be equal to 25%. Consequently, an increase of only 0.5% in the area of the membrane surface corresponds to many times that increase in the free space. Thus, when the membrane undergoes deformation it acts as a nonspecific structure, which in this case is inevitably subjected to depolarization. How, then is the specific nature of the information on the force and character of the mechanical stimulus conveyed? There is no answer to this question. It does not help to refer to the presence of ATPase in the membrane (MIRKIN, TUCHKOV, and MASHANSKII, 1967; MASHANSKII and MIRKIN, 1969), since ATPase is found in any kind of membrane, and its function is to provide an energy supply for the structure of the membrane and all processes taking place in this membrane, sometimes even intensifying these processes. Recently, synaptic structures revealing the activity of acetylcholinesterase were demonstrated between the inner bulb cells and the nerve endings of Vater-Pacini corpuscles. These findings seem to testify to cholinergic (mechanochemical-) processes taking place during stimulation of the Vater-Pacini corpuscles (CHERNIGOVSKII, MIRKIN, and MASHANSKII; pers. comm.).

In our opinion, particular specific proteins must be built in into the plasma membrane of every mechanoreceptor and changes in the conformation of these proteins under the effect of a transformed or direct mechanical stimulus would constitute the trigger mechanism that causes the subsequent depolarization of the receptor cell in the sensilla. Now, the chordotonal and tympanic organs of insects appear to be mechanoreceptor structures, capable of picking up acoustic frequencies, that have been progressively modified during the process of evolution. There is thus no reason to exclude the presence in the peripheral processes of these organs of some kind of specific molecular mechanism, at least in the region of the cap cells discovered by us in Corti's organ of vertebrates. Future investigations will, we hope, disclose the character of the specific molecular processes that occur not only in the hearing organ of insects but also in mechanoreceptors in general.

## 3. Theories of Hearing

Contemporary theories of hearing attempt to answer the question: in what manner does the direct stimulation of hair cells in the organ of Corti take place as the result of a complex cycle of energy transformations of an acoustic stimulus, occurring in the outer, middle and inner ear?

As mentioned above, the mechanoelectrical theory of DAVIS (1958) postulates that the movement of the basilar and tectorial membranes induced by a sound effect causes bending of the stereocilia of the hair cells as a result of the appearance of shearing forces. Davis thinks such bending is quite sufficient to cause a change in membrane permeability, i.e. a change in the ionic equilibrium of the plasma membrane coating the stereocilia[1]. As a result of the depolarization

---

[1] Our objections concerning a possible bending of stereocilia (VINNIKOV and TITOVA, 1961, 1964) must be rejected in view of the fact mentioned above, that the apices of the stereocilia are attached to the lower surface of the tectorial membrane. Naturally, the movement of this membrane must be transmitted somehow to the stereocilia; however, this movement cannot be observed visually.

of the stereocilia of the receptor cell a bioelectrical reaction takes place, and this may cause direct electrical stimulation of the nerve endings near the hair cell. DAVIS (1960, 1961) does not exclude the probability of discharge of a mediator into the synaptic cleft under the effect of a receptor potential, although he tends to favor an ephaptic mechanism. Thus, DAVIS's mechanoelectrical theory assumes a dual transformation of energy during the perception of a sound stimulus: 1. transformation of mechanical into electrical energy in the stereocilia region of receptor cells, and possibly 2. transformation of electrical into chemical energy in the synapse region.

The cytochemical theory (VINNIKOV and TITOVA, 1961, 1963, 1964) postulates that the movement of the basilar and tectorial membranes due to the appearance of shearing forces caused by sound effects leads to the penetration of acetylcholine into the stereocilia region, i.e. into the apex of the receptor cell, which is located under the tectorial membrane washed by what is called Corti's lymph. The presence of acetylcholine in the endolymph, as already mentioned, has been detected by a number of investigators (MARTINI, 1941; DACHA and MARTINI, 1942; GISSELSON, 1950; PLUZHNIKOV and YANTAREVA, 1971; KIBYAKOV et al., 1973). It is still not clear to us which cells of the organ of Corti secrete the acetylcholine which is dissolved in the endo- and perilymph, although acetylcholine ore GABA (FLOCK, 1974) is no doubt synthesized in the inner hair cells and involves the processes in the afferent synapses. It is conceivable that this occurs beyond the limits of the space occupied by Corti's lymph, for the constant presence of acetylcholine here is hard to imagine from a physiological standpoint. It appears that quanta of acetylcholine are released into the stereocilia region and into the cavity occupied by Corti's lymph (which is bounded by the inner surface of the tectorial membrane and the outer surface of the hair cells) during adequate sinusoidal vibrations of the basilar and tectorial membranes (BÉKÉSY, 1952c, 1958a), and during movements of the endo- and perilymph under the effect of vibrations of the stapes and other middle ear ossicles, occurring during the action of a sound wave on the outer ear.

According to present concepts, the secreted acetylcholine must react with a specific choline receptor, which is apparently localized in the plasma membrane of stereocilia, after which it is hydrolyzed by acetylcholinesterase, which is also located, as was established cytochemically, in the stereocilia (VINNIKOV and TITOVA, 1961; VINNIKOV and TITOVA, 1961, 1964; KANEKO and DALY, 1969). When we first published our theory (VINNIKOV and TITOVA, 1961, 1964), we assumed, along with some other investigators (KARASIK, 1946; ZUPANČIČ et al., 1958), that the receptor centers for acetylcholine are bound to acetylcholinesterase. However, there is now no doubt that acetylcholine is primarily bound to an independent cholinoreceptive protein located in the postśynaptic membrane, and that the role of the acetylcholinesterase located alongside the acetylcholine is limited merely to its hydrolysis (BARLOW, 1955, 1960; NACHMANSON, 1958; MIKHELSON and ZEIMAL, 1967, 1970). Thus, the interaction of acetylcholine from the endolymph, transferred into the region of Corti's lymph, with the choline receptor present in the stereocilia of hair cells, constitutes the primary trigger mechanism which causes a change in the ionic permeability of the membrane, i.e. induces depolarization. At the same time, this interaction is the starting point for triggering a number of enzymic reactions in the cytoplasm of hair cells, which finally lead to the release of another quantum of acetylcholine mediator into the synaptic membrane region of nerve endings, where it again interacts with a corresponding choline receptor and, after undergoing hydrolysis by the acetylcholinesterase localized here, constitutes the energy source for the action currents arising along the course of nerve fibers. Thus, the plasma membrane of stereocilia in the organ of Corti is comparable to a synaptic membrane.

In this section, we are not discussing the chemical characteristics of acetylcholine and acetylcholinesterase, since a detailed discussion is given in our book (VINNIKOV and TITOVA, 1961, 1964). We shall just consider briefly the molecular organization of the choline receptor. At the present time, the majority of researchers believe that the choline receptor is a protein (EHRENPREIS, 1960; TURPAEV, 1962; TAKAGI, AKAO, and TAKAHASHI, 1965; DE ROBERTIS, 1970). The interaction of the choline receptor with acetylcholine takes place mainly at the expense of the anionic group (the active center of the choline receptor) with which the cationic head of acetylcholine interacts, and also with some kind of polarized group in the choline receptor, reacting with the ester portion of the acetylcholine molecule according to the dipole–dipole interaction principle (Fig. 21) (BARLOW, 1955, 1960).

We believe that contemporary concepts concerning the mutual arrangement of individual molecules of the choline receptor on the postsynaptic membrane are of great importance (Fig. 22). According to one hypothesis, for instance, neighboring molecules of the choline receptor are arranged on the postsynaptic membrane of skeletal muscles in such a way that their anionic sectors are separated by a distance corresponding to the length of a polymethylene chain containing 10 atoms (about 14Å) (WASSER, 1959) or 16 atoms (BARLOW, 1960). It is possible that the qualitative characteristics of a cholinoreceptive protein in the plasma membrane of stereocilia, as against its synaptic characteristics, are associated with the special way this protein is built into the membrane; this may impart to the cholinoreceptor protein some kind of energetic or kinetic advantages that enable it to effect a transforming, i.e. encoding, function with respect to the sound stimulus. It should be noted that MIKHELSON (1967) was the first to draw attention to the presence of evolutionary laws governing the distribution and organization of cholinoreceptive protein molecules in the postsynaptic membrane.

One way or another, the converion of the acoustic stimulus is finally realized by the interaction of acetylcholine with the choline receptor. This interaction, in turn, is regulated by the enzymic activity of acetylcholinesterase. This process, in our opinion, is the primary trigger mechanism, specific for receptor cells in the organ of Corti. It is important to emphasize that, under the conditions present in Corti's organ, the interaction between acetylcholine and cholinoreceptor molecules occurs in exactly the same way as in any synaptic membrane. However, we still do not know what amounts of acetylcholine molecules, cholinoreceptive protein and acetylcholinesterase have to be supplied to effect the transformation and perception of the energy of a single sound-wave molecule or, more likely, of some kind of acoustic frequency. We can only hope that future research will allow us to understand the processes taking place in the plasma membrane region of stereocilia. In this respect, NAFTALIN's (1966) research appears very encouraging.

At first glance, the mechanoelectric and cytochemical theories of hearing, thought both resting on more or less reliable facts, appear to be mutually exclusive. In fact, we believe that they supplement each other. According to the cytochemical theory, the molecular interaction of acetylcholine with the choline receptor takes place at the moment when shearing forces appear between the bending stereocilia and the tectorial membrane, thus causing a disruption of the ionic equilibrium. And indeed, KOICHEV (1969a, 1969b) in our laboratory, employing the electron cytochemistry method of KOMNICK (1962), has shown that $Na^+$ cytochemical reaction products, represented by $NaSb(OH)_6$ granules, are present in the hair cells of Corti's organ when they are in a state of relative rest, mainly in the plasma membrane region of the stereocilia (Figs. 95 and 96). Under acoustic effect and in accordance with the frequency reception gradient in the cochlea, a sharp increase is observed in the size and number of granules present in the plasma membrane of stereocilia. These granules increase in size up to 1,500—2,500 Å.

It is believed that $Na^+$ enters the cell from Corti's lymph and the endolymph. Because of the low concentration of $Na^+$ in the endolymph this seems improbable. However, as stated above, the potential difference between the receptor cell and the endolymph may be as much as 150 mV (BÉKÉSY, 1960a). Thus, the equilibrium concentration of $Na^+$ in the cell must be approximately 400 times that in the endolymph, so that the electric gradient would permit $Na^+$ to enter the cell. Unfortunately, nothing can yet be stated about the movement of $K^+$ ions during the stimulation of hair cells. However, it was found that when the endolymph is replaced by the perilymph, i.e. when the $K^+$ concentration falls in the stereocilia region, a noticeable suppression of the microphonic potential sets in (TASAKI, 1960; KONISHI, KELSEY, and SINGLETON, 1966). Under the light microscope a change was observed in the nature of the cytochemical reaction to $K^+$ in the receptor cells of the organ of Corti following a sound stimulus (KAWATA, TAKEDA, and HAYATA, 1963).

As mentioned above, certain authors (TONNDORF, DUVAL, and RENEAU, 1962; RAUCH, 1964) assume that the space between the hair cells and the tectorial membrane is completely separate from the endolymph and represents the "subtectorial" lymph. It is also assumed that the composition of this lymph is close to that of the intercellular fluid and that it contains a large amount of $Na^+$ (RAUCH, 1964). However, according to the data of KOICHEV (1969a, 1969b), granules of the reaction product are never found in the subtectorial space, although we cannot rule out the possibility that they may be washed out in the course of preparation of the specimen.

Thus, with the aid of electron cytochemistry it is possible to detect and localize the changes in the ionic equilibrium that occur during acoustic stimulation (at least for $Na^+$) primarily in the stereocilia region of receptor cells; these changes must be accompanied by depolarization of the membrane and the appearance of a receptor microphonic potential. This shift in the ionic equilibrium and the appearance of biopotentials is, in our opinion, preceded by a primary molecular interaction of acetylcholine in the endolymph with a choline receptor and with acetylcholinesterase in the plasma membrane region of stereocilia. Thus, the appearance of biopotentials and subsequent changes in the ultrastructural and cytochemical organization of hair cells are secondary processes, which in turn lead to the appearance of a nerve impulse in the synaptic region and of action currents in the acoustic nerve. Thus, acoustic reception includes two steps: 1. molecular interactions between acetylcholine and cholinoreceptive protein in the plasma membrane of the stereocilium, i. e. the encoding of the transformed sound wave into information; 2. transmission of the encoded information in the form of a biopotential through the synapses to the central nervous system.

Thus it will be seen that the cytochemical and mechanoelectric theories of hearing supplement each other very well. In the light of these theories, it is advisable to examine the structural and cytochemical organization of receptor hair cells in vertebrates and insects, both under relative rest and acoustic stimulation conditions.


# 4. Structural and Cytochemical Organization of Hair Cells in the Organ of Corti in Birds*

Birds and mammals represent two independent evolutionary branches of warm-blooded animals, which became separated a short while before the start of the Upper Carboniferous period, i.e. 250 million years ago. Therefore, it is not surprising that there are a number of differences in the structure of the hearing organ of birds and mammals, although this organ developed on the basis of a common ancestral receptor sector in the labyrinth, known as the papilla acustica, which was already present in amphibians and well developed in lower reptiles (DE BURLET, 1934). It is characteristic of the anatomical structure of the hearing organ in birds (and higher reptiles) that in the sacculus region the labyrinth forms a long sac-shaped outgrowth—the cochlear duct. This is homolog of the cochlea in mammals, the only difference being that its distal portion contains a lagenar macula not found in mammals (Fig. 85). Along the length of the cochlear duct, the elongated Corti's organ is located on the basilar membrane, attached by means of a skeletal frame. It consists of supporting and receptor hair cells their surface being coated with a tectorial membrane. The cochlear duct is bounded from above by the so-called tegumentum vasculosum, which plays the role of the stria vascularis and Reissner's membrane in the cochlea of mammals.

Recently, TITOVA (1968) carried out a special investigation by cytochemical and electron microscopic methods on the embryonic development of the organ of Corti in birds. The cochlear duct in the chick could be first recognized separately from the sacculus on the 7th day of incubation. It represents a blind closed sac, carrying at its anterior end the basis of the lagenar macula.

---

* There are not data on the ultrastructural and cytochemical organization of the organ of Corti in reptiles (e.g. crocodile).

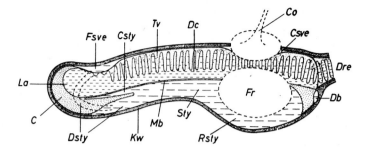

Fig. 85. Diagram of longitudinal section through the inner ear of birds (SCHWARTZKOPFF, 1963). *C* cartilage; *Co* columella; *Csty* Cavum scale tympani; *Csve* cisterna of scale vestibuli; *Db* ductus brevis; *Dc* ductus cochlearis; *Dre* ductus reunion; *Dsty* ductus scale tympani; *Fr* fenestra ovalis; *Fsve* Fossa scale vestibuli; *Kw* osseous wall; *La* lagena; *Mb* basillar membrane; *Rsty* Recessus scale tympani; *Sty* scale tympani; *Tv* tegmentum vasculosum

In the receptor epithelium of the organ of Corti, a subdivision into receptor and supporting cells can be already observed. The future receptor cells are situated in the upper portion of the receptor layer, and the supporting cells extend from its free surface to the basilar membrane. On the summit of many cells distinguished by their polymorphism, the electron microscope reveals a kinocilium developing from the centrosome and containing $9 \times 2 + 2$ fibrils. In the cellular cytoplasm, elements of the rough endoplasmic reticulum and individual ribosomes, as well as circular mitochondria can clearly be seen. On the summits of individual cells, initial development stages of stereocilia can also be observed; these are formed by a protrusion (bulging of the cytoplasm of the microvilli type) and are characterized by high electron density. The cytoplasm in this region has a finely fibrous or granular character which is also typical for the cytoplasm of stereocilia of definitive forms. The plasma membrane of the cell extends continuously over the stereocilia. At these stages, the receptor epithelium exhibits an intense reaction to nucleic acids (RNA and DNA), as well as to total protein and functional groups of protein molecules. On the 8—9th day of incubation large numbers of nerve fibers become attached to the rudiment of the receptor epithelium; these fibers grow into the epithelium and on the 10th day reach the base of the future receptor cells. However, on the 9th day of incubation, the concentration of nucleic acids in the cells drops, as well as the total protein content. Differentiation processes in the cochlear duct of birds do not take place at the same time along its entire length; they start at the base and gradually move toward the summit. In the base of the cochlear duct, there is already a clearcut subdivision of cellular elements into receptor and supporting elements. The receptor cells have a cubical shape and a tapered summit (apex), which is connected to neighboring cells by means of desmosomes. Stereocilia and a single kinocilium branch out from the apex (the future cuticula). The cytoplasm of the receptor cell has high electron density and is rich in organoids; the nucleus is round. The RNA content is high in the apical region. Supporting cells have lower electron density and are not as rich in organoids; their nucleus is oval.

On the 13th day of incubation, the tectorial membrane appears over the receptor cells in the base region of the cochlear duct. This membrane has insignificant electron density and appears to be composed of an amorphous or weakly granular substance. Over the apices of the receptor cells the membrane forms dome-shaped protrusions, the "helmet-shaped spaces" of HELD (1926). Above the microvilli of supporting cells, on the contrary, a concentration of membrane substance is observed. The structural and cytochemical differences between receptor and supporting cells continue to increase. From the 15th day, and especially on the 18—19th days of incubation, the receptor cells of Corti's organ appear to be fully differentiated.

The activity of oxidative enzymes (succinate dehydrogenase and cytochromoxidase) in mitochondria of receptor cells in the organ of Corti increases steeply as the organ becomes more and more differentiated.

It should be pointed out that the activity of acetylcholinesterase, already observable on the 4—7th days of incubation, can be traced for the first time on the 8th day in the bud of the cochlear ganglion, then from the 12th to the 19th day in the region of the synapses of nerve endings with the receptor cells. During the same stages, the enzymic activity of acetylcholinesterase is simultaneously observed in the stereocilia region.

The histological structure of the definitive organ of Corti in birds was investigated mainly by HELD (1928). VINNIKOV, OSIPOVA, TITOVA, and GOVARDOVSKII (1965) and GOGNIASHVILI (1967a—1967c) and recently TAKASAKA and SMITH (1971) have studied it with the aid of the electron microscope in hens and pigeons. The organ of Corti consists, as mentioned, of receptor and supporting cells (Fig. 86). All receptor cells have an identical structure. The number of receptor cells in birds is considerably greater than in mammals. Up to 40 cells may be counted in a transverse section through the organ of Corti, which is covered by a coarsely fibrous tectorial membrane. The receptor cells are arranged in one row and are shaped like short cylinders with a rounded base and a more or less expanding apex. The surface of these cells is limited by a cuticular platelet from which stereocilia and one kinocilia branch out. A circular nucleus is located closer to the base of the cell. Cytochemical studies disclose a high content of RNA, total protein and functional groups of protein molecules in the cellular cytoplasm; the latter are particularly distinct in the cuticula and in the hair. The cuticula and the hairs (antennae) of the receptor cells are in fact separated from the lumen of the cochlear duct by a tectorial membrane that lies on top of them and is characterized by a high content of total protein and functional groups. The bases of the hair cells are located on supporting cells, which adhere firmly to the hair cells at the sides and emerge with their narrowed round heads onto the surface of the organ, forming the so-called phalangeal bridges. The phalanges are characterized by a high content of protein and functional groups. Thus, the hair cells, having a lining of supporting elements, do not come into direct contact with the basilar membrane.

A high activity of acetylcholinesterase is observed in the synapse region, thus indicating that a cholinergic system takes part in conducting a nerve impulse in the organ of Corti in birds (TITOVA and VINNIKOV, 1964). The same enzyme is found in the region of the antennae under the tectorial membrane. It should be noted that there is exceptionally high activity of oxidizing enzymes, especially cytochromoxidase, in mitochrondria of receptor cells in the organ of Corti of birds. The receptor cells are also characterized by a high content of nucleic acids.

In the electron microscope the plasma membrane of receptor cells and the structure of antennae branching off from the cuticula are clearly seen. These antennae constitute a bundle of 50–60–80–90–120–150 stereocilia. Near this bundle, a single kinocilium, in which 9 pairs of peripheral and as a rule 2 central fibrils are present, branches off in all cells directly from the free cuticula of the apical cytoplasm. At their proximal end the stereocilia are equipped with a characteristic basal body. Most cells are polarized in a direction parallel to the transverse axis (pointing to the inferior edge) but some on the dotted

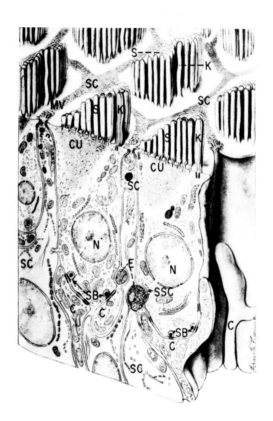

Fig. 86. Schematic drawing showing three-dimensional view of hair cells and supporting cells pigeon's basilar papilla (TAKASAKA and SMITH, 1971). Three hair cells are sectioned across the front to demonstrate their intracellular structure. On the right, whole cells have been removed to show the contour of sensory cells plus nerve endings. The microvillous tufts (MV) on the supporting cell surfaces (SC) form thick angular borders about each sensory cell. Each hair bundle is composed of a large number of stereocilia (S), which show a stepwise increment in height, and one long kinocilium (K). Cochlear nerve endings (C) are finger-like, with one or two processes (two cells at right) or clublike, with membrane thickenings and synaptic balls (SB). Efferent terminals are small (E). SSC subsynaptic cisterna; N nucleus; CU cuticula

area (above the fibrocartilaginous plate), have a more diagonal polarization (TAKASAKA and SMITH, 1971). The stereocilia are connected to the cuticula at their proximal ends by means of a radicular filament; at their distal ends, they terminate in small blunt heads, the apex of which has high electron density. The stereocilia heads fit into special niches located on the inner surface of the coarse-grained tectorial membrane. A clear homogeneous interlayer is present between the substance of the membrane and the head of the stereocilium and can be considered as the cement by which the stereocilium is securely attached to the tectorial membrane. Three types of receptor cells can be distinguished: tall, short and intermediate, and they differ in their localization on the basilar membrane. The length of the tall hair cells ranges from 11 to 25 µm with diameter 5 µm. They occupy the area over the superior fibrocartilaginous plate plus a small part of the free basilar membrane. The short hair cells are located on the free basilar membrane but are present only in the proximal 3 mm of the papilla; they range in height from 7—11 µm, and in surface diameter from 10 to 17 µm. The intermediate cells are intermediate in height as well as position, being from 10 to 23 µm high (TAKASAKA and SMITH, 1971).

Adjacent to the base of a receptor cell are nerve endings, which form synaptic contacts with this cell. The nerve endings are button-shaped and of two types: large ones having a "clear" neuroplasm and containing rod-shaped mitochondria and a small number of synaptic vesicles, and fine "dark" ones, poor in mitochondria and filled with synaptic vesicles. Apparently, the fine "dark" nerve endings are efferent endings (BOORD, 1961). In the synapse region the presynaptic membrane is usually greatly thickened. The synaptic structures were studied for the first time by CORDIER (1964) and recently by VINNIKOV et al. (1965) and TAKASAKA and SMITH (1971).

Thus, the structure of the organ of Corti in birds, as we shall see below, greatly resembles the lateral-line organ and the cristae and maculae of the vestibular labyrinth. This is due to the presence of a single polarized kinocilium along with a bundle of stereocilia. In all probability this polarization also reflects the direction of the stimulus, i.e. its propagation along the basilar and tectorial membranes. As we know, the appearance of shearing forces is assumed to occur here, with endolymph streams taking part along with membranes. This phenomenon is accompanied by the onset of biopotentials, i.e. a microphonic or receptor potential in receptor cells and action currents in the nerve fibers. By analogy with other sense organs of the labyrinth, we can assume that action currents are enhanced if the direction of the stimulation is toward the stereocilia, and inhibited if the stimulation is toward the kinocilium (FLOCK and WERSÄLL, 1962a, 1962b; WERSÄLL and FLOCK, 1963; FLOCK, 1965a, 1965b). However, accurate experimental data are needed in this respect.

As already mentioned, birds can perceive frequencies within the range 40 to 20,000 cps (KNECHT, 1939, 1940). Exactly where the cells capable of perceiving low and high frequencies are located in the organ of Corti of birds has still not been clarified. According to MAZO's (1955, 1958) hypothetical data, receptors capable of perceiving low tones are situated near the apex of the organ of Corti and receptors capable of perceiving high tones at its base. However, the presence of a location gradient for the perception of high and low frequencies in the organ of Corti of birds has been demonstrated in our laboratory in a sufficiently reliable manner by GOGNIASHVILI (1967 a—1967 c), using histochemical methods. He was able to establish that after both high- and low-frequency sound stimulation changes are observed in the organ of Corti of birds in the

A

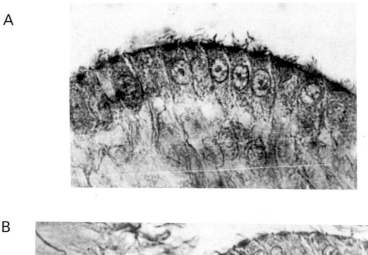

B

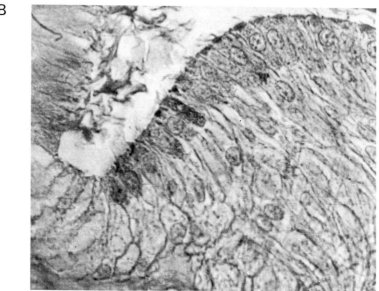

distribution and content of a number of biologically active chemical substances: nucleic acids, total protein and functional groups of protein molecules (COOH, SH, SS-SH) (Fig. 87 A, B). Under the effect of low frequencies (300 cps, 95 db) changes occurred throughout the length of the cochlear duct, whereas under the effect of high frequencies (1,500 cps, 95 db) changes occurred nearer to its base. Following stimulation of the organ, the most characteristic changes were observed in the distribution of nucleic acids. These changes consisted in the disappearance of RNA granules previously observed in the cytoplasm, and in the appearance in the cytoplasm of the basal portion of the cell of a fine, rod-shaped or circular formation, containing RNA and adhering to the outside of the nuclear membrane. This phenomenon represents the exit of nuclear RNA into the cytoplasm (Fig. 87 C). In addition, during short periods of adequate stimulation, there is an increase in the concentration of protein and its functional groups (SH, SS-SH, COOH) in individual receptor cells. No distinct shifts in the enzymic activity of acetylcholinesterase could be detected in the stereocilia region.

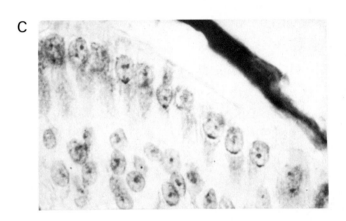

Fig. 87 A—C. Variation in the content of biologically active compounds in receptor cells of the hen's organ of Corti under the effect of sound (GOGNIASHVILI, 1967a—c). A. Total protein distribution under relative rest conditions; B. Same, in the cochlear base region subjected to the effect of sound (1,500 cps, 25 db) for 30 min; C. RNA distribution in the receptor cell, following exposure to sound (300 cps, 95 db) for 30 min. Escape of RNA from the nucleolus into the cytoplasm. For A and B treatment according to DANIELLI, for C according to BRACHET. Immersion, objective 60, eyepiece 7

The cytochemical data are supported by the pattern of shifts observed in the ultrastructural organization of the hair receptor cells along the length of the cochlear duct, depending upon the frequency and the duration of the sound stimulus applied. These shifts are manifested in a rounding and migration of mitochondria into the apical portion of the cell under the cuticula and into the region of the nucleus and the base of the cell, where they exhibit the phenomenon of adherence to the nuclear or pre-synaptic membrane. In this region there is intensive formation of rough endoplasmic reticulum membranes; mitochondria may also adhere to this rough endoplasmic reticulum. In the nucleus, migration of the nucleolus toward the inner surface of the nuclear membrane and the passage of individual ribosomes through the pores of the nuclear membrane into the cytoplasm are observed. In both afferent and efferent nerve endings there is a sharp increase in size and a rounding of individual mitochondria, as well as a decrease in the number of synaptic vesicles in the neuroplasm of efferent endings.

We must note that the above cytochemical and ultrastuctural shifts in the receptor cells are observed when birds (hens and pigeons) are subjected to both low-frequency (300 cps, 95 db) and high-frequency (1,500 cps, 95 db) sound. In the first case these shifts are observed in the organ of Corti at the distal end of the duct, and in the second case at the proximal end, thus clearly demonstrating the presence of a gradient in the perception of sound frequencies along the length of the duct. However, in both cases during sound stimulation, one observes among the receptor cells showing distinct shifts in their cytochemical and ultrastructural organization individual cells whose organization is the same as that of control cells, i.e. the receptor cells of the organ of Corti in a state of relative rest.

## 5. Structural and Cytochemical Organization of Hair Cells of the Organ of Corti in Mammals

The organ of Corti of mammals has been rather fully investigated in regard to its structural, cytochemical and in part biochemical organization, as well as its functional organization (ENGSTRÖM, 1955, 1958, 1960a, 1960b, 1961; SMITH, 1954, 1957; IURATO, 1960, 1961, 1962a, 1962b, 1962c; SMITH and SJÖSTRAND, 1961; VINNIKOV and TITOVA 1961, 1963, 1964; RAUCH, 1964; ENGSTRÖM and ADES, 1960; ENGSTRÖM, ADES, and ANDERSON, 1966; WERSÄLL, FLOCK, and LUNDQUIST, 1965; TITOVA et al., 1968). Of particularly great importance is the method of *in vitro* isolation of the cochlea, which made it possible to carry out direct observations of the structure of Corti's organ *in vivo* (VINNIKOV and TITOVA, 1959, 1961, 1964).

The embryonic development of the organ of Corti in mammals has been studied by TITOVA (1968). In goat and sheep embryos of 9 mm head-to-coccyx length and in 17-day-old rabbit embryos, the cochlear duct is an oval, blindly closed tube; its base consists of a pseudostratified epithelium. In 11-mm-long goat embryos the cochlear duct starts to bend. The nuclei of cells in the pseudostratified epithelium move toward the base of the cells, the cytoplasm becomes vacuolated, and a cuticular border is formed on the apical surface. These cells have a high content of RNA, DNA and protein. The mesenchyma surrounding the duct becomes thickened, although the process of cartilage formation does not yet take place. The spiral ganglion is still poorly differentiated; however, in its dorsocaudal portion it is possible to detect, by silver impregnation, nerve fibers extending toward and growing into the pseudostratified epithelium.

It was noted long ago that processes involving a differentiation of all the components of the cochlear duct, including the receptor cells, begin in its basal portion and gradually move towards the apex (BOETTCHER, 1869; VAN DER STRICHT, 1918; ALEXANDER, 1926; HELD, 1926; KOLMER, 1927; WEIBEL, 1957). In 40-mm-long embryos the cochlear duct already has 1.5 coils, and in 60-mm-long embryos 2.5 coils. At different levels, i.e. coils, of the cochlear duct we find different degrees of differentiation of the cellular elements.

On an apical section across the posterior end of the basal coil we can see that the pseudostratified epithelium of the base forms two hillocks with a small groove between them, namely the start of the formation of the tunnel. Under this groove, a large blood vessel is located in the connective tissue. The cells forming the hillocks are characterized by their basophilic cytoplasm. The irregular apical surface of the cells expands slightly and located on top of it is a dark, homogeneous film, representing the initial stage of formation of the tectorial membrane. Attention is focused on two divergent cells with a light cytoplasm, large nuclei, and a small vacuole; these represent the initial stage of formation of the tunnel and of pillar cells. Located on the surface behind these cells are three large cells with large oval nuclei and a well-developed nucleolus — the future outer hair cells. According to the electron microscope data of NAKAI and HILDING (1968), in a 22-day-old rabbit embryo the future organ of Corti (on its apical coil) consists of a 2- or 3-layer epithelium, located on the basal membrane. At their summits, the cells are connected by desmosomes. The above authors were unable to observe any receptor or supporting cells. However, at the summit of each cell, a pair of centrioles without kinocilia can be detected. Microvilli are present, but the tectorial membrane is absent, as well as the nerve fibers and nerve endings. The lower coil in the cochlea of the same embryo is well advanced in its development. Here, hair cells and clear efferent endings are well differentiated, although distinct patterns of synapse formation cannot yet be seen. On the apical surface short, thick stereocilia, differing from microvilli, are already visible, while thin kinocilia containing $9 \times 2 + 2$ fibrils branch off from the marginal, more transparent portion of the cell. A cross-striated rootlet can branch off from the basal body; the outline of the tectorial membrane can already be seen. In a 27-day-old rabbit embryo, it is possible to observe the penetration of clear efferent nerve fibers deep into the cytoplasm of hair cells; after the birth of the animal the usual synaptic contact is observed here. NAKAI and HILDING draw the unexpected conclusion that the differentiation of hair cells takes place independently of the synaptic contacts with nerve endings, although they had previously described how nerve endings grow into the cytoplasm of future hair cells.

The inner and outer hair cells grow with their axes at an angle to each other. On the apical surface of these cells intensely staining cuticular platelets are observed (HELD, 1926) and from these branch out a bundle of hairs as was observed under the light microscope (VAN DER STRICHT, 1918), that is stereocilia and one kinocilium containing $9 \times 2 + 2$ fibrils as has been now confirmed under the electron microscope (Fig. 88) (KIMURA, 1968; SHIRO and KYOZO, 1967). As already mentioned, the kinocilium is lost in the definitive stages and only its basal body is preserved (Fig. 82 B). Both the cuticula and the hair cells, according to the data of TITOVA (1968), have a low RNA content. The hair cells are rich in total protein and thiol groups and poor in carboxyl groups. The nuclei of the cells are shifted into their basal portions. The subnuclear portion gradually narrows down and the cell assumes its typical shape. RNA is present in the cytoplasm in a moderate concentration.

Leaving aside a description of the cytochemical organization of supporting cells in the organ of Corti, the role of which would require a special investigation, we shall only mention that much greater concentrations of nucleic acids, protein and protein carboxyl groups are found in the cytoplasm and in the nucleus of neurons of the spiral ganglion, during these stages.

We believe that the appearance of acetylcholinesterase (see below), and of cholinoreceptive protein, in stereocilia corresponds not only to the appearance

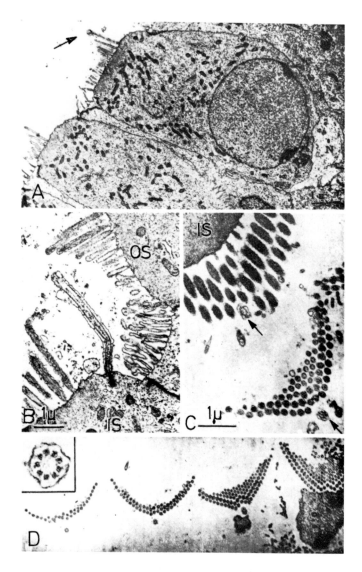

Fig. 88 A—D. Organ of Corti of a one-day-old mouse (R. KIMURA, 1966). A—B. Cilium and centriole in the inner (*IS*) and outer (*OS*) hair cells. C. Cilia (arrows) of both inner (*IS*) and outer (*OS*) sensory cells oriented in the same direction. D. Cross section of 4 outer hair cells. The bundle of stereocilia is shaped like the letter "W" with the kinocilium located at its base. Numerous microvilli can be seen. The magnification is shown by the scale bar

of acetylcholine in the endolymph but also to the synthesis of acetylcholinesterase and cholinoreceptive protein in the postsynaptic membranes of nerve endings. The synthesis of this protein and its localization in stereocilia can be considered as a special mutation that enables the auditory cell to act as transducer of the information carried by acoustic frequencies.

The differentiation of hair cells is accompanied by a marked increase in the activity of oxidizing enzymes in the axoplasm and in the mitochondria, and also in the numerous afferent and efferent nerve fibers running close to the base of the cells and forming synaptic contacts with them. According to the data of DEL BO and CONTI (1961), immediately after birth acetylcholinesterase activity is found only in the basal coil; after several days it is found along the entire length of the cochlear duct.

Thus, studies of the structural and cytochemical differentiation of the auditory cell in the organ of Corti of mammals, as well as of birds, have enabled us to trace the development of the molecular receptive mechanism in the region of the stereocilia, where the first mechanochemical transformation of a sound stimulus takes place.

In newborn animals which are born blind (mice, rats, kittens, rabbits, etc.) various stages of differentiation of the organ of Corti can be observed in different coils of the cochlea. The differentiation of the organ of Corti in the basal coils of the cochlea coincides with the beginning of its function. In a series of morphological and physiological studies on fetuses of a marsupial rat species ( *Didelphis virginiana* ) MCCRADY et al. (1937, 1938), LARSELL et al. (1944) were able to demonstrate convincingly the complete conformity of the course of histological differentiation of the cochlea with the ability of the fetus to perceive given sound frequencies; the latter was determined by recording biocurrents through a round window. Thus, by the time Corti's organ has developed the fetus, starting from its 2nd and up to its 59th day of life in the pouch, is capable of receiving on the lower coil sound frequencies ranging from 500 to 6,000 cps. From the 59th day on, after development of the middle and upper coils, the fetus can receive sound frequencies from 300 to 10,000 cps, and on the 68th day frequencies from 200 to 20,000 cps. Thus, reception of sound frequencies in the organ of Corti is extended in step with the development of the structural, cytochemical and molecular organization of its receptor cells.

The organ of Corti of adult mammals, situated in the cochlear duct, consists of hair (receptor) and supporting cells (Fig. 82 A). The inner hair cells are arranged in one row nearer to the axis of the cochlea; the laterally positioned outer hair cells are arranged in 3 to 4 rows. Supporting elements of the organ of Corti include inner supporting cells, inner phalanx cells, inner and outer pillar cells, and Deiters, Hensen, and Claudius cells.

Among the auxiliary elements of the organ of Corti which are of great functional and trophic importance, we might mention cells of the inner and outer spiral sulcus of the spiral limbus and of the vestibular lip, as well as the stria vascularis, and the basilar, tectorial and Reissner's (vestibular) membranes.

The inner and outer hair cells differ in their organization. In man the number of inner hair cells is approximately 3,500; in the cat it is 2,600; in the rabbit,

1,000 (ENGSTRÖM and WERSÄLL, 1958a, 1958b). The corresponding number of outer hair cells is in man 12,000—20,000; in the cat, 9,700; in the rabbit, 6,100—6,200 (RETZIUS, 1881, 1884). Inner hair cells are generally slanted and form an angle of 140° with the long axis of the modiolus (TONNDORF et al., 1962). The upper portion of the cell is in direct contact with the terminal cells of the inner spiral sulcus and with the inner supporting phalanx cells (Fig. 89). The apical portions of the cells are connected with each other by desmosomes. The usual intercellular spaces are present between inner hair cells and neighboring supporting cells. In the apical portion of the hair cell a cuticular platelet is found under the plasma membrane, and from this platelet 30 to 40 stereocilia branch out into the subcuticular cavity; these stereocilia are arranged in two rows, parallel to the axis of the cochlear duct (ENGSTRÖM, 1961; IURATO, 1961, 1967; DUVALL, FLOCK, and WERSÄLL, 1966). The number of stereocilia varies with the animal species (KOLMER, 1927). The stereocilia of inner hair cells are twice as thick as those of outer hair cells, and have a diameter of 0.35 μm. and a length of 4—5 μm. The stereocilium is coated by an extension of the plasma membrane and is located above the cuticular platelet, while its apex is joined to the tectorial membrane by means of an osmiophilic cementing substance (KIMURA, 1966; KOICHEV, 1969a). At the point where the stereocilium emerges from the cuticula it tapers down to 0.05 μm. An axial fibril runs through the center of the stereocilium; it is formed by a compact bundle of thin fibrils of diameter 20—30Å, which also fill up the remaining portion of its body

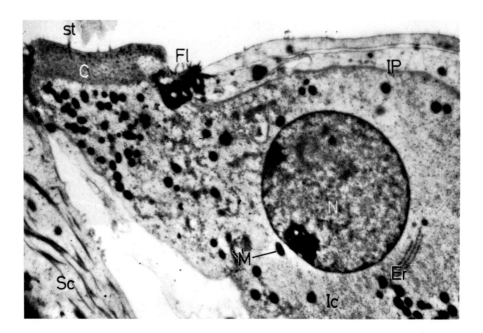

Fig. 89. Inner hair receptor cell (*Ic*) in the organ of Corti of the guinea pig (×12,000) (KOICHEV, 1969a). *C* cuticle with stereocilia rootlets; *M* mitochondria; *N* nucleus; *Er* sectors of the endoplasmic reticulum; *Fl* phalanx; *IP* inner cells-pillars; *Sc* supporting cell; *st* stereocilia

(ENGSTRÖM and WERSÄLL, 1958a; 1958b; SPOENDLIN, 1957; IURATO, 1961, 1967; WERSÄLL et al., 1961; ENGSTRÖM, ADES, and HAWKINS, 1962, 1965; KOICHEV, 1969a). Recently, excellent micrographs which illustrate the distrubution of stereocilia and kinocilia on the surface of hair cells of organ of Corti were obtained with the aid of the scanning microscope (BREDBERY et al., 1970; ENGSTRÖM et al., 1970).

The cuticular plate consists of electron-dense granular material, and it does not cover the entire surface of the inner hair cell. On the side facing the modiolus there is a free sector containing the basal body, from which, as was noted above, a kinocilium branches off during embryonic and postnatal stages (ENGSTRÖM et al., 1962; IURATO, 1967; SMITH, 1967, 1968a; KOICHEV, 1969a). Numerous vesicles, fine canaliculi of the endoplasmic reticulum, osmiophilic granules, individual lysosomes and Golgi's apparatus are found in the subcuticular zone of the hair cell. The presence of a large number of circular mitochondria is also characteristic for this zone. The nucleus is round and is located in the basal portion of the cell. The paranuclear zone is relatively poor in mitochondria, but contains quite a large number of rough endoplasmic reticulum elements and ribosome clusters. In the basal zone mitochondria are found, as well as microtubules and synaptic vesicles in the vicinity of synapses.

The outer hair cells are cylindrical and located more laterally from the outer pillar cells; they form 3 to 4 and sometimes even 5 rows. The apical surface of the cells is coated with a cuticle (Fig. 90), and the base of the cuticle is submerged into a calyx of Deiter's cells. In their apical area hair cells are in contact with the lateral surfaces, or phalanges of Deiter's cells. Outer hair cells, located on the basal cochlear coil, are slightly larger and longer than the hair cells of upper coils (ENGSTRÖM et al., 1962). The axis of the cell forms an angle of 110—115° with the cuticle surface, and the open side of this angle faces the modiolus (ENGSTRÖM, 1960a). The stereocilia of outer hair cells, coated by an extension of the plasma membrane, have the same structure as the stereocilia of inner cells; their length is 4—5 µm, but their diameter only half that of the inner cells, namely 0.15 µm (SMITH, 1961; IURATO, 1967). The stereocilia are arranged in 3 to 4 rows, which together form a letter W (ENGSTRÖM et al., 1962). In the embryonic stages, a kinocilium is located in the central part of the base of this letter (Fig. 88); as was noted above, only the basal body is preserved from this kinocilium in definitive stages (KIMURA, 1966; SHIRO and KYOZO, 1967). Already KOLMER (1927) had noted that the stereocilia of each outer hair cell are of different lengths, the tallest being located in the vicinity of the basal body. The apices of stereocilia seem to be held together at the point of contact with the lower surface of the tectorial membrane by means of an osmiophilic substance (Fig. 91) (IURATO, 1960; KIMURA, 1966; SMITH, 1967, 1968a, 1968b; KOICHEV, 1969a).

The subcuticular zone of the outer hair cell is rich in organoids, such as circular mitochondria, granules, elements of the smooth and rough endoplasmic reticulum, and individual ribosomes. As a special element of the smooth endoplasmic reticulum, found only in outer hair cells, Hensen bodies should be mentioned (HENSEN, 1863; HELD, 1926; ENGSTRÖM and ADES, 1960; KOICHEV, 1969a, 1969b); these bodies consist of 3 to 8 layers of interrupted membranes arranged

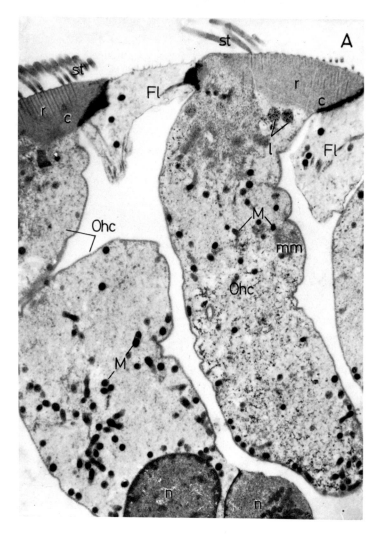

Fig. 90 A—D. Outer hair cells of the organ of Corti of the rat. A. Body of the outer hair cell and its connection with phalanxes (× 10,000); B. Apex of the outer hair cell (× 30,000); C. Apical portion with basal body (× 25,000); D. Complex of membranes (× 25,000) (KOICHEV, 1969). *Ohc* outer hair cells; *Fl* phalanxes of Deiters' cells; *st* stereocilia; *r* stereocilia rootlets; *c* cuticle; *bb* basal bodies; *mm* complex of membranes, located parallel to the plasma membrane of the lateral side of the sensory cell; *l* lysosomes; *M* mitochondria; *n* nucleus

concentrically, like an onion. Isolated mitochondria may be found in the center and at the periphery of this formation. It is assumed that Hensen bodies are specialized and modified Golgi apparatuses (ENGSTRÖM and WERSÄLL, 1958a, 1958b; ENGSTRÖM, ADES, and HAWKINS, 1962; IURATO, 1967; SMITH, 1967).

In Corti's organ of guinea pigs there is an entire system of 10 to 13 interrupted membranes, arranged in several rows along the side walls of the cell, next

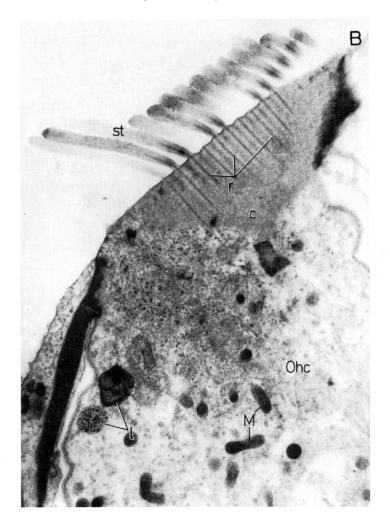

to the external plasma membrane (ENGSTRÖM, 1955; IURATO, 1967; SPOENDLIN, 1958; KOICHEV, 1969a, 1969b) (Fig. 90). In the nuclear region these membranes are gradually reduced and vanish near the synaptic contacts. In white rats, elongated vesicles about 200—300 Å in diameter are found at this spot instead of membranes (IURATO, 1967; KOICHEV, 1969a, 1969b). Membranes and vesicles are accompanied by elongated mitochondria. NAKAI and HILDING (1967) assume that these membranes constitute intracellular paths along which information (most probably of a chemical nature) is transmitted from stereocilia to synapses.

Thus, the organization of inner and outer hair cells exhibits a number of peculiar features, which can be associated with their function. This fact is also underscored by the character of their innervation.

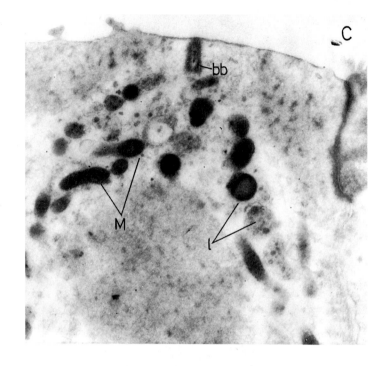

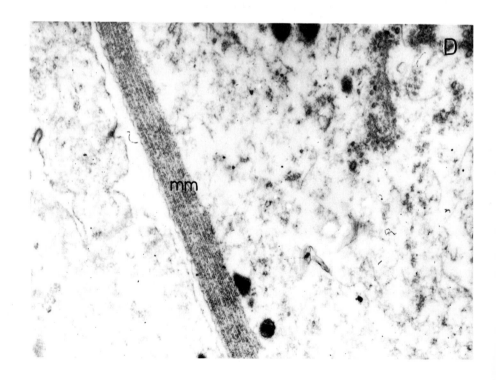

The nerve endings are button-shaped; they terminate at the base of inner and outer hair cells and, as well as in birds, can be divided into two types: dark or granular, and light or agranular (ENGSTRÖM and WERSÄLL, 1958a; SPOENDLIN, 1959; IURATO, 1961, 1964; SMITH, 1961, 1967, 1968a, 1968b; SMITH and SJÖSTRAND, 1961; SPOENDLIN and GAČEK, 1963; RODRIGUEZ-ECHANDIA, 1967; KOICHEV, 1969a, 1969b). The dark or granular nerve endings are filled with vesicles, 200—400Å in diameter, resembling the synaptic vesicles found in other nerve endings of the central nervous system (PALADE and PALAY, 1954; DE ROBERTIS and BENNETT, 1955; PALAY, 1956; DE ROBERTIS, 1958;

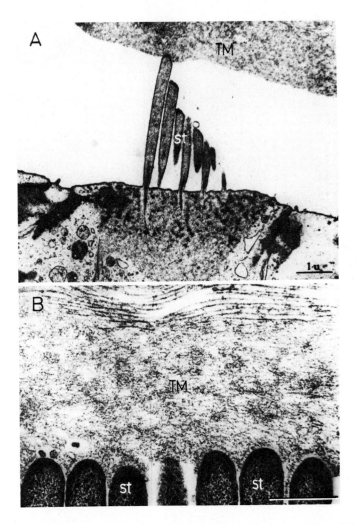

Fig. 91 A and B. Attachment of stereocilia (*st*) of hair cells to the inner surface of the tectorial membrane of the monkey (KIMURA, 1966). A. Typical position of stereocilia; B. Longitudinal section through stereocilia (*st*) of the peripheral row. Insignificant spaces are located between stereocilia. Thin and narrow membranous structures are visible at the top of stereocilia, as well as granules of the tectorial membrane (*TM*). The magnification is shown by the scale

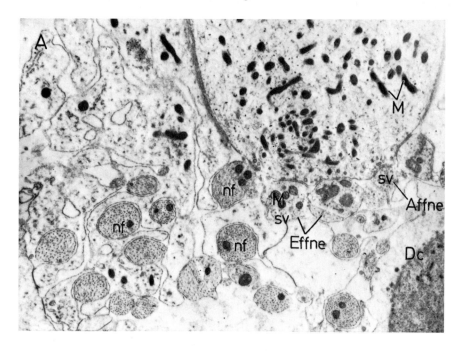

Fig. 92 A and B. Nerve fibers of an outer hair (receptor) cell in the organ of Corti of the guinea pig (KOICHEV, 1969a). A. Section through outer spiral plexus fibers, nerve endings, the synapse (× 15,000); B. Base of the outer sensory (*Orc*) cell (× 20,000); dark efferent (*Effne*) and light afferent (*Affne*) nerve endings; *Dc* Deithers' cells; *M* mitochondria; *n* nucleus; *sv* synaptic vesicles; *nf* nerve fibers with tubules

DE ROBERTIS and IRALDI, 1961). These endings form typical synapses with the base of hair cells (Fig. 92). The synaptic cleft is about 250Å wide; the postsynaptic membrane is often duplicated. Elongated mitochondria are found in the nerve ending region furthest away from the synaptic cleft. In the synapse region, mitochondria, microtubules and small canaliculi of the endoplasmic reticulum are found in the cytoplasm of the hair cell; synaptic vesicles are absent. Experiments involving the cutting and subsequent degeneration of Rasmussen's olivo-cochlear bundle have shown that the dark granular nerve endings are efferent endings (IURATO, 1962b; KIMURA and WERSÄLL, 1962; IURATO et al., 1968, etc.). The light agranular nerve endings are characterized by their small size and small number of vesicles of varied shapes and dimensions; they also contain mitochondria. Light nerve endings usually penetrate slightly into the body of the receptor cell; they can come close not only to the base, but also to the lateral surface of the inner hair cell. Occasionally, light nerve endings are enveloped by the larger dark endings, and synaptic structures are visible at the point of contact of such fibers. In the cytoplasm of the hair cell, near light endings, are found synaptic vesicles and synaptic bodies surrounded by a group of synaptic vesicles. At the point of synaptic contact, the membrane is noticeably thicker, particularly on the postsynaptic side. In sectioning experi-

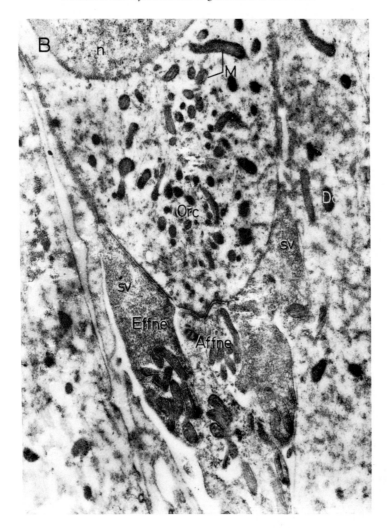

ments, light nerve endings are not damaged, which indicates their afferent nature.

Thus, along with afferent nerve endings, terminals of efferent nerve fibers of Rasmussen's olivo-cochlear bundle come close to the base of inner and outer hair cells (RASMUSSEN, 1946, 1953, 1960). The function of efferent nerve endings is mainly an inhibitory; it consists in regulating the susceptibility of the cochlea and seems to perform the role of modulator of the flow of auditory information to the central nervous system (HERRICK, 1948; BOCCA, 1954; CALAMBOS, 1956; DESMEDT, 1960; FEX, 1962; SMITH, 1968a, 1968b). Thus, the function of hair cells in Corti's organ is regulated by descending impulses according to the feedback principle. In other sense organs, for example in the retina of the eye, such regulation usually occurs at a higher level of the analyzer system.

In the opinion of many investigators, the presence of synaptic vesicles entitles us to believe that synaptic transmission in afferent and efferent nerve endings

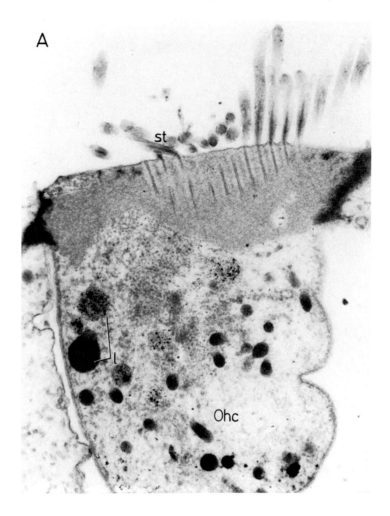

Fig. 93 A—C. Ultrastructural shifts in hair cells of the organ of Corti under the effect of sound (KOICHEV, 1969a). A. Apex of the outer hair cell (*Ohc*) in the lower turn of the organ of Corti of the rat, following exposure to sound (10,000 cps, 95 db for 30 min). Bending stereocilia (*st*) and an increase in the number of lysosomes (*l*) can be seen (× 20,000). B. Doubling of Hensen bodies (*Hb*) in an outer hair cell (*Ohc*) of the middle turn of the organ of Corti of the guinea pig under the effect of sound (2,000 cps, 95 db for 30 min) (× 20,000). C. Increase in number and dissociation of endoplasmic membranes (*mm*) in the outer hair cell (*Ohc*) of the middle coil of the organ of Corti of the guinea pig following exposure to sound (1,000 cps, 95 db for 30 min) (× 22,000)

is associated with a cholinergic mechanism, since it is assumed that these vesicles are filled with acetylcholine. However, some workers believe that cholinergic mechanisms must be attributed only to the efferent nerve endings originating in Rasmussen's olivo-cochlear bundle (SCHUKNECHT et al., 1959; ROSSI, 1961; ROSSI and CORTESINA, 1962a, 1962b, 1963, etc.). Other published data indicate that adrenergic nerve fibers, the origin of which is still unclear, are found in

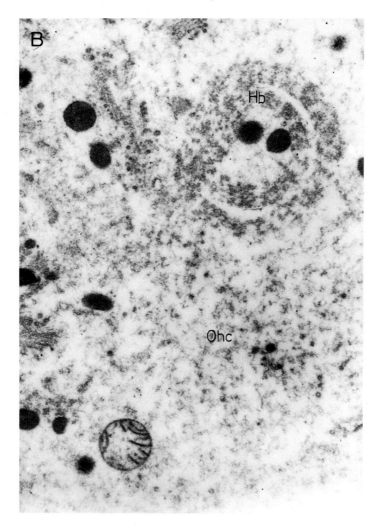

Corti's organ, at least in the region of the inner spiral plexus. Under the electron microscope, granular vesicles, presumably adrenergic, have been observed in the nerve fibers of both the inner and outer spiral plexus (RODRIGUEZ-ECHANDIA, 1967, 1968). Adrenergic fibers can be detected in the inner spiral plexus also by means of cytochemical methods (VINNIKOV et al., 1966; TERAYAMA, HOLZ, and BECK, 1966). These data raise the question about the still not quite clear connections between the receptor cells of Corti's organ and the sympathetic nervous system.

Under acoustic stimulation conditions the ultrastructural organization of hair cells undergoes a series of regular shifts (SPOENDLIN, 1958, 1962; ENGSTRÖM and ADES, 1960; ENGSTRÖM et al., 1970; BREDBERG et al., 1970). Usually, high-intensity noise was used as the acoustic stimulus, and its effect was investigated only in hair cells of the lower cochlear coil. In our laboratory, KOICHEV

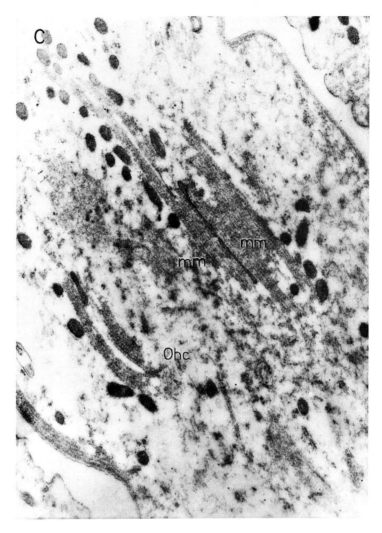

(1969a) subjected guinea pigs to the effect of noise of frequency 350 cps (95 db) for a period of 30 minutes and observed shifts in the ultrastructural organization of hair cells, mainly at the level of the upper coil but also is other cochlear coils. Under the effect of noise of 1,000—2,000 cps (95 db), shifts were observed at the level of the middle cochlear coils, and with noise of 4,000 cps (95 db) at the level of the lower cochlear coil. In rats subjected for 30 minutes to noise of 200 cps (95 db), ultrastructural shifts were observed in hair cells of the upper coil, and also in other cochlear coils; with noise of 5,000 cps (95 db), shifts were observed at the level of the middle coil, and with noise of 10,000 cps (95 db) at the level of the lower basal coil. Thus, the site of ultrastructural shifts in the hair cells located at different levels of the cochlear duct in various animals was in strict accordance with the frequency perception gradient. The most characteristic shifts were observed in outer hair cells.

The most striking features of acoustic stimulation are the inclination of the stereocilia in outer hair cells and the increase in the number of Hensen bodies in the cytoplasm. Whereas in controls the number of such bodies does not exceed 2, in experimental animals there are 3 to 5 (Fig. 93, B). Sometimes, these bodies are duplicated and resemble a figure eight. SPOENDLIN (1958, 1962) and ENGSTRÖM and ADES (1960) were the first to draw attention to an increase in the number of Hensen bodies caused by acoustic effects. In the Hensen bodies 8 to 10 rows of interrupted membranes can be clearly seen; an increase in the number of mitochondria accompanying such bodies, and frequently a swelling of mitochondria and an increase in the size of the structures of the Golgi apparatus is also noteworthy. Numerous membraneous aggregates also appear, often separated and surrounded by mitochondria; these aggregates consist of a large number of interlaced and superimposed membranes of the type that make up Hensen bodies, and of other membranes located parallel to the plasma membrane of the lateral surface of the hair cell (Fig. 93, C). The appearance of osmiophilic structures of a double type is noted in the subnuclear part of the cell (Fig. 93, A). These structures may represent 1. an accumulation of relatively small osmiophilic granules bounded by a common membrane and immersed in a somewhat lighter substance, and 2. osmiophilic granules of larger size, lying freely in the cytoplasm. Apparently, these formations are linked in their genesis and represent different stages in the formation of lysosomes (KOICHEV, 1969a). The nuclei of outer hair cells often have a peripheral arrangement of small chromatin lumps.

The presynaptic region of the hair cell under acoustic stimulation shows an accumulation of synaptic vesicles, both wrinkled and swollen (Fig. 94). One can also observe the deformation of the presynaptic membrane, its "drawing in" to the cellular cytoplasm; there may be analogous invaginations of the postsynaptic membrane into the neuroplasm of the nerve ending that correspond to this. Vesicles of afferent nerve endings also exhibit similar changes, and their mitochondria swell to a considerable extent. A light, finely granular zone, free of vesicles, is seen in efferent nerve endings in the presynaptic membrane region; adjacent to this zone are either wrinkled vesicles, or vesicles with a very light contour (vesicle "shadows"). Mitochondria also swell non-uniformly.

Generally similar shifts, although not quite so pronounced, are observed in the inner hair cells and their nerve endings under the effect of acoustic stimulation. Hensen bodies are not formed in these cells.

KOICHEV (1969a) in our laboratory was unable to fix distinct ultrastructural shifts in auxiliary structures in Corti's organ. The sole exception was Hensen's cells, in which vacuolization processes, characteristic for these cells in a state of relative rest, are greatly intensified under acoustic stimulation conditions.

Thus, under the action of an acoustic stimulus the hair cell undergoes a series of shifts, which make it possible to characterize its functional state. These shifts have already been noted during the course of supravital observations of hair cells under analogous conditions. Changes in the shape of the body, rounding, swelling and contraction of the nucleus, vacuolization of the cytoplasm and changes in the character of dye deposition during intravital staining were observed (VINNIKOV and TITOVA, 1961, 1963, 1964; VINNIKOV and SOKOLOVA,

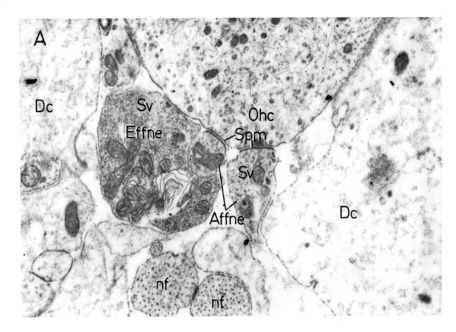

Fig. 94 A and B. Structural changes in the organ of Corti under the effect of a sound stimulus. A. Guinea pig (× 24,000) and B. rat (× 30,000) (KOICHEV, 1969a, b). *Ohc* outer hair cell; *Affne* afferent nerve endings; *Effne* efferent nerve endings; *Sv* synaptic vesicles; *n* nucleus; *M* swollen mitochondria; *Dc* Deiters' cell; *spm* synaptical membrane; *nf* nerve fiber; Sound effect for 30 min, 95 db, 2,000 cps (for A) and 5,000 cps (for B)

1961). Obviously, a study of the ultrastructural shifts allows us to form a much clearer picture of the effect exerted by an acoustic stimulus on the hair cell. This effect is accompanied by a change in the slant of stereocilia, the appearance of characteristic membrane complexes (expressed in the new growth of Hensen bodies), the rearrangement of mitochondria, the abutment of the nucleolus upon the inner surface of the nuclear membrane, the modification of synaptic membranes and a change in the character of synaptic vesicles, etc. Unfortunately, even electron microscopy does not enable us to determine what kind of molecular shifts take place inside the stereocilia and the plasma membrane that envelops them. However, from the entire complex of ultrastructural shifts in the hair cell, we can reach some conclusion regarding its total reaction to an acoustic stimulus.

The ultrastructural organization of a hair cell and its shifts under the effect of acoustic stimulation appear in an entirely new light if we study the biologically active chemical compounds, including enzymes, located in these structures when they are in a state of relative rest, and when they are subject to an acoustic effect.

Cytochemical investigations have shown the presence of acetylcholinesterase activity in Corti's organ. It was impossible not to correlate this fact with the

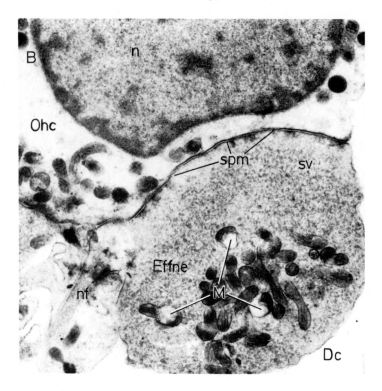

previously mentioned data on the presence of acetylcholine and the increase in its content in the endolymph, particularly after the animal (pigeon and cat) was subjected to an acoustic stimulus (GISSELSON, 1950; PLUZHNIKOV and YAN-TAREVA, 1971; KIBYAKOV et al., 1973). Since acetylcholinesterase inhibitors affect currents in the cochlea, i. e. they prolong the latent period of the microphonic potential and action currents, the assumption was made that a cholinergic system is involved in the genesis of bioelectric potentials of the cochlea, a hypothesis made earlier by some investigators (DERBYSHIRE and DAVIS, 1935a). Histochemical methods demonstrated the localization of the enzymic activity of acetylcholinesterase in the synaptic region of hair cells (SCHUKNECHT, CHURCHILL, and DORAN, 1959; KAWAMOTO and KANEKO, 1959; VINNIKOV and TITOVA, 1958b, 1961, 1963, 1964; ROSSI, 1961; WERSÄLL, HILDING, and LUNDQUIST, 1961; HILDING and WERSÄLL, 1962; ISHII, MURAKAMI, and BALOGH, 1967, etc.).

The studies of VINNIKOV and TITOVA (1958a, 1961, 1963, 1964) on the enzymic activity of acetylcholinesterase in Corti's organ of guinea pigs, in a state of relative rest and after exposure to acoustic effects of different frequency and duration, demonstrated acetylcholinesterase activity both in stereocilia of receptor cells (Fig. 95, A) and in the region of the inner spiral plexus along the entire spiral of the cochlea, as well as in the region of the outer spiral plexus at the level of the lower and middle coils. KIMURA (1966), using the electron microscope, discovered in the apical region of the stereocilia an electron-

A

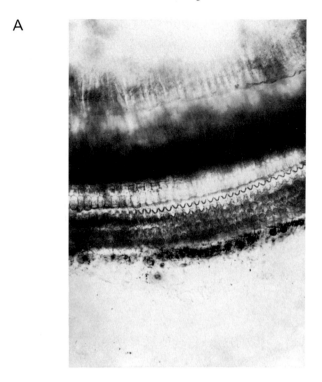

B

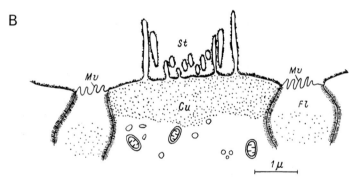

Fig. 95A—D. Acetylcholineesterase activity (A, B) and distribution of products of the histochemical reaction used to detect (*arrow*) Na⁺ (C, D) in hair cells of the organ of Corti of the cat (A) and guinea pig (B, C) under relative resting conditions (VINNIKOV and TITOVA, 1961; KANEKO and DALY, 1969; KOICHEV, 1969b). A. Localization of acetylcholinesterase is detected in stereocilia of inner and outer hair cells at the level of the lower coil of the cochlea. Treatment according to KOELLE and FRIEDENWALD (immersion, objective 60, eyepiece 10). B. Acetylcholinesterase activity is observed on the surface of the plasma membrane of stereocilia and of the apex of the hair cell facing the subtectorial space. The enzyme is absent on the surface of phalanxes. Treatment according to KARNOVSKIY (magnification shown by the scale). Na⁺ reaction products are detected (C) in the stereocilia and in the plasma membrane ($\times$15,000), and (D) in the region of the hair cell base and nerve endings ($\times$15,000). *Ohc* outer hair cell; *Fl* phalanx; *St* stereocilia; *M* mitochondria; *pm* plasma membrane; *Affne* afferent nerve endings; *Effne* efferent nerve endings. *Nf* nerve fibers; *Mv* microvilli; *Cu* cuticle. *Arrows* show the distribution of Na pyroantimonate

dense substance, the location site of which may correspond to the acetylcholinesterase activity reported by us (VINNIKOV and TITOVA, 1961, 1964). KANEKO
and DALY (1969), using Karnovskiy's method, discovered acetylcholinesterase
activity on the surface of outer hair cells of the guinea pig facing the membrana
tectorialis. The enzyme is absent on the surface of phalanges. The location
of the enzyme activity is limited strictly to the plasma membrane covering
the stereocilia and the cuticle of hair cells. It is noteworthy that the location
site of acetylcholinesterase coincides with the location site of sodium ions, as
described above. Thus, our observations under the light microscope were confirmed by means of the electron microscope.

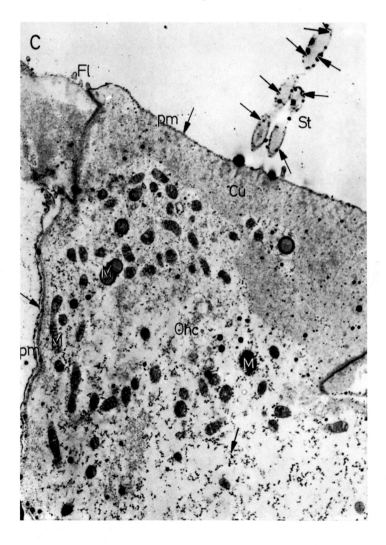

VINNIKOV and TITOVA (1961, 1964) observed under the effect of an acoustic
stimulus first a frequency-dependent increase in acetylcholinesterase activity in

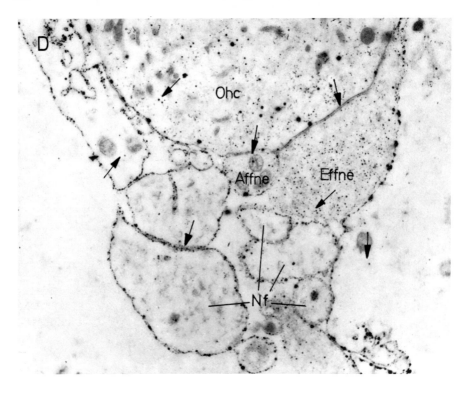

the corresponding cochlear coils of Corti's organ, followed by a decrease in this activity, apparently due to depletion of this enzyme in the receptors. Similar results were obtained in our laboratory by ANICHIN (1964, 1965), who investigated cholinesterase activity in Corti's organ of rats under the effect of intermittent noise.

According to our concepts, as already mentioned, the plasma membrane of the stereocilia of the hair cell contains a cholinoreceptive protein and acetylcholinesterase. During the movement of the basilar and tectorial membranes, when the plasma membrane of stereocilia is subjected to the action of quanta of acetylcholine which had penetrated into the cavity filled with Corti's lymph, this membrane performs the role of a presynaptic membrane. Following the interaction of acetylcholine with the cholinoreceptive protein, which is regulated by acetylcholinesterase, the membrane permeability changes, and it becomes depolarized and generates a microphonic or receptor potential. The energy liberated during this trigger mechanism leads to the stimulation and corresponding structural and cytochemical shifts of all systems present in the hair cell, i.e. to its excitation. As a result of this excitation, a further release of acetylcholine takes place in the synapse region, where another sector of the cholinergic system is located, and this causes the generation of action currents in the acoustic nerve. We have already pointed out that, under the electron microscope, it is possible to detect sodium ions and to show how the distribution of these ions in the stereocilia of hair cells changes under the effect of an acoustic stimulus (Figs. 95 and 96) (KOICHEV, 1969a; VINNIKOV and KOICHEV, 1969). It is thus possible to visualize the phenomenon of depolarization taking place under the effect of the cholinergic mechanism. Unfortunately, in regard to $K^+$ such data are not yet available. Granular products of the cytochemical reaction for $Na^+$, sodium pyroantimonate, are deposited mainly on the surface of the plasma membrane of stereocilia and of the cuticle, and to a lesser extent in the cytoplasm, mitochondria and nucleus. The deposition of these granules has a different character in afferent and efferent nerve endings. Reaction products are also deposited in the cavities filled with Corti's lymph and perilymph. After exposure to acoustic effects, a large increase in the number and size of granules of $Na^+$ reaction products is observed, mainly on the surface of the plasma membrane of stereocilia and the cuticle (Fig. 96). In nerve endings, shifts in the content and distribution of reaction products are less striking. Sodium can be supplied to the receptor cell by Corti's lymph, where, as already pointed out, it is present in a high concentration.

Thus, the cholinergic mechanism, when applied to stereocilia of hair cells, indeed increases the permeability of their plasma membrane for $Na^+$, and probably also for $K^+$; this is accompanied by a depolarization of the membrane and the appearance of a receptor (microphonic) potential.

Histochemical studies have shown that the hair cells of Corti's organ are extraordinarily rich in substrates and enzymes. Thus, hair cells have a high content of glycogen, apparently their main energy substrate; we believe that this is responsible for the anaerobic phase of the microphonic effect (VINNIKOV and TITOVA, 1957a, 1963, 1964). The glycogen is located primarily in the outer hair cells, in the stria vascularis, and in Hensen's cells (BELANGER, 1953, 1956; VINNIKOV and TITOVA, 1957a, 1961, 1963, 1964; FINZI, 1958; ZORZOLI and BORIANI, 1958; TAKAHASHI, 1961; VOSTEEN, 1964). Under the effect of an acoustic stimulus of different frequency, glycogen present in outer hair cells of the corresponding coil is converted from a granular into a diffuse form (VINNIKOV and TITOVA, 1957a). The absence of glycogen in inner hair cells of the guinea pig emphasizes the difference in sensitivity and reaction type between the inner and outer hair cells (VINNIKOV and TITOVA, 1961). Biochemical studies have shown that a rapid change occurs in the ratios of glycogen fractions during acoustic stimulation, and that the total amount of glycogen is increased. Biochemically it is possible to establish that the amount of glycogen firmly bound to protein also increases (LEIBSON, VINNIKOV, and ZHELUDKOVA, 1961). Some 2 to 6 hours following acoustic stimulation the concentration of glycogen present in Corti's organ decreases (VINNIKOV and TITOVA, 1957a).

VINNIKOV and TITOVA (1961, 1962, 1964) studied the distribution of phosphorylase in Corti's organ of the guinea pig in order to clarify its possible participation in the synthesis and resynthesis of glycogen under conditions of relative rest and adequate load. It was found that the localization of phosphorylase coincides with that of glycogen, although the method used in our study did not allow us to detect any changes in the activity and location site of the enzyme during acoustic stimulation.

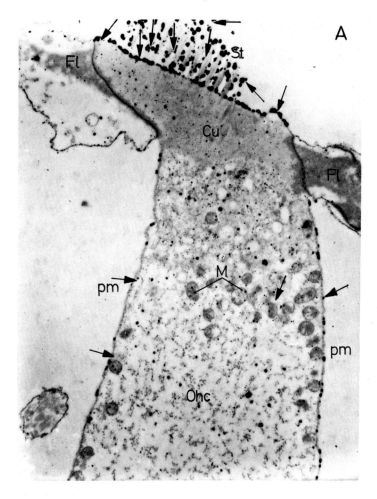

Fig. 96 A and B. Distribution of products of the chemical reaction for the detection of Na$^+$ (*arrows*) under effect of sound on the organ of Corti in rats (outer hair cell—*Ohc*—from the middle coil of the cochlea) (KOICHEV, 1969b). A. Apex of the outer hair cell ($\times$ 14,000); B. Afferent (*Affne*) and efferent (*Effne*) nerve endings on the base of the outer hair cell ($\times$ 20,000). *St* stereocilia; *Cu* cuticle; *pm* plasma membrane; *Fl* phalanx; *M* mitochondria. Sound stimulation: 5,000 cps, 96 db, 30 min

A high activity of alpha-glycerophosphate dehydrogenase, lactate dehydrogenase and glutamate dehydrogenase can be detected by cytochemical methods in Corti's organ, mainly in outer hair cells; this indicates that these cells are able to utilize the energy of anaerobic metabolism (VOSTEEN, 1958; SPOENDLIN and BALOGH, 1963a, 1963b). Biochemical methods show that the activity of lactate and malate dehydrogenase is relatively high in the stria vascularis cells, particularly in the basal coils (KÜRSCHNER, 1968).

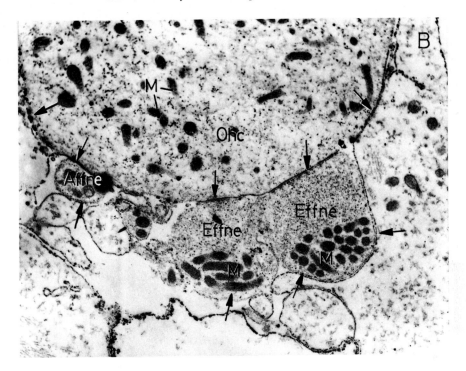

Thus, hair cells of Corti's organ exhibit the localization of enzymes and substrates involved in anaerobic metabolism; this metabolism supplies ATP during the performance of functional activities.

Particularly revealing were cytochemical studies of the activity displayed by oxidative enzymes of the succinoxidase system, in particular of succinate dehydrogenase and cytochromoxidase, which take part in dehydrogenation and associated phosphorylation processes (MIZUKOSHI, KONISHI, and NAKAMURA, 1957; VOSTEEN, 1958; VINNIKOV and TITOVA, 1958d, 1961, 1962a, 1962b, 1963, 1964; GERHARDT, 1961, 1962; KAWAMOTO and KAKIZAKI, 1962; SPOEN-DLIN and BALOGH, 1963a, 1963b; KOIDE, HANDO, and YOSHIKAWA, 1964). The activity of enzymes of the succinoxidase system can be detected primarily in mitochondria of hair cells and in spiral plexus endings. During acoustic stimulation, depending upon the frequency, it is possible to observe in hair cells and nerve endings of appropriate coils increased enzymic activity, then a decline in activity during more prolonged stimulation, as well as rearrangement and swelling of mitochondria (SPOENDLIN, 1959, 1962; ENGSTRÖM, 1960a; VINNIKOV and TITOVA, 1961, 1963, 1964).

During an investigation of $NAD^+$-diaphorase and $NAD-H^+$-diaphorase (enzymes taking part in the Krebs cycle) in Corti's organ, it was found that $NAD^+$-diaphorase displays a high activity in outer hair cells, while $NAD-H^+$-diaphorase activity is high in nerve endings (VOSTEEN, 1958; GERHARDT, 1961, 1962).

Monophosphoesterases (acid and alkaline) taking part in dephosphorylation processes have been studied in Corti's organ (VINNIKOV and TITOVA, 1957b, 1958a, 1961, 1963, 1964). These enzymes display a rather high activity in the stereocilia of hair cells, whereas the activity of alkaline phosphatase is predominantly observed in the cytoplasm of hair cells. Following an acoustic stimulus, increased activity of monophosphoesterases, particularly of the acid enzyme, is first observed, possibly connected with the appearance of lysosomes (KOICHEV, 1969a); after a longer period of time, a gradual decline in this activity is observed. On the other hand, the activity of acid phosphatase was preserved and even increased in the neuroplasm of the outer spiral plexus.

In stereocilia of hair cells in Corti's organ it was possible to detect with the light microscope the presence of adenosine triphosphatase, an enzyme characterizing the intensity of energy processes (MIZUKOSHI, KONISHI, and NAKAMURA, 1957). With the aid of the electron microscope, very high ATPase activity can be detected primarily in stereocilia membranes, on the apical surface of receptor cells, and at the boundary between receptor and supporting cells (Fig. 97).

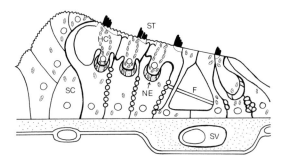

Fig. 97. Diagram showing the distribution of adenosine triphosphate activity in receptor cells of the organ of Corti of the guinea pig (NAKAI and HILDING, 1967). The heavy line shows the location site of the enzymatic activity. *HC* hair cells; *ST* stereocilia; *SC* supporting cells; *F* nerve fibers; *NE* nerve endings; *SV* spiral vessel

Some enzymic activity can also be detected in mitochondria and in the Golgi apparatus also in the plasma membrane of supporting cells (NAKAI and HILDING, 1967). Thus, peak ATPase activity is found in the plasma membrane of stereocilia of hair cells, the first cells to encounter the converted acoustic stimulus; this is associated with the need to intensify conversion processes, and primarily to supply energy to effect the transport of $Na^+$ and $K^+$ across the plasma membrane, i.e. its depolarization. Very high ATPase activity is always observed in the plasma membranes of stereocilia in hair cells.

Thus, oxidative enzymes, alkaline and acid phosphatases, and finally ATPase characterize the general energy system of the hair cell, which is localized both in its mitochondria and membranes, but mostly in the plasma membrane of stereocilia. We have already encountered a similar phenomenon in photoreceptor disk membranes (SCARPELLI and CRAIG, 1963) and in the plasma membrane of the antennae of olfactory cells (BRONSHTEIN and PYATKINA, 1969a, 1969b).

Studies of mucopolysaccharides, which, according to some concepts, play a definite role in the transformation of mechanical into electric energy, has shown them to be present in the tectorial membrane, between stereocilia, in the stria vascularis and in cells of the spiral limbus, i.e. practically wherever microvilli are present (DOHLMAN, 1959a, 1959b; MANGABEIRA-ALBERNAZ, 1961; ORMEROD, 1961; VILSTRUP and JENSEN, 1961; CHRISTIANSEN, 1962; BELANGER, 1953; WISLOCKY and LADMAN, 1954; PLOTZ and PERLMAN, 1955; FERRERI and GRIFO, 1956; IURATO, 1960; KURATA et al., 1963). Thus, we should remember that mucopolysaccharides always accompany microvilli and most likely characterize their permeability function (ITO, 1965; BOYD and PORSONS, 1969).

Investigations of nucleic acids have a special significance, since regular changes in the shape and size of hair cell nuclei under the effect of an acoustic stimulus had long been observed. A relationship was noted between the sound frequency and the location site of these changes in the cochlear coils (RUEDI and FURRER, 1947; MERKLE, 1953; NEUBERT and WÜSTENFELD, 1955). Statistical studies showed that the surface area and volume of nuclei in the outer hair cells undergo a frequency-dependent change: the average increase in the surface area is 28 %, and in volume 40 %. At the same time, the volume of the nuclei of the inner hair cells remains practically unchanged (WÜSTENFELD and SPRENGER, 1958). Therefore, it was interesting to compare the change in the size of nuclei with the change in nucleic acid content (BECK, 1955, 1959, 1965; BECK and MILLER, 1960). VINNIKOV and TITOVA (1958b, 1961, 1963) showed that acoustic stimulation (1,500 cps, 95 db) produced after 15 minutes an increase in the size of nuclei in outer hair cells and a contraction in others; this result was enhanced after 1 hour, according to the gradient of frequency perception along the spiral of the cochlea. In nuclei whose dimensions had increased DNA was found to occupy a marginal position, while the nucleolus simultaneously moved to the periphery of the nucleus (later confirmed under the electron microscope: KOICHEV, 1969a). The RNA concentration in the cytoplasm decreases, and this is apparently associated with its depolymerization. In nuclei which have contracted, clusters of DNA are distributed more or less uniformly throughout the entire nucleus, while RNA is distributed diffusely and in a rather high concentration through the entire karyoplasm. In the cytoplasm, RNA can be detected in the paranuclear zone, where its concentration is much increased, indicating apparently that processes involving a resynthesis of nucleic acids take place in cells with contracted nuclei. Similar results were obtained in our laboratory by ANICHIN (1964, 1965, 1968) on rats and guinea pigs after exposure to an intermittent acoustic stimulus, and have also been confirmed by autoradiographic methods (MEYER ZUM GOTTESBERGE, 1960; KOBURG, 1961; MEYER ZUM GOTTESBERGE and PLESTER, 1961; and others). Thus, nucleic acids, at least those found in outer hair cells, exhibit a number of regular shifts in response to an acoustic stimulation. Since nucleic acids are connected with protein synthesis, it was interesting to correlate them with the distribution and content of the "total protein"[2] and functional groups of protein molecules (carboxyl and thiol

---

[2] The term "total protein" usually designates the three simultaneously identified aromatic amino acids found in every protein molecule: histidine, tryptophan and tyrosine.

groups) in the hair cells of Corti's organ under conditions of relative rest and acoustic stimulation (YAKOVLEV *et al.*, 1961; VINNIKOV and TITOVA, 1961, 1963, 1964). The histochemical pattern of the conversion and distribution of "total protein" and functional groups of protein molecules revealed that what occurs during acoustic cell stimulation is a process involving all protein structures. Only 10—15 minutes after an acoustic stimulus a large increase is detected in the concentration of total protein and thiol and carboxyl groups in structures of the cytoplasm of hair cells, corresponding to the increase in the number of Hensen bodies (KOICHEV, 1969a) and in the nucleus. After 1, 2, 4, and 6 hours, however, there was a fall in the concentration of protein and functional groups of protein molecules. These changes were observed in the outer hair cells of particular cochlear coils, depending upon the frequency of the acoustic stimulus. We believe that the processes involving the synthesis and subsequent decline in protein content during stimulation of hair cells reflect the function of their nucleic acids, as observed by means of electron microscopic, cytochemical and autoradiographic studies.

Although in general changes in the ultrastructural and cytochemical organization could be assigned to all outer hair cells of the relevant coil, there were always some cells included in the field of vision that did not exhibit any changes whatsoever. The same observation also applies to all inner hair cells along the entire spiral of the cochlea.

Summarizing our study of the development and ultrastructural and cytochemical organization of hair cells in Corti's organ in birds and mammals, we shall attempt to combine our observations into a coherent whole. In our opinion, the quantum emission of acetylcholine from the endolymph into Corti's lymph, and into the region of bending stereocilia during the appearance of shearing forces, results in the interaction of acetylcholine with cholinoreceptive protein and acetylcholinesterase, localized in the plasma membrane. This changes the ionic equilibrium between $Na^+$ and $K^+$ and causes depolarization of membranes, accompanied by the appearance of a receptor microphonic potential. Thus, the appearance of the potential results from the action of a mediator, which induces a number of metabolic and ultrastructural changes, first in the stereocilia membranes, then in the body of the cell; the system ATP-ATPase also contributes to these changes. During an acoustic stimulus, rearrangement of mitochondria, endoplasmic reticulum membranes, nuclear structures, etc. takes place in the body of the cell, accompanied by changes in the metabolic processes. These metabolic processes involve interaction between anaerobic and oxidative metabolisms, a series of interconnected enzymic reactions, and a change in the nucleic and protein regimes. These processes produce energy, which leads to a further emission of acetylcholine in the synapse region, where it interacts with cholinoreceptive protein and acetylcholinesterase located in the post-synaptic membrane and induces electric impulses, i.e. action currents, in the nerve fibers that transmit the encoded information to the central nervous system. Thus, the electrical phenomena recorded on the surface of the hair cell are in reality the physical reflection of complex ultrastructural and biochemical changes involving all the structures of the cytoplasm.

# 6. Structural Organization of Receptor Cells of Chordotonal Sensilla of Insects

We have already examined the general principles of the structural and functional organization of the chordotonal sensillae, which are part of the tympanic organs of a number of insects (Acrididae, Grillididae, etc.), and we have seen that the equivalent processes of transformation of an acoustic stimulus in tympanic organs are very similar to the processes that occur in the middle and inner ear of vertebrates. Insects can perceive oscillations ranging from low-frequency vibrations to sounds of moderately high frequency. In some insects chordotonal organs are present but are not connected with the tympanic membrane; these organs are usually located on flexible sectors of the cuticle, in particular between abdominal segments (MCINDOO, 1922). All these organs are capable of perceiving low-frequency vibrations (in beetles and flies), and some of them even higher-frequency sounds. Such organs include, for example, Johnston's organ located on the second antennal segment of mosquitos or the tympanal organs located on the tibia of orthopterans.

Every chordotonal organ, whether it forms a part of the tympanic organ or not, is made up of a number of sensilla. The sensillum consists of a distal cap cell into which the peripheral process of a primary sensory receptor cell penetrates; the central process of this cell, coated with Schwann cells, is directed into the central nervous system.

A few words now about the embryonic development of sensilla. Whether the sensillum is mechano- or chemoreceptive, its elements are formed from hypodermal cells (STOSSBERG, 1938; KRUMINS, 1952; RÖNSCH, 1954; PETERS, 1963). After repeated divisions of a hypodermal cell, one or more bipolar receptor cells arise, also trichogen and tormogen cells, which take part in the formation of the cuticular section of the sensillum. Hairs (if formed) develop from trichogen cells, and connecting or articular membrane from tormogen cells. Thus, the definitive sensillum consists of one or more receptor, trichogen, tormogen and Schwann cells, plus a cuticular sector modified in a special way (SNODGRASS, 1926, 1935; DETHIER, 1963; BULLOCK and HORRIDGE, 1965).

Johnston's organ (JOHNSTON, 1885) has been studied under the light microscope in representatives of all the principal orders of insects (CHILD, 1894; ZAWARZIN, 1912; EGGERS, 1923). It consists of several chordotonal sensilla, stretched out parallel to the long axis of the antenna. Chordotonal sensilla form a ring round the central zone of the antennal segment and the neural and tracheal stipes are located in this segment. The distal ends of sensilla are attached to the articular membrane connecting the second (pedicel) and third antennal segments, and their proximal ends to the antennal nerve. The number of chlordotonal sensilla may vary with species or sex.

In our laboratory, IVANOV (1968) has studied the structural organization of Johnston's organ in Coleoptera *(Acilius sulcatus)* (Fig. 98). In these beetles, Johnston's organ is located in the pedicel of the antennae. The distal ends of the sensilla terminate in the articular membrane connecting the second (pedicel) and third antennal segments, and the proximal ends, consisting of central processes of receptor cells, enter the antennal nerve and proceed to the central nervous system as part of this nerve.

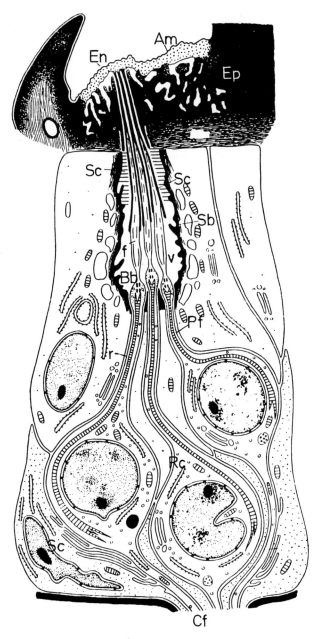

Fig. 98. Structural diagram of the chordotonal sensilla of Johnston's organ of the beetle *Acilius sulcatus*, based on electron microscopic data (IVANOV, 1968). *Rc* receptor cell; *Cf* central process; *Sc* Schwann cells; *r* rootlet; *Pf* peripheral process; *Bb* basal body; *Am* articular membrane; *v* vacuole; *f* fibrils of flagellum; *Sb* scolopoid body; *Sc* scolopoid sheath; *En* endocuticle; *Ep* epicuticle

Each chordotonal sensillum consists of several receptor and enveloping cells, probably analogous to the trichogen and tormogen cells found in other insect sensilla. The cuticular section is common to all sensilla of an organ and consists of an elastic membrane connecting neighboring antennal segments. The articular membrane, to which are attached the peripheral processes of receptor cells, consists of four layers. On the outside, this membrane is coated with a thin, electron-dense layer, corresponding to the epicuticle of the outer integuments of the body. In ultrathin sections, the epicuticle of the membrane has a wavy outline. Located under the epicuticle is the interlayer of the exocuticle 0.5 to 1 µm thick; this in turn rests on the thick layer of the spongy cuticle, which has a characteristic structure, being perforated with a large number of pores, apparently communicating with each other. Finally, the innermost layer of the articular membrane consists of a layer of densely packed, thin fibrils lying parallel to each other.

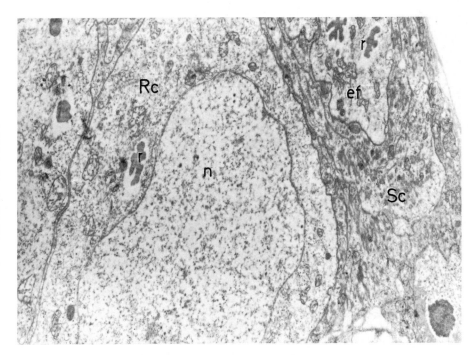

Fig. 99. Sector of receptor cell in Johnston's organ of the beetle *Acilius sulcatus* (×22,000) (IVANOV, 1968). *Rc* receptor cell; *n* nucleus; *r* rootlet; *ef* peripheral process; *Sc* enveloping cell

The receptor cell (Fig. 99) consists of an oval body, containing a nucleus, and two thin processes, a peripheral and a central process. The nucleus is round and is characterized by a compact granulated nucleolus, with a diameter of 0.6 µm, often pressed tightly against the inner leaflet of the nuclear membrane.

Large numbers of rods-daped mitochondria and elements of rough endoplasmic
reticulum are located in the paranuclear zone, as well as isolated ribosomes,
elements of Golgi's apparatus, multivesicular corpuscles and electron-dense
granules of diameter 0.3 to 1 µm. Vesicles with a diameter of about 200Å and
fibrils with a thickness of 150—200Å are found throughout the entire cytoplasm.
The peripheral process has an average diameter of 2 µm, and consists of a
proximal and a distal segment. Approximately 30 µm from the body of the
cell is a pair of centrioles, from which a flagellum containing 9 pairs of peripheral
fibrils branches out distally. A rootlet with a striation period of 650Å branches
off from the basal body and runs deep into the body of the cell. The proximal
segment contains mitochondria, polyribosomes and a large number of small
vesicles or vacuoles. The distal segment contains flagellum fibrils and oval vacuoles
up to 400Å in diameter. In the vicinity of the articular membrane, the narrowing
process enters a canal running through the cuticle of the membranes and terminates without reaching the spongy endocuticle. Thus, the distal end of the
process is enclosed within a peculiar cuticular tube, known as the scolopoid
(cuticular) sheath, which is an extracellular derivative of the cell surrounding
the peripheral process. This sheat continues to the top of the process, where
it turns into a thin cord or terminal filament. The terminal filaments are arranged
in the pores in groups of 3, 5, 9 or more and are attached to the exocuticle
of the articular membrane. The central process, branching off from the receptor
cell, is thin and has a diameter of 1—2 µm, it is relatively poor in organoids.

A Schwann cell, with its nucleus lying near the body of the receptor cell,
is located in the basal portion of the sensillum. The cytoplasmic membrane
of the cell has outgrowths in the form of thin leaflets that cover the body
of the receptor cell in one, two or three layers. The most characteristic feature
in the structure of the cytoplasm of the Schwann cell is its high concentration
of glycogen granules; it is also rich in organoids. Located further distally from
the Schwann cell is an enveloping cell, which encompasses the peripheral process
of the receptor cell in the form of a ring. The basal portion of the enveloping
cell contains large numbers of fibrils with a diameter of up to 150Å, mitochondria,
elements of Golgi's apparatus, granules, etc. The middle and apical sections
of the enveloping cell are strongly vacuolized. These vacuoles, from 0.1 to 3 µm
in diameter, are filled with a cottonlike substance, which is the dry residue
of compounds dissolved in the vacuoles. The vacuoles are particularly well
developed in the portion where the enveloping cell borders the distal section
of the receptor. Here, the cytoplasm between vacuoles is filled with fibrils about
200Å in diameter. The fibrils, merging together, form columellae surrounding
on all sides the distal segment of the peripheral process; these columellae, according to IVANOV (1968), correspond to the scolopoid body of chordotonal sensilla,
described under the light microscope. The scolopoid body originates in the
vicinity of the bulb of the peripheral process, tightly enveloping it from all
sides, and terminates at the level of the inner surface of the articular membrane.

So far, no data are available concerning changes in the ultrastructural organization of receptor and sustentacular cells of Johnston's organ under the effect
of acoustic stimulation, nor are there data on the cytochemistry of Johnston's
organ.

Among the tympanic chordotonal organs investigated, IVANOV (1968) has studied the tympanic organ of the grasshopper *Decticus verrucivorus* under the electron microscope. This organ is located in the proximal region of the tibia of the forelimbs and communicates with the outer environment through a narrow slit, lying open on the surface of the tibia, or covered by a special outgrowth of cuticle. The tympanic organ includes several score of chordotonal sensilla, attached at their distal ends to the membrane. The proximal ends of these sensilla are connected to a branch of the tympanic nerve running into the third thoracic ganglion.

Each sensillum consists of one bipolar receptor cell and enveloping cells (Fig. 100). Located in the basal portion of the sensilla is a Schwann cell, encasing the body of the receptor cell and its central process. The peripheral process is surrounded by a distal enveloping cell. Finally, the apical region of the sensilla contains a small cap cell, by means of which the entire receptor complex is attached to the membrane.

The receptor cell consists of a nuclear-plasmatic body, from which branch off a central and a peripheral processes. The peripheral process is divided into a proximal and a distal segment, formed by a modified flagellum containing $9 \times 2 + 0$ fibrils, branching off from the basal body. The apex of the process forms an apical expansion with several outgrowths (Fig. 101). A rootlet, branching off from the basal body and having a striation period of 650Å, is located in the proximal segment. The rootlet branches off in the form of 9 thin fibrils, which merge together proximally to form a tube of circular cross-section. The opening of the tube narrows as it approaches the body of the cell, and the rootlet finally assumes the appearance of a shaft, with a thickness of about 0.7 µm, which is then subdivided into individual lobes having a fibrous texture. In the body of the cell the rootlet appears to be subdivided into individual microtubules, large numbers of which can be observed in this area.

The distal segment of the peripheral process contains 9 pairs of fibrils extending up to the apical expansion, where a special subterminal expansion can be found, containing tubular fibrils arranged parallel to each other and elongated in a longitudinal direction. Thus, fibrils of the flagellum can be detected all the way up to the cap cell. The peripheral process is surrounded by an enveloping cell. The nucleus of this cell is oval and has a characteristic nucleolus with a vacuole in the central zone. According to data obtained by IVANOV (1968), the cytoplasm (which is poor in organoids) contains a special structure, known as the scolopoid body, located near the inner surface of the cell (Fig. 101, A). This scolopoid body can be observed extending from the bulb of the peripheral process to the apex of the enveloping cell; it has a tubular structure, the walls of which are formed by seven equidistant columellae consisting of densely packed fibrils. These columellae fit tightly against the inner surface of the enveloping cell, protruding slightly into the vacuole cavity. Desmosome structures are observed in the area of the base and apex of the scolopoid body, i.e. where the plasma membrane of the enveloping cell adjoins the surface of the receptor and cap cells. IVANOV (1968) assumes that such pictures indicate that the apex of the scolopoid body is firmly attached to a cap cell, whereas its base is connected to the bulb of the peripheral process of the receptor cell. Numerous vacuoles and mitochondria, accumulating in the vicinity of the scolopoid body, can be observed in the cytoplasm of the enveloping cell.

The cap cell is located in the apical portion of the sensillum. A relatively narrow intercellular space filled with a large number of fibrils separates the cap cell from the tracheal stipes. The most striking and distinctive morphological sign of the cap cell is the presence of a specialized structure, called the scolopoid cap; it has an oval shape and is located in a recess on the basal surface of

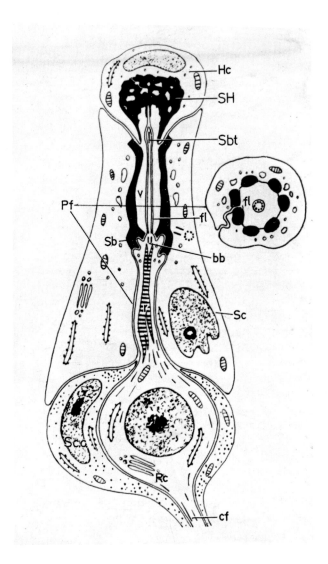

Fig. 100. Structural diagram of the chordotonal sensillum in the tympanic organ of the grasshopper, based on electron microscopic data (IVANOV, 1968). *Hc* cap cell; *SH* scolopoid cap; *Sbt* subthermal dilatation; *v* vacuole; *fl* modified flagellum; *Sb* scolopoid body; *r* rootlet; *Sc* enveloping cell; *Pf* peripheral process; *Rc* receptor cell; *Sc.c* Schwann cell; *cf* central process; *bb* basal bodies

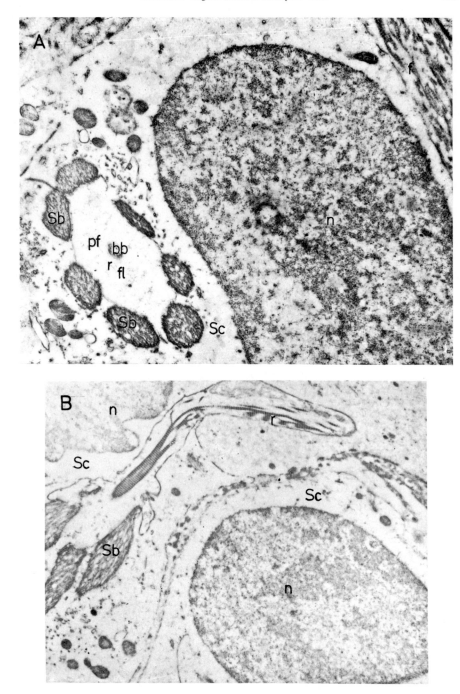

Fig. 101 A and B. Chordotonal sensilla of the tympanic organ of the grasshopper *Decticus verrucivorus* (IVANOV, 1968). A. Transverse section through modified flagellum (*fl*) and scolopoid body (*Sb*) (× 12,000). B. Sensilla sector (× 9,000). *n* nucleus; *f* fibril; *Sc* enveloping cell; *pf* peripheral process; *bb* basal body; *r* rootlet

the cap cell. A small pit is observed in the base of the cap; located inside this pit is the apex of the distal segment, i.e. of a modified cilium (flagellum) of the receptor cell. A tubular structure, analogous to the scolopoid (cuticular) sheath of other sensilla extends from the upper wall. In the same way as the scolopoid sheath, this structure surrounds the apex of the modified cilium, which thereby is firmly fixed with respect to the cuticular section of the sensillum, i.e. the scolopoid cap.

The Schwann cells coating the base of the body of the receptor cell and its central process are characterized by their wealth of organoids. A comparison of the structural organization of Johnston's organ and of the tympanic organ shows that the latter has a higher and more complex organization. Perhaps, this is associated with the fact that, whereas the tympanic organ is indeed capable of perceiving definite acoustic frequencies within the range, for example, of 800 to 45,000 cps (long-horned grasshoppers), Johnston's organ is also able to perceive vibrations along with acoustic stimuli, and can perform the function of an equilibrium organ, i.e. it is characterized by certain rather primitive features (PROSSER and BRAWN, 1967). However, the ultrastructural organization of the tympanic organ in the grasshopper is not basically different from that of the tympanic organ in locusts, studied by GRAY (1960), although these organs developed independently and on different parts of the body. This is presumably a sign of their common origin from chordotonal sensilla.

Unfortunately, in contrast to vertebrates, no data are at present available on ultrastructural shifts in receptor cells of insect tympanic organs during acoustic stimulation. The cytochemical organization of these organs also has not been investigated at all so far.

# 7. Electrophysiological Studies

Potentials of the cochlea in mammals have been studied most thoroughly. When a microelectrode is inserted into the scala tympani, a positive potential difference of about 5 mV can be detected between the scala tympani and an indifferent electrode inserted into the body of the animal. After passage of the electrode through the basilar membrane, a resting potential of 50 to 80 mV is recorded in cells of Corti's organ. When the microelectrode penetrates the cavity of the cochlear duct, the potential exhibits a jump of up to +75 to +85 mV (BÉKÉSY, 1951a, 1951b, 1951c). This potential, called the endocochlear potential, does not depend upon the ionic composition of the endolymph and is the result of the metabolic activity of the stria vascularis (TASAKI and SPYRO-POULOS, 1959). The extreme sensitivity of the endocochlear potential to oxygen shortage leads us to believe that the onset of this potential is associated with oxidative processes (TASAKI, DAVIS, and ELDREDGE, 1954; DAVIS et al., 1955). After penetration of the electrode from the cochlear duct across Reissner's membrane into the scala vestibularis, a small positive potential of the order of 5 mV is again recorded. The microphonic potential is the receptor potential of a hair cell (TASAKI, DAVIS, and ELDREDGE, 1954; DAVIS, 1960) and depends upon the integrity of Corti's organ. The shape of the potential reflects the shape of the stimulus and reflects the mechanical movement of structures in Corti's organ (DAVIS, FERNANDEZ, and McAULIFFE, 1950; DAVIS, 1958, 1961).

The microphonic potential consists of two components: the first is very sensitive to lack of oxygen and disappears immediately upon the death of the animal; the second component is the smaller fraction (5—20 %), persists after the death of the animal, and is apparently anaerobic (DAVIS et al., 1934). We think that from the energy standpoint the anaerobic fraction of the microphonic potential is maintained at the expense of the huge glycogen reserves found in hair cells (VINNIKOV and TITOVA, 1961, 1963, 1964). BÉKÉSY (1960a, 1960b) has shown that the phase and magnitude of the microphonic potential depend upon the direction in which the tectorial membrane is displaced. This direction is determined by the morphological polarization of hair cells, which is in turn connected with the position of stereocilia and basal body (ENGSTRÖM, ADES, and HAWKINS, 1962; FLOCK et al., 1962).

The summation potential was described for the first time by DAVIS, FERNAN-DEZ, and McAULIFFE (1950). It is a constant potential, arising during static displacement of stereocilia in a definite direction. The larger negative component is connected with inner hair cells, while the small positive component is induced by outer hair cells (DAVIS, 1958; DAVIS et al., 1958; DAVIS and ELDREDGE, 1959).

The endocochlear potential is not absolutely necessary for the onset of the microphonic and summation potentials, but it considerably increases the amplitude of these potentials (TASAKI and FERNANDEZ, 1952; DAVIS et al., 1958; DAVIS, 1961).

The action potential is recorded from the auditory nerve in the modiolus region of the inner auditory meatus (DAVIS, TASAKI, and GOLDSTEIN, 1952; TASAKI, 1957a, 1957b). At frequencies below 200 cps, all cochlear structures undergo phased oscillations, which give synchronized discharges in the auditory nerve. For sound frequencies above 500 cps, the propagation time of mechanical vibrations along the cochlea is comparable with the oscillation period. As we have seen, the transmission of stimulation in the synaptic region of hair cells, which leads to the onset of action currents, is effected by a mediator mechanism. DAVIS (1961), however, suggested that stimulation of a hair cell can be transmitted to nerve endings both by ephaptic means and with the aid of a mediator.

Thus, potentials in the cochlea can be assigned to definite structures of Corti's organ, and primarily to hair cells; the genesis of these potentials can be explained more or less satisfactorily, and they can even be linked with definite biochemical cycles.

The situation is quite different in regard to the study of biopotentials of chordotonal (tympanic) organs in insects. Recording of action potentials from the tympanic nerve and observation of behavioral reactions during acoustic stimulation have shown that tympanic organs are relatively insensitive to low frequencies; however, at frequencies of 1,000 cps and above, their sensitivity is close to or even higher than the sensitivity of the human ear (PROSSER and BROWN, 1967). Two insects registered a reaction in the frequency range 800 to 45,000 cps: in the cricket Gryllus at frequencies over 10,000 cps, and in the locust Locusta—at frequencies from 300 to over 10,000 cps (WEVER and VERNON, 1959). As recordings of electric reactions of the tympanic organs show, sensitivity rises to a maximum at a frequency of 1,000 cps, drops slightly with a further increase in frequency, and then rises again. The upper boundary of the auditory range is approximately 9,000 cps. When the crista of the tympanic organ is damaged, the insect loses its ability to perceive high frequencies. At frequencies over 10,000 cps the audibility threshold may reach 0.04 microbar or 0.04 dyne/cm$^2$, which is considerably lower than the threshold of the human ear at this frequency. In the grasshopper *Paroxia*, at frequencies below 200 cps nerve impulses are in step with the frequency of acoustic vibrations, whereas at frequencies of 4,500 to 10,000 cps this synchronism is disrupted (WEVER and VERNON, 1959). In a number of other members of the locust family the synchronism of impulses in tympanic nerves is preserved only up to a frequency of 90 cps. When the frequency is increased, the synchronism is disrupted, and at a frequency of about 120 cps the reaction in general suddenly van shes (HAS-KELL, 1956a, 1956b). According to the data of POPOV (1969), the tympanic organ of cicads contains a number of receptor cells (up to 1,500), but all of them are connected to the same sector of the membrane and are therefore tuned to the same frequency range (2,000 to 8,500 cps in the initial phase and 6,000—10,000 cps in the final phase); this corresponds exactly to the maximum energy region in the spectrum of male calling songs. These receptors are able to synchronize their discharge at the moment when the sound intensity increases sharply. Because of this, the powerful currents of the total discharge repeat the precise rhythm of the insect song (PRINGLE, 1953).

In the locust, different clusters of sensilla on the tympanic membrane are characterized by different ranges of perceived frequencies. For example, according to the data of POPOV (1965), receptor cells of the pear-shaped body can perceive frequencies in the range 12,000 to 20,000 cps, while receptor cells of the rod-shaped body can perceive frequencies in the range 3,000 to 10,000 cps. According to POPOV (1965), the different specialization of these cells is associated with their different location and mode of attachment to the tympanic membrane, and this is reflected in the position of the peripheral process of the modified flagellum (GRAY, 1960). It is assumed that the tympanic membrane possesses a different displacement amplitude maximum, depending upon its structure and, as in Corti's organ of vertebrates, this is responsible for the spatial localization of the acoustic frequencies perceived. High-frequency sounds cause a maximum displacement of the thinnest and most rigid parts of the membrane, while low-frequency sounds cause a displacement of the thicker and softer parts (POPOV, 1965).

Thus, in all orthopterans studied the tympanic organ contains two types of receptor cells: low-frequency and high-frequency cells. Usually, one of these groups is sharply tuned to the frequencies that occur most frequently in the spectrum of communication signals (POPOV, 1969).

Chordotonal organs, which do not have tympanic membranes and are located on the tibia of orthopterans, cockroaches, moths and certain true bugs (Hemiptera), react to vibrations of frequencies up to 8,000 cps (SCHNEIDER, 1950). The tympanic organ on the leg of locusts and grasshoppers also reacts to vibrations of the substrate within the range 1,500 to 2,000 cps. The threshold at this frequency is determined by the mechanical displacement, which is equal to $3.6 \times 10^{-9}$ cm (AUTRUM, 1941; AUTRUM and SCHNEIDER, 1948).

Johnston's organ in the male mosquito *(Aedes aegypti)* reacts to the sound emitted by the flying female and induces the mating reaction. Young female mosquitos can perceive vibrations in the frequency range 400 to 525 cps, while old females perceive vibrations in the range to 250 to 700 cps (ROTH, 1948). POPOV (1969) points out that the high efficiency of sound recognition in insects is achieved in all cases studied by means of a very small number of receptor and neural elements making up the auditory system. Thus, the auditory organ of moths contains only two receptors, that of locusts about 70, but that of cicads some 1,500 receptors (SCHWALBE, 1906; VOGEL, 1923; EGGERS, 1928). As regards the central neurons, these are found in very small numbers, and so far we know nothing about the cytochemical and molecular organization of the receptor cells responsible for the auditory function of insects.

# 8. Conclusion

A sound stimulus exerts a direct mechanical effect on the cell and induces a nonspecific reaction, probably determined by the character of the acoustic "resonance", i.e. a change occurs in the conformation of the protein molecules in the protoplasm of animal cells. This original reaction is preserved in auditory cells, since otherwise sound sensation would not reflect reality. In the process of animal evolution structures developed can carry to hair cells mechanical vibrations that are strictly equivalent to the acoustic stimulus; this is achieved by means of similar energy transformations (in vertebrates in the structures of the inner ear, in insects in the chordotonal and tympanic organs). Thus, the hair cell is in direct contact with the acoustic stimulus; information about this stimulus is indirect, i.e. it is the result of a series of adequate energy transformations.

To sum up: the hair cell, at least in Corti's organ of vertebrates, is stimulated by shearing forces that arise in the region of the stereocilia in connection with the movement of the basilar and tectorial membranes, which in turn is caused by the movement of ossicles in the inner ear under the effect of synchronous impacts of molecules of air or water on the tympanic membrane. According to the mechanoelectric theory (DAVIS, 1958), the bending of the stereocilia under the effect of shearing forces is sufficient to cause deformation and changes in permeability, i.e. changes in the ionic equilibrium of the plasma membrane of the stereocilia, accompanied by the appearance of potentials (microphonic potential in hair cells) and then of action currents in the auditory nerve, following ephaptic or chemical switching of the potential in the synaptic region. According to the cytochemical theory (VINNIKOV and TITOVA, 1961, 1963, 1964), the bending of the stereocilia and deformation of the plasma membrane are associated from the first with the triggering of substrates and enzymes of the cholinergic system. Acetylcholine, supplied from the endolymph into the region of Corti's lymph, reacts in a quantum ratio with molecules of cholinoreceptive protein present in the plasma membrane of stereocilia. Acetylcholine is then hydrolyzed by acetylcholinesterase, which is also localized in the plasma membrane of stereocilia. It is still not clear what purpose is served by the kinocilium in birds, containing

$9 \times 2 + 2$ fibrils, or the basal body in mammals, with respect to auditory cells.

As a result of the preliminary triggering of the cholinergic system mediator a change occurs in the ionic permeability of the plasma membrane of stereocilia (in particular, a change in membrane permeability to $Na^+$) leading to depolarization and the appearance of a receptor (microphonic) potential. Thus, the interaction of acetylcholine with a cholinoreceptor and a change in the conformation of the latter constitute the primary trigger mechanism for a whole series of secondary processes: first, a change of ionic permeability, i.e. depolarization and genesis of a potential, and then regular shifts in substrates and enzymes of both anaerobic and aerobic metabolism and associated phosphorylation. Intensifying energy processes apparently start at the moment when acetylcholine quanta are released onto the plasma membrane of the stereocilia; this membrane is characterized by a very high ATPase activity (NAKAI and HILDING, 1967). Cytochemical changes proceed along with rebuilding of the ultrastructural organization of the hair cell, rearrangement of mitochondria and endoplasmic reticulum membranes, the appearance of additional Hensen's bodies, etc. Finally, as a result of this stimulation of the hair cell, another quantum of acetylcholine is released into the region of the postsynaptic membrane of afferent nerve endings; in this region acetylcholine interacts with the cholinoreceptor and, on undergoing hydrolysis by the acetylcholinesterase located in this region, modifies the permeability of the postsynaptic membrane of the nerve ending, thus causing depolarization of this membrane and the appearance of action currents along the fibers of the eighth nerve. Analogous mediator (may be GABA, FLOCK, 1974) processes also take place in the efferent nerve endings, in relation to which the plasma membrane of the hair cell acts as a postsynaptic membrane.

Thus, the hair cell of Corti's organ possesses a molecular mechanism, located in the stereocilia area, which is triggered by equivalent transformations of the acoustic stimulus. This mechanism consists, on the one hand, of acetylcholine (the quantum emission of molecules of acetylcholine in the area of the plasma membrane of stereocilia must somehow reflect the synchronous movement of air molecules, which in aggregate constitute the given acoustic frequency) and on the other hand, of a corresponding number of molecules of a cholinoreceptive protein located in the plasma membrane of stereocilia. The interaction of these molecules with acetylcholine, which is regulated by the hydrolyzing function of acetylcholinesterase, leads to a depolarization of stereocilia and constitutes the basis of the primary molecular mechanism of stimulation of hair cells by the acoustic stimulus.

Consequently, reception of an acoustic stimulus, at least in vertebrates, takes place according to the same molecular principles that have been established for vision and taste and are probably applicable to smell as well. The electrophysiological and cytochemical processes that take place in the receptor cells of Corti's organ are not really mutually exclusive. One can hardly agree with DAVIS (1970), the author of mechano-electrical theory of hearing, when he said during his final speech at the Symposium on the biochemical mechanisms of hearing and deafness that biochemical and electrophysiological data on mechanisms of hearing are so much in contradiction with one another that the contrast reminded him of a line from Kipling: "East is east and West is west, and never the twain shall meet." However, as explained here, the cytological, biochemical and electrophysiological data complement one another.

The embryology of Corti's organ in vertebrates makes it possible to observe to a certain extent the development of a molecular cholinergic mechanism in the ontogenesis of hair cells. Thus, if we take the appearance of the activity of acetylcholinesterase as a test for this mechanism, we can indeed oberserve the localization of acetylcholinesterase in the area of hair cell synapses and stereocilia in the lower coils of the developing cochlea of prematurely born animals; these lower cochlear coils begin to function early, while the upper apical cochlear coils still appear undifferentiated (TITOVA, 1968; DEL BO and CONTI, 1961). The adaptation of the cholinergic synaptic mechanism to act as a molecular trigger mechanism for the hair cells of Corti's organ is the result not only of a protein mutation, i.e. synthesis of new proteins (cholinoreceptive protein and acetylcholinesterase) in onto- and phylogenesis, but also—and this is equally important—of a spatial rearrangement of these proteins in the cell and their displacement into the stereocilia area, where they are able to perform such a trigger function. As we shall explain in the following chapter, the receptor cells of the other organs of the acoustic-lateral system have not, apparently, undergone such an evolution.

In conclusion, a few words about the organization of the auditory receptor in insects. As in vertebrates, it is the outcome of evolution of the universal mechanoreceptors, which become grouped together and increase the complexity of their cuticular structures and so are ultimately transformed into the chordotonal and tympanic organs. The morphological characteristics of these organs show that they are always based on a bipolar receptor cell equipped with a central and a peripheral process, the latter being modified flagellum with $9 \times 2 + 0$ fibrils. The structural organization of both chordotonal and tympanic organs indicates that the stimulation of a receptor cell is effected, in spite of the presence of a permanent scolopoid body, by means of a cap cell crowning the apex of the peripheral process. This cap cell transmits to the receptor cell the encoded information concerning the acoustic stimulus. How does this transmission take place? Is it effected by means of mechanical deformation of the plasma membrane of the peripheral process, which would be sufficient for its polarization and the appearance of a biopotential, or by a mediator, as it is in Corti's organ of vertebrates? Special investigations are required to resolve this puzzle.

# Chapter VIII

# Gravity Reception

## 1. Introduction

The orientation of animals with respect to the direction of the Earth's gravitational field is effected, no matter how high their organizational level, with the aid of the otolith apparatus. In invertebrates, this apparatus is generally represented by statocysts, while in vertebrates its functions are performed by the vestibular portion of the labyrinth. A gravitational stimulus is associated with the function of mechanoreceptor cells, which at the lower levels of evolution consist of cells containing in their cytoplasm a concretion; this cell is known as a lithocyte. As the organizational level rises, the mechanoreceptor cells can perceive movements of the otolith by means of the flagella or stereocilia, with which the primary sensory cells in the labyrinth of vertebrates are equipped. The flagella of primary sensory cells in the statocysts of invertebrates contain $9 \times 2 + 2$ fibrils in which ATPase is located, but the movement of these flagella is apparently inhibited under normal conditions. In vertebrates, the secondary sensory cells of the labyrinth retain only a single mobile kinocilium, which is "opposed" to a whole bundle of immobile stereocilia; the latter can move, but only under the effect of the shearing forces generated by the otolith when the animal changes its position in the gravitational field of the Earth.

By studying the development in phylogenesis of the structure and function of the otolith apparatus at the organic, cellular, subcellular and, if possible, molecular level of organization, we can come fairly close to understanding how it functions as a gravity receptor. We can observe how natural selection, given the laws governing the Earth's gravitational field, is finally able to create by "trial and error" a universal model of gravity receptor which, though similar for all animals, becomes more complex with increasing level of organization, and is finally transformed into a true organ of equilibrium in representatives of three phyletic lines: arthropods (decapoda), molluscs (cephalopods), and vertebrates.

## 2. Gravitational Stimulus

All organisms that have lived in the past or are now living on Earth have developed under conditions in which they were exposed to the force of gravity, in other words, under the effect of the Earth's gravitational field. During the course of evolution organisms developed a whole series of devices without which life in a gravitational field would have been impossible (for example, the bony skeleton, muscles, etc.). The presence of the gravitational field forced living organisms to assume a definite position with respect to the force of gravity, i.e. a vertical line. If the animal was not able to maintain this position, it was threatened with rather serious consequences, particularly if it was a large animal.

Indeed, many systems in organisms are adapted to work in a definite position with respect to a vertical line (bloodcarrying systems, digestive systems, etc.). These systems can also function normally when the position of the body is subjected to considerable deviation, but if the animal is turned upside down for a time, the operation of these systems will be greatly disturbed.

In the majority of organisms, the need to maintain a definite position with respect to the Earth's gravitational field was opposed to the need for coordinated motor activity (obtaining food, protection against enemies), which frequently requires considerable deviation of the body's position from the normal. This led to the development of sensory motor systems, which allowed animals not only to determine "ups" and "downs" and the magnitude of the deviation of the body's position from the normal, but also to correct the setting of the body by maintaining it within the necessary isophysiological limits. In other words, the Earth's gravitational field became for animals a means of orientation (or plumb line) in the three-dimensional space surrounding them.

The orientation of animals in the Earth's gravitational field differs from orientation according to any other kind of physical or chemical characteristics of the environment perceived by animal sense organs. This difference is associated with the fact that, while both chemical and physical environmental characteristics change and frequently disappear for short periods (sounds, odors, illumination, etc.), the gravitational field possesses two special characteristics: 1. it is practically constant both in magnitude and in its direction relative to the Earth's surface; 2. it is "all-pervading", i.e. it acts on any body on the Earth, and one cannot "shield oneself" from its effect. It is perhaps because of these properties of the gravitational field that it has acquired such great importance not only for the orientation of animals, but also for their navigation.

For orientation with respect to the Earth's gravitational field most animals are equipped with a "body-position transducer", i.e. the special otolith organ. This organ has reached a lesser or greater degree of perfection during the evolutionary process but is nevertheless built according to the same principle, one which can be easily understood on the basis of elementary physical concepts. The important thing is that the equilibrium organ consists of two parts: a "standard mass", i.e. the otolith (sometimes of nonbiological origin), possessing a certain freedom of movement within the limits of the organ (Fig. 102), and a system of receptors capable of perceiving the position or movement of this mass within the organ (the position of the organ is, of course, "rigidly" related to the position of the body). Any deviation in the position of the body is accompanied by displacement of the "standard mass" (otolith, otoconia, otolith membrane), which stimulates the corresponding group of receptors in the equilibrium organ. The signal emitted by these receptors is processed by the central nervous system, which sends off a command to the muscles to correct the position of the body. Thus, we are dealing here with the restoration of a strictly static equilibrium, in which the effect of the so-called "gravitational" mass of the otolith is manifested.

As the speed of transportation has increased, human equilibrium organs sometimes emit "false" signals, i.e. signals which contradict normal experience, for example, visual sensations. These "false" signals are associated with the

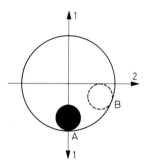

Fig. 102. Diagram of the otolith organ (V. BUDDENBROCK, 1952). *A* and *B* Deflected "standard mass" (otolith or otoconium) during change in the position of the organism in the gravitational field. *1, 2* Direction of principal axes

fact that, at high accelerations of movement, the "inertial" mass of the otolith begins to exert its effect. In other words, the effect of constant acceleration ceases to be distinguishable (for the organism) from the effect of the gravitational field. The equilibrium organ can hardly be blamed for this, since under normal conditions movement at constant acceleration (comparable in magnitude with the acceleration of gravity, i.e. $9.81 \, m/sec^2$) is noncharacteristic for an animal or man, and is simply impossible during the course of at least several tenths of a second. A possible exception here is birds, which are able to move at great speeds along curvilinear trajectories. For this reason, the equilibrium organ has historically been an organ of static equilibrium, and hence we can say that the organism possesses special gravity receptors or "gravireceptors". When using this term, we must keep in mind that the cells of the equilibrium organ do not in themselves perceive "gravity"; they perceive only the magnitude and direction of the force exerted on them by the "standard mass" under the effect of the Earth's attraction. In other words, the perception of gravity is in essence the measurement of the weight of the otolith during inclinations and this measurement can only be made when an appropriate organ is present. In other cases, when an animal or a man moves with a certain acceleration (including angular acceleration), systems of inertial orientation ("inertia receptors") operate in the organism, and these systems (for example, the semicircular canals) are capable of "measuring" both angular and linear accelerations.

As already mentioned above, the "secret" of the operation of gravity and inertia receptors can be understood by starting from simple physical concepts.

Newton's universal law of gravitation states that bodies are attracted to each other with a force directly proportional to their mass and inversely proportional to the square of the distance separating them, i. e.

$$F = G \frac{M_1 M_2}{d^2}$$

where $F$ is the attractive force, $G$ is the gravity constant, $M_1$ and $M_2$ are the gravitational masses of two bodies, and $d$ is the distance between the bodies (more precisely, between their centers of gravity).

For bodies located near the surface of the Earth (at a distance h from it), the above law takes on the form:

$$F = G \frac{M_1 M_3}{(r + h)^2}$$

where $M_1$ is the gravitational mass of the body, $M_3$ the gravitational mass of the Earth, $r$ the Earth's radius, and $h$ the height of the body over the surface of the Earth.

Since for all animals present in the biosphere of the Earth h does not exceed several kilometers, and this is very much less than the Earth's radius (6,370 km), the value of $h$ is negligible in comparison with $r$. The attractive force exerted by the Earth on the body is then equal to:

$$F = G \frac{M_1 M_3}{r^2}$$

Thus it is clear that the attractive force exerted by the Earth on the body depends only on the gravitational mass of the body.

The acceleration acquired by the body under the action of the force $F$ can be determined in accordance with Newton's second law as:

$$\alpha = \frac{F}{m_1},$$

where $\alpha$ is the acceleration of the body and $m_1$ is its inertial mass. Therefore, the mass of the body $m_1$ serves as a measure of the resistance of the body to the effect of the external force $F$, i.e. as a measure of the body's inertia (the mass $m_1$ is called the inertial mass of the body). The acceleration imparted to a body of gravitational mass $M_1$ and inertial mass $m_1$ in the gravitation field of the Earth is equal to:

$$\alpha = G \frac{M_1}{m_1} \frac{M_3}{r^2}.$$

Thus, we find that the acceleration with which a body falls onto the Earth depends upon the ratio between its gravitational and inertial masses $M_1/m_1$. Careful tests have shown that all bodies fall onto the Earth with the same acceleration. From this fact, two important conclusions can be derived. First, that the gravitational mass of a body $M_1$ is proportional to its inertial mass $m_1$, i.e., if $M_1$ and $m_1$ are expressed in appropriate physical units, then $M_1/m_1$ = 1 (precisely this conclusion was drawn at one time by NEWTON). Second, that the acceleration of a freely falling body is a constant magnitude, characterizing in this case the gravitational field of the Earth (this magnitude is normally designated by the letter $G$ and is equal to approximately 9.81 m/sec$^2$.

EINSTEIN later showed, while elaborating his general theory of relativity, that in small areas of space (where the gravitational field can be considered uniform, i.e. constant in magnitude and direction) it is impossible in principle to distinguish the movement of a body under the effect of gravitational forces from the movement of a body with constant acceleration induced by the action of any other kind of force. In other words, an effect which cannot be distinguished from the action of the gravitational field can be the result of motion with constant acceleration, although the nature of the forces acting upon the body is different in the two cases. From the above statements it should be clear that when a "standard mass" (e.g. an otolith) is present in the existing equilibrium organ, then if there is static deviation[1] of the body from the equilibrium position, the organ, if we may put it this way, "operates on the gravitational mass" of the otolith. When movement is involved, the organ "operates in the inertial mass" of the otolith. If the deviation of the otolith is the same in both cases, the animal is unable to discern what is causing the deviation of the otolith: Is it due to a change in position, or to motion with acceleration? This explains some well-known errors in orientation when the equilibrium organ, instead of giving us the true position of the horizontal plane, gives us the position of the plane perpendicular to the resultant force (vector sum). This is the sum of the weight of the otolith plus its inertial pressure on the receptor epithelium of the equilibrium organ, and is what occurs in the case of motion with acceleration, for example, during turns.

The fact that (as stated in EINSTEIN's equivalence principle) gravitational effects are sometimes indistinguishable from purely mechanical effects is widely utilized in experimental studies, ranging from the creation of overloads with the aid of special centrifuges to experiments in nearer space and with weightlessness. This does not mean there is no effect on the part of the Earth's gravitational field; the Earth's attractive force is simply counterbalanced by centrifugal forces arising during the movement of a spacecraft along a circular orbit around the Earth. It is natural that a biophysical models of this instrument should have been built on the same principle in all animals during the process of evolution because of the laws governing the Earth's gravitational field, described above. Any defects or deviations in the construction of such a model would have been eliminated by natural selection.

## 3. Evolution of the Structural and Functional Organization of the Gravireceptor of Unicellular, Invertebrate and Protochordate Organisms

The infusorians *Loxodes* and *Holotricha* are equipped with special organelles known as Muller's vesicles, 8—10 µm in diameter and filled with round mineral

---

[1] "Static deviation" is such an infinitely slow deviation that acceleration can be disregarded.

concretions or otoconia (Fig. 103). It is assumed that these forms possess a miniature statocyst-like organelle which, thanks to the movement of the concretions, can perceive their position in the gravitational field and regulate it with the aid of flagella (PÉNARD, 1922; DOGIEL, 1929). However, there is so far no experimental confirmation of the accuracy of such a viewpoint. In other infusorians, which do not possess a statocyst-like organelle, it has proved possible to detect the gravitational field and to study it experimentally. In this case, apparently, a digestive vacuole acts as the statocyst. If a *Paramecium* is fed finely ground iron, it reacts to the action of a strong, single-pole magnet as it would to gravitational forces, by turning towards the magnet with the aid of the flagella on the lower part of its body (KOEHLER, 1922; MERTON, 1935).

If we can prove that the statocyst-like organelle of protozoa indeed performs the role of receptor, then it will be clear that, in the course of evolution, this function was already structurally designed in an appropriate manner in unicellular animals. As pointed out above, such a phenomenon is known to occur with respect to visual function, for example, the eyespot of *Euglena* (Diflagella). It is interesting that both organelles perform their locomotor function indirectly with the aid of flagella containing $9 \times 2 + 2$ fibrils. This structural and functional link with the flagellum is preserved in multicellular animals, both in the photoreceptors (VINNIKOV, 1964, 1965a, 1965b, 1966a, 1966b) and in the statocysts and the vestibular apparatus (VINNIKOV et al., 1971).

It is believed that the development of the two main branches of the animal world starts with the dissymmetrical descendants of the Coelenterata: Protostomia and Deuterostomia. In coelenterates it is indeed possible to observe all variations in the development of the gravity receptor. Jellyfish (medusae) have gravireceptors that can be divided into two types: true statocysts and lithostyles; these are found both in true medusae (Scyphomedusae) and in hydromedusae (BULLOCK and HORRIDGE, 1965). Statocysts exhibit all transitional forms ranging from a small impression to a closed vesicle (Fig. 104). Lithostyles are flask-shaped; they appear to have developed from tentacles but differ in size and degree of structural complexity. An example of a large lithostyle is the rhopalium or marginal organ of medusae. The merging of the lithostyle into the statocyst is a tendency frequently observed, for example in the Trachinemidae family (DOGIEL, 1937).

Two types of cells constitute the structural basis of the gravity organ in medusae: a special cell known as lithocyte and a little-known receptor cell equipped with hairs. Lithocytes are usually of endodermal origin and receptor cells of ectodermal origin. The lithocytes has inside its cytoplasm a round concretion, believed to be mobile, known as the otoconium, consisting mostly of calcium carbonate or sulfate and organic compounds. These cells in lithostyles and rhopalia must be considered as the carriers of the "standard mass".

In Scyphomedusae, which often attain a very large size, the gravireceptors are located in the rhopalia, the rhopalium represents essentially a giant lithostyle. The number of rhopalia may vary: in *Obelia* and *Alginopsis* there are always 8, in *Carmarina* and *Getionia* 12, and in *Cunina* and *Mitrocoma* from 4 to 80. Rhopalia are an expansion in the edge of the umbrella, in the base of which runs an extension of the radial gastric canal. The free end of the rhopalium

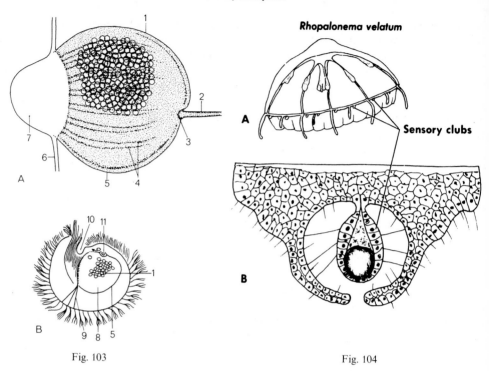

Fig. 103                                                Fig. 104

Fig. 103 A and B. Concretion vacuole or "statocyst" in infusorians (V. A. DOGIEL, 1929). A. Vacuole in *Blepharoprosthium pireum*, viewed from the side. B. Transverse section of the front end of the body with a concretion vacuole in *Paraisotricha colpoidea 1* concretion cluster; *2* centripetal fibril; *3* pore; *4* parietal fibrils; *5* vacuole wall; *6* pellicule of body wall; *7* pellicular cap; *8* vacuole cavity; *9* overhanging fibril; *10* peristome; *11* opening for the passage of concretions

Fig. 104 A and B. Diagram of rhopalia or marginal organs in *Rhopalonema velatum* (HICKMAN, 1967). A. Body of medusa with marginal organs. B. Rhopalium with single lithocyte

is a static cone, the lithostyle, which contains in its endodermal layer the lithocyte with a larger mineral concretion or otolith. Some Scyphomedusae contain clusters of lithocytes instead of a single lithocyte. The entire rhopalium is usually enveloped by lobed outgrowths of the umbrella edge in the form of a tube (Fig. 104). Eyespots may develop in the endoderm of the main portion of the rhopalium. We should point out the "roof" filled with mesogloea, formed at the expense of the gastric canal, which thrusts above the rhopalium in *Cotilorhiza* and *Rhizostoma* (BOZLER, 1926; FRÄNKEL, 1925). On the subumbrellar side a receptor epithelium is also present, usually identified as the inner receptor fossa. There is also a cluster of ganglion cells located in the nerve plexus at the base of rhopalia; this cluster apparently acts as the nerve center for the rhopalium (BOZLER, 1926). Thus, the gravireceptor in medusae is a system consisting of the rhopalium, the inner receptor fossa and the rhopalium ganglion. Whereas it is assumed that the functional mechanism of a gravireceptor of the lithostyle type is associated with otoconia, which are deflected under the effect of the gravitational field like the needle of a metronome or a pendulum when the animal changes its body position, a number of functional characteristics of rhopalia have not yet been clarified. Some authors have even reached the conclusion that rhopalia in general are not gravireceptors (VON UEXKULL, 1901; VETO-KHIN, 1926a, 1926b; BETHE, 1935); however, studies performed by FRÄNKEL (1925) and BOZLER (1926) demonstrated the gravitational role of rhopalia in medusae. Very careful removal of all parts of the marginal organs, including adjacent ganglions, resulted in a complete cessation of spontaneous movement of the medusa. At the same time, it was established that the normal movement of a medusa does not require impulses on the part of the receptor portion of the rhopalium, but is effected automatically, in all probability through the ganglion in the marginal organ (BOZLER, 1926). However, compensatory movements of the medusa depend upon position of marginal organs. The nature of the contraction of the animal's musculature varies with a change in the position of marginal organs (FRÄNKEL, 1925).

According to our data (VINNIKOV et al., 1971), the cytochemical organization of ectodermal and endodermal cells in the rhopalium of the medusa *Aurelia aurita* is characterized to a sufficient extent by a high content of RNA, and also of total protein and functional groups of protein molecules, both in the cytoplasm and in the nucleus. In the apical region of the rhopalium, it is possible, with the aid of the electron microscope, to determine the structural organization of lithocytes, which represent a product of the transformation of endoderm. The lithocytes are separated by a plasma membrane and are arranged in the form of a complex, multirow cluster, apparently in a state of continuous new growth and development. After osmium fixation, the concretion or otoconium

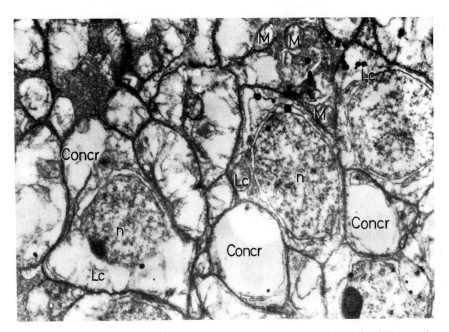

Fig. 105. Lithocytes (*Lc*) in rhopalia of *Aurelia aurita* (× 11,000) (VINNIKOV *et al.*, 1971). *n* nucleus; *Concr* concretions; *M* mitochondria. In the lithocytes were concretions, dissolved during treatment of the material

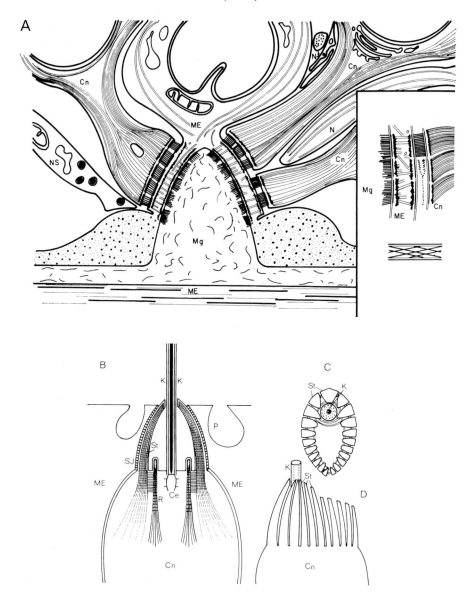

in every lithocyte is dissolved; the general organization of the cell is thus preserved intact. Lithocytes are polygonal cells of comparatively small size with an expanded apex and are coated with a clearly defined plasma membrane. A large nucleus of round or oval shape with coarse-grained chromatin, a large nucleolus, and a distinct double porous membrane occupies the central position. The cytoplasmic rim around the nucleus is small. The outer membrane of the nucleus is connected by passages to the rough endoplasmic reticulum, which is clearly defined. Large mitochondria are found in the cytoplasmic rim between the nucleus and the

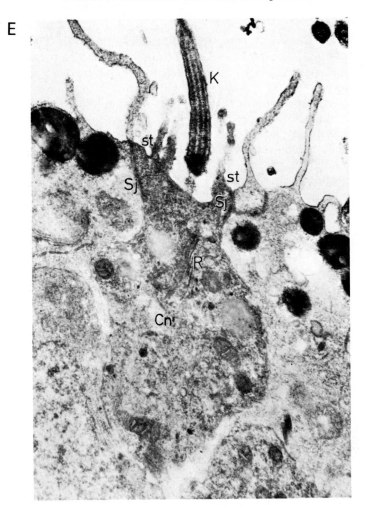

Fig. 106 A—E. Structural diagram of cnidoblasts in the hydra (SLAUTTERBACK, 1967). A. Diagram showing connections of the cnidoblast with other cells in the hydra. B. Diagram of cnidocil, seen in longitudinal section. C. Same, in transverse section. D. Reconstruction of cnidocil. E. Apex of cnidoblasts from the ectoderm of rhopalia of *Cyanea arctica* (VINNIKOV *et al.*, 1971) (×40,000). *Cn* cnidoblast; *Ce* centriole (basal body); *R* rootlet; *ME* musculoepithelial cell; *SJ* desmosomes; *st* stereocilia; *K* kinocilium; *Mg* mesogloea; *N* neuronal processes; *NS* neurosecretory cells; *P* pits

cytoplasmic membrane of the cell. The otoconium occupies a special position in the cytoplasm of the lithocyte; a single otoconium is found on one side in all lithocytes (Fig. 105). The otoconium or concretion is oval and constricted at one end, or square with rounded corners; it is coated with a rather thick membrane, from the surface of which a number of fibers branch out, entwining it from all sides. In some spots, mitochondria may be adjacent to the outer surface of the otoconium membrane. Apparently, otoconia grow continuously. In view of the compact packing of otoconia, the presence of a surface membrane and its connection with the membrane of the original cell, we must view with some scepticism the suggestion of vibrational movements of the otoconium inside the lithocyte, by means of which the latter is supposed to be stimulated (BULLOCK and HORRIDGE, 1965). Further more, nerve plexuses are absent in endoderm sectors containing lithocytes, therefore it is not clear where such a vibration could be transmitted. Although the numerous lithocytes in the rhopalia of medusae are completely independent cells, each with its own plasma membrane, these cells nevertheless function as a total mass. In coelenterates the "standard mass" (i.e. the otoconia) is still connected directly with the cytoplasm of the lithocyte, in which the otoconia develop.

What, then, are the receptor cells like? They are equipped with hairs, which must be able to perceive deflections of the standard mass enclosed in the lithocyte of the rhopalium when the medusa changes its position in the gravitational field. Are specialized receptor cells present in the ectoderm of rhopalia of coelenterates in general, and in the region of the receptor fossa of marginal organs in particular? If we use electron microscopic data as a basis, we are confronted with a number of difficulties in our attempts to distinguish special receptor cells in the endoderm of coelenterates, along with myoepithelial and interstitial cells, also cnidoblasts, which are present in different stages of development. So far, no convincing pictures are available showing the presence of such special cells (LENTZ and BARNETT, 1955; HORRIDGE, 1969). A striking feature is the presence of a large number of cnidoblasts, both on the surface of the endodermal layer of rhopalia and in the receptor fossa region, although their protective role in this region is rather problematical. However, if we recall that cnidoblasts act simultaneously as receptor and effector cells, connected by means of synapse-like structures with neighboring myoepithelial cells and also possibly with nerve cells, we are moved to ask: Is it possible that these cnidoblasts assume the function of perceiving the deflection of rhopalia?

Cnidoblasts and their mutual relations with myoepithelial and nerve cells have recently been investigated by SLAUTTERBACK (1967) in the hydra (Fig. 106) and by us (VINNIKOV et al., 1971) in the rhopalium region of *Aurelia aurita* and *Cyanea arctica*. In general, the subcellular organization of cnidoblasts was found to be similar. The cnidoblast is a cylindrical cell with a nucleus at its center; a special organoid, known as a cnidocil (SLAUTTERBACK, 1961, 1963, 1967) or "stiff rod", as it was previously designated by HYMAN (1940), projects from the apical surface (shaped as a constricted end) of the cnidoblast. This cnidocil is crowned with a characteristic curved flagellum-kinocilium, slightly to one side of center and surrounded by 18–21–22 stereocilia. Only 2 or 5 of the surrounding stereocilia are about the same length as the flagellum and are in contact with it. The remaining stereocilia are shorter and are located at a certain distance from the flagellum (Fig. 106, b—d). In cross-section the flagellum exhibits a structure consisting of 9 peripheral fibrils and groups of modified central fibers, among which it is difficult to distinguish the 2 central fibrils that characterize motile flagella or cilia. The stereocilia, which are modified microvilli, consist of a bundle of many fine fibrils with a striation period of 200Å, coated by an extension of the plasma membrane (Fig. 106). The stereocilia fibrils, in the same number (18–21–22), extend deep into the cytoplasm of the cnidoblasts as far as the nematocyst, an organoid filled with a secretion capable of paralyzing the victim stung by the flagellum. The modified flagella is connected to the centriole, or basal body, from which extends a powerful ramified rootlet with a striation period of 400Å, surrounded laterally by stereocilia rootlets.

An extraordinary similarity has been noted by a number of authors in the organization of a cnidocil and of the surface of the receptor hair cells found in lateral-line organs and in the vestibular apparatus (utricle, sacculus and semicircular canals), and even in Corti's organ of vertebrates (WERSÄLL, FLOCK, and LUNDQUIST, 1966; SLAUTTERBACK, 1967). The apices of cnidocil receptor hair cells are also crowned with a single kinocilium with 9 pairs of peripheral fibrils and 2 central fibrils; located opposite this kinocilium is a bundle of 50—70 stereocilia of very similar structure. Stimulation of the hair cells occurs when the stereocilia are deflected toward the kinocilium during the movement of covering structures; inhibition occurs when the deflection of stereocilia proceeds from the kinocilium. Thus it appears that the onset of stimulation in the cnidoblast is also associated with a morphological polarization of the kinocilium, but stimulation can occur with every deflection of the stereocilia, since they surround the kinocilium on all sides. In the course of evolution stereocilia appear for the first time in coelenterates (SLAUTTERBACK, 1967; HORRIDGE, 1969; VINNIKOV et al., 1971). Analogous relationships are found in the maculae and cristae of statocysts in cephalopod molluscs, where the kinocilium is surrounded on all sides by stereocilia similar to microvilli (VINNIKOV et al., 1967, 1968). Therefore, it is possible to establish a mechanoreceptor parallel between the organization of the cnidocil in the cnidoblasts of coelenterates, and the distribution of stereocilia and kinocilia in the hair cells of the vestibular apparatus and of the hearing organ in vertebrates or of statocysts in cephalopod molluscs.

The cytoplasmic organization of the cnidoblast of rhopalia in the hydra seems to differ somewhat from that found in medusae, in particular as regards the structure of the nematocyst. In the hydra, the nematocyst may be oval or shaped like a truncated pyramid and coated with a membrane but it communicates with the matrix of the cell; it is usually located near the nucleus or may even displace the latter toward the base of the cytoplasm. Elements of the rough endoplasmic reticulum and of Golgi's apparatus take part in the development and differentiation of the nematocyst, as well of its membranes and secretion of its content (SLAUTTERBACK and FAWCETT, 1959). In the rhopalium ectoderm of medusae, in contrast to the hydra, the nematocyst present in cnidoblasts has an undifferentiated character. Usually, several nematocysts are present in a single cnidoblast; they are located both in the upper part of the cell, in the region containing the system of rootlets branching off from the kinocilium, and in the base of the cell. Nematocysts take the form of a round or oval, closed or semi-closed body, coated on the surface with a powerful system of membranes and tubules with a granular content, dark against a light matrix or having the character of a dark granule with very high electron density.

Nematocysts, after reaching the peak of their differentiation, are subjected to a regression after a certain time. In the course of this regression they are transformed into hyaline bodies of irregular shape with an electron-dense granular content (SLAUTTERBACK and FAWCETT, 1959). A careful study of the nematocysts in cnidoblasts in the rhopalium region (Fig. 106), suggests underdevelopment rather than regression, since the hyaline substance is not found at their location site. The strategic position of the rhopalium between the sensitive lobes of the umbrella and the velum, where it would be difficult for an enemy or prey to land, raises doubts as to whether these cells require large stocks of poison and an excessive development of the nematocyst. We believe that contact stimulation of the cnidocil during deflection of the rhopalium is not accompanied by the secretion of poison. However, additional studies are needed in this respect, since we may simply be dealing here with different development stages of the nematocyst.

Thus, the structural organization of the gravireceptor in coelenterates is characterized by the fact that the standard mass in (lithostyle or rhopalia) is a lithocyte, while the receptor cell is a cnidoblast. The cnidocil of the cnidoblast consists of a kinocilium and surrounding stereocilia and hardly differs from the corresponding structures found in the labyrinth of vertebrates.

The organization of the aboral organ of Ctenophora undoubtedly represents a considerable advance over the coelenterates, since Ctenophora are a more progressive and independent evolutionary branch of the animal world. The high level of differentiation and functioning of the nervous system of Ctenophora accounts for their great mobility and the ability of their body and tentacles to contract significantly as a result of the operation of their locomotor apparatus, consisting of combs made up of agglutinated cilia. The aboral (apical) organ of Ctenophora is the principal sense organ and coordinates the structure and function of the nervous system. We shall understand the structural organization of the aboral organ better if we examine its development. In the young ctenophore the aboral pole is uniformly coated with ciliated cells. The hairs of special cells girdling the aboral pole in the form of a crown, increase considerably in length, bend over the aboral pole and stick together to form a thin, glass-like cap or dome over this pole. As a result of this process, a cap-shaped formation is formed over the aboral pole, which is sometimes incorrectly called the cupule (KOMAI, 1922). Inside the dome are long flagella twisted in the shape of the letter "S" and adhering together (but slightly separated in some crawling ctenophores); these flagella, known as balancers, extend from the four symmetrical epithelial portions of the ciliated bottom lining and run toward the center of the dome in the form of four radial bundles, the free ends of which are almost in contact with each other. In time, fine circular concretions, apparently consisting of calcium phosphate, accumulate in some cells lithocytes otoconiablasts; they are deposited in the cavity of the dome where they crystallize and become attached to the tips of the balancers. These concretions agglutinate and together form the complex otolith. Thus, in contrast to coelenterates, the ctenophores were the first organisms to "invent" the excretional method for the synthesis of otoconia, which adhere together to form the otolith that acts as the standard mass. The extracellular formation of an otolith can be observed in the gravitation organs of higher animals.

The receptor cells of the aboral organ of Ctenophora have recently been studied both cytochemically (VINNIKOV et al., 1971) and under the electron microscope (HORRIDGE, 1965a, 1965b; VINNIKOV *et al.*, 1971; TITOVA *et al.*, 1973) (Fig. 107). The receptor epithelium of the aboral organ is characterized by a rather high content of total protein and functional groups of protein molecules. Nucleic acids are present in the usual distribution. An electron microscopic study performed in our laboratory has shown that the balancers, which, as stated above, are fused flagella (HORRIDGE, 1965a, 1965b) generally contain $9 \times 2 + 2$ fibrils. It is of particular interest that these flagella originate deep in the cytoplasm of the receptor cell, where they are present in the form of tightly packed formations of hexagons; closer to the apical sector of the cell, they exhibit a less ordered arrangement. After emerging onto the free surface of the cell, these flagella carry on along a thin layer of cytoplasm, which frequently forms a sort of additional membrane on the balancer.

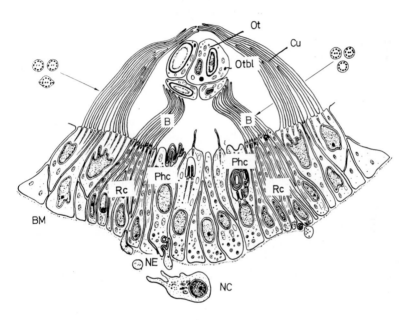

Fig. 107.  Diagram of ultrastructural organisation of the gravity receptor (aboral organ) in Ctenophora (TITOVA *et al.*, 1973). *Rc* receptor cell of gravity receptor; *Phc* photoreceptor cells; *B* balansers; *Cu* cupula; *Ot* otolith; *NC* nerve cells; *NE* nerve endings; *BM* basal membrane; *Otbl* otoconiablasts

Our observations have shown that flagella from at least 9 cells can take part in the formation of a single balancer. Long, stretched out receptor cells extend from a rather well-developed basal membrane. A relatively small nucleus, characterized by high electron density and having a large, dark nucleolus, is located in the basal part of these cells. Mitochondria are found in the cytoplasm of the receptor cell, as well as numerous basal bodies ($9 \times 2 + 0$ fibrils) connected with the highly developed rootlet system of the flagella; the rootlets, as also pointed out by HORRIDGE (1965a), branch off from the base of the flagellum at right angles. The rootlets are cross-striated, with a striation period of 400Å.

A clearly expressed basal foot branches off from the basal body in a direction opposite to the rootlet. In some cases, two basal feet were seen branching off from one basal body, parallel to each other or at an angle of about 60 °. About 0.4 μm from the lower border of the basal body is a basal plate above which the fibrillar apparatus of the flagellum assumes its normal appearance (9 × 2 + 2 fibrils) (Fig. 107).

Our results make it possible to be more precise about the observations recorded by HORRIDGE (1964, 1965a, 1965b); at the same time we succeeded in showing that there is synaptic contact between the base of receptor cell and the nerve fibers which penetrate the basement membrane and run off from the nerve cell of the aboral ganglion. Thus, the cells that contribute to the balancers in ctenophora can be considered the prototype of the secondary sensory cells (ARONOVA, in press) that appear later in the lateral-line and labyrinth organs of vertebrates. It must be pointed out that the aboral sense organ also represents a polyvalent receptor because it contains photoreceptor cells of peculiar organization (Fig. 107).

How is the excitation of the gravity organ transmitted to the motor system of a ctenophora? There is an intimate connection between the aboral organ and the meridional rows of combplates. A ciliated comb, starting at the base of the cells taking part in the formation of the balancer, runs along the surface of the body; this comb soon splits off into two branches in such a way that each branch approaches the starting point of the two nearest rows of combs. *In vivo* observations established (HORRIDGE, 1965a, 1965b) that at definite time intervals one of the flagella in the balancer exhibits a sudden beat which is transmitted to the central parts of the balancer, whose flagella respond by means of a reversible rapid phase. Since the flagella of the balancer are located at the top of the line of cilia branching off from the cells forming the ciliated groove at the bottom of the combplates, every deflection of the balancer is transmitted along the ciliated comb to the corresponding rows of comb plates and induces in these plates a beat wave, which travels from the aboral to the oral pole. It has been shown that ciliated movements of comb plates take place under the control of the nervous system (BAUER, 1910; GÖTHLIN, 1920; FEDELE, 1926; CONFIELD, 1934). Studies performed a long time ago have shown that the movement of a single comb plate takes place according to the type of metachronal waves, which are synchronous to the movements of other comb plates as long as the integrity of the meridional grooves is not disturbed, or as long as the aboral gravireceptor is not removed (CHUN, 1880; EIMER, 1880; VERWORN, 1889, 1881; PARKER 1905). From the gravireceptor, impulses are propagated to all rows of meridional comb plates responsible for the movement of the animal. Even after *in vitro* isolation of one of the rows of comb plates, the beat in such a plate can take place synchronously with that of plates left *in vivo;* moreover, any lower sector in the row of a comb plate is capable of such a beat. These facts are in agreement with data implying that all cilia possess autonomy of movement and are controlled by the nervous system only during inhibition, restoration, and change relative to the oral beat time. Transmission of pulsation is usually possible only from the aboral to the oral pole. This fact, by the way, was one of the examples of Child's apicobasal sensitivity gradient (CHILD, 1933). Inhibition and restoration of the act of beating, as well as its speed, is controlled by the nervous system. The direction of movement is changed by means of differential inhibition of comb plates on one side, which enables the animal to turn. The corresponding impulses originate from the gravireceptor and are probably associated with the asymmetric movement of the otolith resulting from the modified position of the animal's body in the gravitational field. In this case, the inhibition wave travels towards the oral pole (BULLOCK and HORRIDGE, 1965).

Thus, in ctenophores, it is the flagellar apparatus that predominates in the ectodermal epithelium coating the animal's body and so constitutes the material which seems to be a precursor of secondary sensory cells, forming the basis for the creation of the structural organization of the gravireceptor. This tendency, as well as the excretional formation of the otolith, is firmly preserved throughout the evolution of higher animals.

A statocyst with a lithocyte is found in early representatives of Protostomia, flatworms and, in particular, in ciliated worms. Electron microscopic studies performed in our laboratory (VINNIKOV et al., 1971; IVANOV et al., 1972) have shown that concepts of the structure of the statocyst formed on the basis of light microscopy require considerable modification. Thus the statocyst wall in *Convoluta convoluta* was found to be formed by a single flattened cell, having a cavity, equipped with a nucleus, mitochondria and other cellular organoids. A thin cuticula can be observed under the cytoplasmic membrane of this cell. The receptor cell forming the statocyst wall is surrounded in turn by numerous leafshaped processes of sustentacular cells, the nucleus-containing cell bodies being located between or under these processes. Membranes of rough endoplasmic reticulum, isolated small granules and vacuoles can be seen in the cytoplasm of these processes. The lithocyte is an oval cell with a concretion at its center, surrounded by a double plasma membrane. The cytoplasm contains a nucleus, mitochondria and other cellular organoids. The lithocyte is attached at its base, by means of a thin pedicle, to the cytoplasmic membrane of the cell that forms the statocyst wall; nerve fibers ends approach this cell. It is still not clear how deflections of the lithocyte are perceived by the cell lining the statocyst when the worm is in motion. Nevertheless, the data obtained so far indicate that, judging from the presence and position of the lithocyte, the gravireceptors of ciliated worms are somewhat similar in their organization to the lithostyle of certain coelenterates and, as we shall see below, of protochordates. The organization of statocysts in nemerteans is apparently similar to that of ciliated worms (BÜRGER, 1895; GERNER, 1969).

The gravireceptor of segmented worms (Annelidae) have a considerably higher level of organization. Usually, they take the form of a statocyst communicating with the environment by means of a narrow duct, which may be obliterated with increasing age. Otoliths or otoconia can be sand particles brought in from outside and agglutinated by means of chitin, or they can be formed entirely by the secretory activity of the statocyst cells (FAUVEL, 1907). A study of the function of statocysts removed from some annelids *(Arenicola)* has shown that they are indeed capable of recording the position of the animal in the gravitational field (BUDDENBROCK, 1912).

According to data obtained in our laboratory (VINNIKOV et al., 1971), the statocysts of *Arenicola* have an irregular rounded shape. The cavity of the statocyst contains numerous otoconia with a thin coating of chitin; they are located between large kinocilia, cut lengthwise and crosswise, and containing $9 \times 2 + 2$ fibrils. The wall consists of a multirow epithelium, with a cuticle on the outside. Branching off from the medial portion of the statocyst is a bundle of fibers, known as the static nerve, running into the corresponding ganglions. The structural organization of the statocyst comprises two types of cells, namely large or light cells, and smaller and more numerous dark cells (Fig. 108). The dark cells are located between the light cells and give off a large number of irregular microvillar processes, approaching the cuticle and apparently forming the latter. The nuclei of the dark cells are small and festoon-shaped. The cytoplasm contains vast numbers of various organoids and inclusions. The most remarkable feature of the dark cells is the presence of numerous filamentous bundles which seem to represent the analog of myelin. The light cells are considerably larger and shaped like pyramids; they taper at the base, from which a central nervous process branches off; their flat apices are just short of the base of the cuticle and send off a number (9—12) of kinocilia containing $9 \times 2 + 2$ fibrils. The kinocilia originate on the basal body, from which a thin rootlet with a striation period of 400—500Å branches off. The kinocilia force apart the microvillar processes of the dark cells and, penetrating through the cuticle into the statocyst lumen, come into contact with otoconia at their apices and perhaps on their side surfaces. The cytoplasm of the light cells, characterized by a large oval nucleus, is rich in mitochondria and in elements of Golgi's apparatus and of rough endoplasmic reticulum. Histochemical treatment of *Arenicola* statocyst preparations reveals high activity of succinate dehydrogenase and other oxidative enzymes in the light cells; the dark cells have a lower activity. Both types of cells, however, have a high content of total protein and functional groups of protein molecules. For reasons of space, we shall not dwell here on the peculiar unicellular statocysts of archiannelids, equipped with kinocilia and containing an otoconium (MERKEL and HARNACK, 1967).

Thus, the statocysts of annelids are the first to display primary sensory cells equipped with kinocilia and stimulated by movements of the otoconia (standard mass), then transmitting the resultant excitation by means of their central process to the central nervous system.

However, the most perfect form of organization of a statocyst, which is transformed into a true equilibrium organ, is observed in arthropods, and in particular in crustaceans (Crustacea). The statocysts of higher crustaceans consist of an invagination of integuments with communication with the environment through a cleft; they can be located in both the head and abdominal parts of the animal's body. Only in the lower crustaceans are statocysts represented by vesicles, which are completely sealed off from the skin. However, in both types of crustaceans the chitin covering of the statocyst is sloughed during every molting period, and the vesicular statocysts are then temporarily also in contact with the external environment. During molting, the statocyst covering is shed together with the sand particles (otoconia) enclosed in it, and fresh sand particles are introduced either by the claws or by repeated borrowing in the sand. The sand particles of statocysts are usually agglutinated into a single mass by means of an organic substance secreted by the glandular cells of the statocyst. Kreidl's classical experiment (KREIDL, 1893) was performed

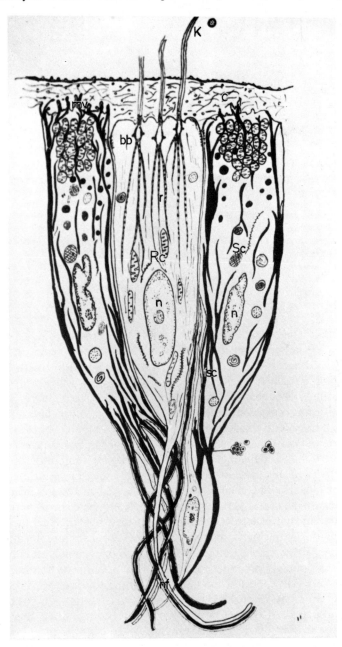

Fig. 108. Diagram showing the organization of receptor cells in the statocyst of *Arenicola marina* (TITOVA *et al.*, 1973); *Rc* receptor cell; *Sc* supporting cell; *n* nucleus; *fsc* cell process; *mv* microvilli; *bb* basal body; *K* kinocilium; *r* rootlet; *c* cuticle; *nf* nerve fibers

on statocysts of the crayfish: iron filings were offered to the animal after molting instead of sand to fill up his statocyst, and the animal was then exposed to a magnet. The effect of the magnetic field stimulated the effect of the gravitational field.

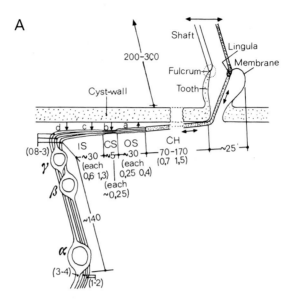

The structural organization of statocysts in Decapoda was studied by COHEN (1955, 1960) in the American lobster *(Homarus americanus)*, by SCHÖNE and STEINBRECHT (1968) in the river crayfish *(Astacus fluviatilis)* with the aid of the electron microscope, and in our laboratory (VINNIKOV *et al.*, 1971) on the Kamchatka crab *(Paralitodes camtschatica)*. The statocyst in the crayfish consists of a semi-translucent chitin sac covered with chitin hairs of caps, the ends of which point into the lumen of the liquid-filled organ. The otolith consists of a mixture of fine sand, picked up from the ground and cemented into a compact mass, and attached in a mobile manner to the statocyst wall by a secretion produced by special glands. The statocyst communicates with the environment by means of a narrow opening located in the anteromedial part of the antenna. The static nerve branches off from the ventral surface of the statocyst wall. The receptor cells are primary sensory cells; their central processes, laid together, form the nerve of the statocyst. The cells are located 0.5 mm from the base of the chitin hairs or caps, which they innervate by means of a distal, or peripheral, process, branching off from one or several cells (Fig. 109 A). This process penetrates the inner wall of the statocyst through a special canal and terminates in the widened base of the chitin hair, designated as the ampulla or cask (COHEN, 1960). Part of the cask wall in the crayfish is reinforced by a sclerotized chitin layer and is called the "tooth". The other wall of the cask has a membraneous character. Located opposite the "tooth" is a bright light-refracting thread, consisting of chitin and called the chorda (KINZIG, 1919); this chorda enters into the cuticular barb, or lingula, of the

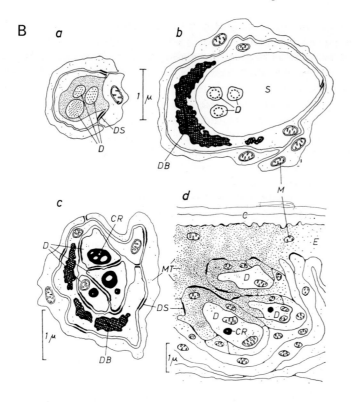

Fig. 109 A and B. Diagram showing the organization of receptor elements in the statocyst of the crayfish *Astacus fluviatilis* (SCHÖNE and STEINBRECHT, 1968). A. Longitudinal section; B. transverse sections. For A: α, β and γ three receptor cells; *IS, CS, OS* inner, ciliary, and outer segments, respectively; *CH* chorda; a—d locations corresponding to transverse sections in B; double arrows show the directions of movement during stimulation. All dimensions are given in microns. Number in parentheses correspond to the diameters of processes. For B: a—d are the transverse sections of peripheral processes, coated by processes of covering (epidermis) cells. *D* peripheral process, containing $9 \times 2 + 0$ fibrils; *DS* desmosomes; *DB* dense bodies; *M* mitochondria; *MT* microtubules; *E* epidermis cells; *C* cyst cuticle; *CR* ciliary rootlets; *S* extracellular space around ciliary segments. In a, b and c only enveloping cells are shown; in d the membrane of the enveloping cell is shown as a line

chitin hair. Attachment at this spot is analogous to the bracings found between different layers of the cuticle. The chorda extends along the lumen of the cask and enters the canal connecting the statocyst with the cask. On leaving the canal, the chorda forms an angle and runs parallel to the statocyst up to the nerve ending. Each chorda in the crayfish is connected to three peripheral processes which run in the same direction until they leave the ectodermal wall of the statocyst, curve round and make contact with the bodies of three receptor cells. The peripheral process of each cell represents a modified flagellum or cilium. It consists of three segments: outer (short), ciliar, and inner. The outer segments of the triplet of the peripheral processes are surrounded and separated by an extracellular granulated substance which becomes denser toward the distal part of the peripheral process and gradually turns into the substance of the chorda. The postciliar segments have no mitochondria but are characterized by numerous hexogonally packed microtubules. More proximally they turn into the short ciliar segment which contains 9 pairs of peripheral fibers. Beyond the ciliar region the peripheral processes become thicker and form the inner segments. At this level they make contact with each other by means of desmosomes and contain a large number of mitochondria. From the basal body of the flagellum a rootlet may originate; this rootlet is well developed in the receptor cells of the statocyst of Kamchatka crab.

The chorda and peripheral processes are surrounded by several layers of enveloping cells (Fig. 109 B), whose processes contain microtubules. Electron-dense bodies of scolopoid type can be detected in the membranes surrounding the ciliary segments. In the inner segment region these membranes are brought into contact with each other and with the peripheral processes by means of desmosomes. Axons are also arranged in groups of three in the static nerve.

Thus, every cap or hair of the statocyst in crayfish is a sensillum consisting of three mechanoreceptor cells. Consequently, the receptor surface of the statocyst is a receptor field with a rather compact arrangement of individual sensilla. Analogous relations are found in the proprioceptors of the crab (HOFFMAN, 1964) and, as discussed in Chapter VII, in the chordotonal and tympanic organs of insects (VINNIKOV et al., 1971).

Stimulating mechanical forces act in connection with shearing movements of the otolith, apparently in the direction of the long axis of the receptor organ. The structure of the receptor element in the statocyst implies the presence of a lever mechanism by means of which the stimulating force is transmitted to the base of the hair. This is confirmed by direct observations of the deflection of the hair immediately after molting and also by behavior tests. If the hair is deflected, usually by the shearing force of the otolith mass, it rotates around the notch between the "tooth" and its extension, the thickened wall of the hair. As can be seen in Fig. 109 A, if this rotation takes place in the direction of the hair symmetry, the hair acts like a lever on the chorda. The side of the cask, or lingula, in which the chorda is immersed can be seen to move up and down in the light microscope (SCHÖNE and STEINBRECHT, 1968). The chorda probably slides around the edge of the wall, thus transmitting mechanical energy to the receptor region. Resistance apparently arises in the postciliary segment by means of its skeleton, consisting of fine tubules of enveloping cells and epidermis. It is not yet clear whether all hairs are stimulated per unit time, or whether some of the hairs are stimulated while the rest are inhibited. Thus, the direction of movement of the otolith is perceived by three receptor cells. Electrophysiological tests involving recording of biopotentials from the hair cap, which represents an individual sensillum, confirm the gravitational function of the majority of receptor cells in a statocyst; these cells can perceive a change in the position of the crab's body (COHEN, 1953, 1955, 1960, 1964; COHEN, KATSUKI, and BULLOCK 1953; COHEN and DIJKGRAAF, 1961). However, receptors capable of perceiving angular accelerations have also been found; the hairs of such receptors are not connected to the otolith mass and can bend freely under the effect of the stream of liquid filling up the statocyst.

Recordings of biopotentials have shown that the hairs of the receptor cells that perceive angular accelerations are arranged in a separate row near the entrance to the statocyst cavity. Finally, hair cells have been found that are capable of perceiving vibration as well, provided it is transmitted along a hard substrate. Action currents are usually recorded against a background of spontaneous activity. As a result of a whole series of investigations of behavior reflexes, it has been established that there is a connection between the function of statocysts and eyes in crustaceans (DIJKGRAAF, 1961), also that their nervous system plays an important role in gravity reception.

Thus, we can see that a very effective model of gravity receptor has evolved in higher crustaceans; this model, indeed, represents a universal organ of both static and dynamic equilibrium. The chitin lining of the statocyst is an original device: for contact between the otolith membrane and the peripheral processes of the receptor cells an additional transformer was needed, and this took the form of the chitin hair cap.

Insects, because of the extreme lightness of their body, do not possess a statocyst. However, insects are capable of good orientation in the gravitational field, and the equilibrium function in flying insects deserves special attention. Flying insects have located behind the eyes a special mechanoreceptor organ, which may be considered as the organ contributing to the maintenance of equilibrium (MITTELSTAEDT, 1950). The head of the insect is connected to the body by a thin neck, and its rather significant mechanical inertia regulates the position of the wings. If the head receptor structures are removed in the dragonfly, it holds its head in an oblique manner, while the position of the wings is normal; on the other hand, if the head is oriented symmetrically with respect to the body, the wings are deflected. As we shall explain below, the mechanoreceptor apparatus in the head of the dragonfly, for example, is in many respects quite similar in its function to the gravireceptor of vertebrates. In vertebrates the head assumes a normal position thanks to the activity of the labyrinth, whereas in the dragonfly the inertial function of the head fulfills a similar purpose. Certain insects, for example flies *(Diptera)*, have a second pair of wings known as balancers (or halters) which are of equal interest. Electrophysiological experiments have shown that the mechanoreceptor sensilla of the balancer are true equilibrium organs (PRINGLE, 1963), but it seems probable that balancers should be considered rather as organs capable of perceiving angular accelerations (BUDDENBROCK, 1952).

Thus, during flight the position of the body of an insect with respect to the gravitational field is regulated by means of a mechanoreceptor mechanism in the head (dragonfly), or as a result of the function of balancer wings *(Calliphora)*. In both cases, reception is effected, as in crustaceans, by modified sensilla which perform very complex, graded mechanoreception processes.

The gravireceptor is particularly well developed in molluscs. In gastropods the statocyst is a small round sac filled with endolymph and containing what appears to be a "free otolith". The statocyst is connected to the cerebral ganglion by means of the static nerve. In the statocyst of *Pterotrachea* it is possible to identify a limited sector of receptor cells, which all together form a macula (TSCHACHOTIN, 1908). The receptor cells are primary sensory cells and are equipped with hair-kinocilia. Electron microscopic studies (VINNIKOV *et al.*, 1971) on the freshwater and land gastropod *Planorbis corneus* have shown that the hairs crowning the giant primary sensory cells of this mollusc are kinocilia, containing $9 \times 2 + 2$ fibrils (Fig. 110). The statocyst of the pteropod, *Cliona limacina*, has a similar structure. It consists of large, mushroom-shaped primary sensory receptor cells, equipped with kinocilia which contain $9 \times 2 + 2$ fibrils.

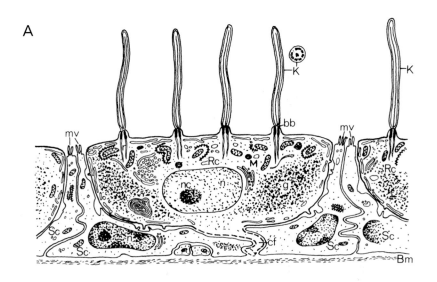

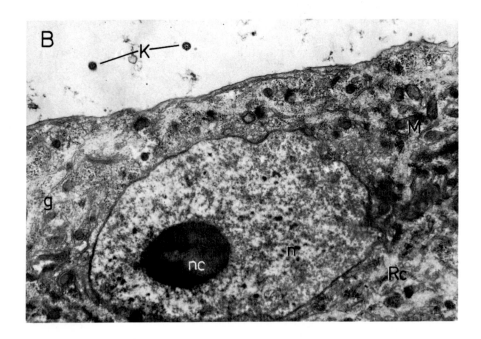

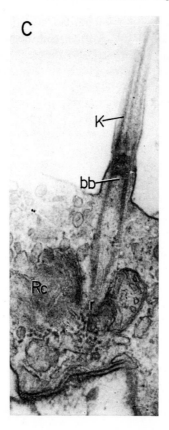

Fig. 110A—C. Structural organization of a statocyst in the pulmonate mollusc *Planorbis corneus* (VINNIKOV *et al.*, 1971). A. Structural diagram of the statocyst wall; B. giant receptor cell (× 11,000); C. longitudinal section of a kinocilium (× 36,000). *Rc* receptor cell; *cf* central process; *Sc* supporting cell; *K* kinocilium; *mv* microvillum; *n* nucleus; *nc* nucleole; *M* mitochondria; *bb* basal body; *r* rootlet; *g* granular content; *Bm* basal membrane

The otoconia are synthesized by the supporting cells and then removed by excretion. GEUZE (1968) was the first to demonstrate this in *Lymnaea stagnalis* (L). The structural and functional organization of the statocyst in Pulmonata (*Limax maximus*, *Limax flavus* and *Arion empiricorum*) is quite similar to that of Pteropoda (QUATTRINI, 1967a, 1967b; WOLFF, 1969). WOLFF succeeded in recording biopotentials in the static nerve: when his preparation was rotated around its longitudinal or transverse axis the frequency curves of the activity gave a typical shape (WOLFF, 1970). Efferent impulses (several units) were observed and spontaneous efferent impulses recorded. The sensilla in the statocysts of these species can be regarded as gravireceptors only; they do not respond to angular acceleration. A similar structure is exhibited by the cells of bivalve molluscs, although the statocysts of these animals do not have cell clusters in the form of maculae. BARBER and DILLY (1969) were the first to study the statocyst in Pecten under electron microscope. We have obtained similar data (VINNIKOV *et al.*, 1971) on the ultrastructural organization of the right and left statocysts in the scallop (Pseudolamellibranchia). The primary receptor cells of both statocysts are equipped with kinocilia containing $9 \times 2 + 2$ fibrils (Fig. 111). The kinocilia found in the right (lower) statocyst are somewhat shorter; in all other details the statocysts do not differ from each other. However, whereas

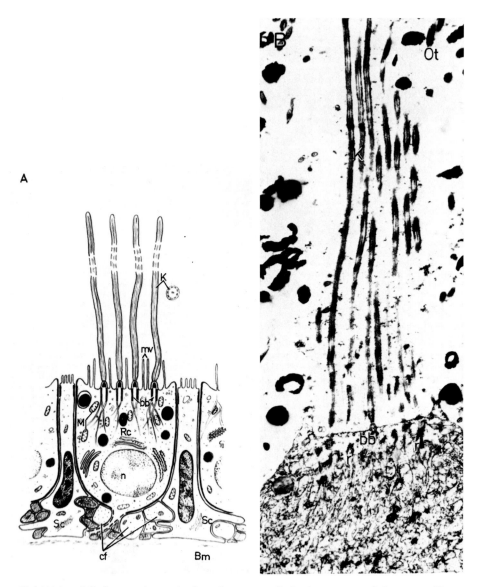

Fig. 111 A and B. Structural organization of receptor cells in the statocyst of the pecten (*Pecten jessoensis* Lay) (VINNIKOV *et al.*, 1971). A. Diagram showing the structure of the statocyst wall; B. apex of the receptor cell ($\times 16,000$). *Rc* receptor cell; *K* kinocilia; *mv* microvilli; *bb* basal body; *r* rootlets; *M* mitochondria; *cf* transversely cut central process; *Bm* basal membrane; *Ot* otoconia; *Sc* supporting cell; *n* nucleus

a well-developed otolith is present in the left (upper) statocyst, the right statocyst contains a cluster of otoconia. Physiological observations show that the function of statocysts consists in regulating the muscular tonus, i.e. thus ultimately regulating the nature of the movement of these molluscs (BUDDENBROCK, 1915). In Pecten we observe a continuous and spontaneous turning to the right, which

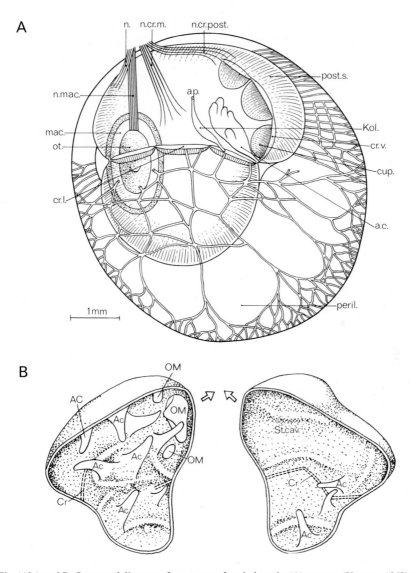

Fig. 112A and B. Structural diagram of statocysts of cephalopods: (A) octopus (YOUNG, 1960) and (B) squid (VINNIKOV *et al.*, 1971). For A: *n.* nerve; *n.cr.m.* nerve of the medial crista; *n.cr.post* nerve of the posterior crista; *ap.* apex of Kölliker's canal; *post.s* posterior sinus; *Kol.* Kolliker's canal; *cr.v* ventral crista; *cup.* cupula; *a.c.* anticrista; *peril.* perilymph; *cr.l.* lateral crista; *ot.* otolith; *mac.* macula; *n.mac.* macula nerve. For B: *Ac* anticristae; *OM* otoliths of maculae; *St.cav.* statocyst cavity; *Cr* cristae

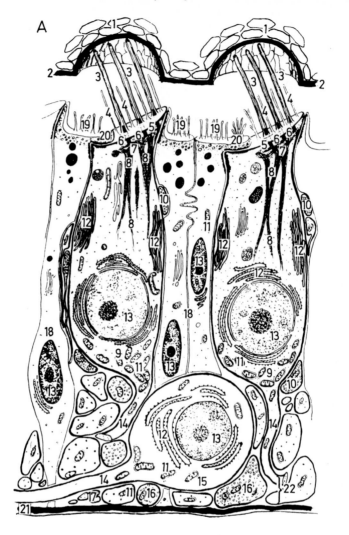

Fig. 113 A and B. Diagram showing the organization of (A) macula and (B) crista of cephalopods (VINNIKOV *et al.*, 1971). *1* otoconia; *2* otolith membrane; *3* kinocilium; *4* stereocilialike microvilli; *5* basal body; *6* pedicles; *7* rootlet plexus; *8* rootlets; *9* receptor cells (I, II, III, IV, and V rows of cells of the crista); *10* efferent nerve ending; *11* mitochondria; *12* membranes of endoplasmic reticulum; *13* nucleus; *14* axon; *15* unipolar nerve cells; *16* efferent fibers; *17* synapses; *18* supporting cells; *19* microvilli; *20* phalanges; *21* basal membrane; *22* nerve fiber layer; *23* crista cupula

is explained by the fact that the right-side statocyst is non-functional. Apparently, this anomaly is associated not so much with the structural organization of the receptor cells as with a weakened effect of the otoconia on the kinocilia of receptor cells in the right statocyst. The mechanism of the contact between kinocilia and otolith (otoconia) in the statocysts of gastropod and bivalve molluscs is still not clear to us, i.e. whether the otoliths are attached to the distal ends of kinocilia or whether they can move "freely" in the endolymph. One

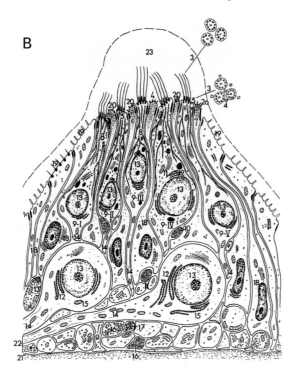

way or another, the deflection of kinocilia of receptor cells is achieved by the
displacement of otoliths when the mollusc changes the position of its body
in the gravitational field. We shall not discuss here our findings on the characteristics of the cytochemical and ultrastructural organization of primary sensory
receptor cells in gastropod and bivalve molluscs, since they are very similar
to the receptor cells of cephalopod molluscs.

It is generally assumed that the different classes of molluscs originate from
a common ancestor; among them, cephalopod molluscs have reached the highest
level of organization. A study of their gravireceptors is of particular interest
for two reasons: the reactive method of their movement, and their extraordinary
similarity to the equilibrium organs of crustaceans and vertebrates. In the octopus,
the statocysts have not only an endolymphatic cavity but also a perilymphatic
space (YOUNG, 1960) (Fig. 112); the latter is not found in the squid. The viscosity
of endolymph fluid from the statocysts of the squid Ommatostrephes sloanei
pacificus is about 1,18 centipoise, that of Octopus sp. 1,14 centipoise, its specific
weight being equal to 1,03 g/me for both animals. Sodium content of the endolymph is about 420 megv/l, that of potassium and magnesium −9,5 and less
than 5 megv/l correspondingly (GOVARDOVSKII, 1971b). In the octopus, only
one anticrista protrudes into the statocyst cavity, whereas there are two anticristae
in the squid and their arrangement represents a complex three-dimensional
system. It is assumed that the presence of anticristae allows the regulation

of the movement of the endolymph when the animal moves about, as do the semicircular canals in vertebrates. Nevertheless, the basic structures in both types of animals are the maculae, equipped with otoliths, and the cristae (appearing for the first time in invertebrates), which are coated with cupulae and are deflected by the movement of the endolymph. The macula of the octopus is located in the mediofrontal cavity; the principal macula of the squid is located in the same cavity but is equipped with two additional maculae, occupying a medial position. Three cristae are located in three orthogonal cavities, so that two cristae are horizontal and one vertical. The fourth crista has recently been found (BUDELMANN and WOLFF, 1973). A series of physiological studies has established that the maculae of cephalopods are gravireceptors (BOYCOTT, 1960; DIJKGRAAF, 1961, 1963a, 1963b; YOUNG, 1964), i.e. receptors ensuring static equilibrium, whereas the cristae are receptors of angular and linear acceleration (BUDELMANN and WOLFF, 1973) i.e. they ensure dynamic equilibrium. Electrophysiological investigations of the nerve of the statocyst in *Octopus vulgaris* showed that spontaneous activity is recorded, in contradiction to the data of MATURANA and SPERLING (1963). A sharp increase in activity is observed during the directional displacement of otoliths. Both maculae and cristae appear to be quite sensitive to vibration (BUDELMANN and WOLFF, pers. comm.). The crista and the macula are represented by primary sensory cells having a very complex cytochemical and ultrastructural organization, which we have studied as carefully as possible (Fig. 113). These cells are crowned with kinocilia containing $9 \times 2 + 2$ fibrils, the distal ends apparently being connected to the otolith membrane. The kinocilia are surrounded by 2 to 5 long microvilli; we identified these, by analogy with vertebrates, as stereocilia-like microvilli (Fig. 114). It should be noted that the apical surface of receptor cells in both the macula and the cristae always inclines towards the center; this apparently determines not only its morphological but also its functional polarization. BARBER (BARBER, 1965, 1966, 1968; BARBER and DILLY, 1969; BARBER and WRIGHT, 1969; BOYDE and BARBER, 1969; BUDEL-MANN, BARBER, and WEST, 1973) considers that the direction in which the pedicle of the basal body branches off determines the polarization of receptor cells in the statocysts of molluscs, since only a deflection of kinocilia in the direction of the basal pedicle is accompanied by depolarization of the cell. Apparently, the direction of the basal body pedicle coincides with the direction of inclination of the receptor cells. A complex system of rootlets with a cross-striation period of 400—500 Å branches out from the basal bodies of kinocilia into the cytoplasm. The ramifications of these rootlets are attached to the inner surface of the plasma membrane by some sort of cementing lining. The cytoplasm of the cells contains a huge number of endoplasmic reticulum membranes, which may form a continuous belt. The cells are exceptionally rich in ribosomes, polysomes, mitochondria, granules, etc. As we have been able to observe, an axon, containing protoneurofibrils and mitochondria, branches off from the base of the cell. These cells also exhibit a high content of nucleic acids, total protein and functional groups of protein molecules. Unipolar neurons, also having a very complex ultrastructural and cytochemical organization, are located under the receptor cells. The bodies and axons of these neurons may reach giant dimensions and may run over into a layer of nerve fibers, where they

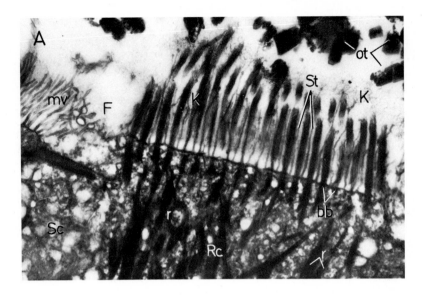

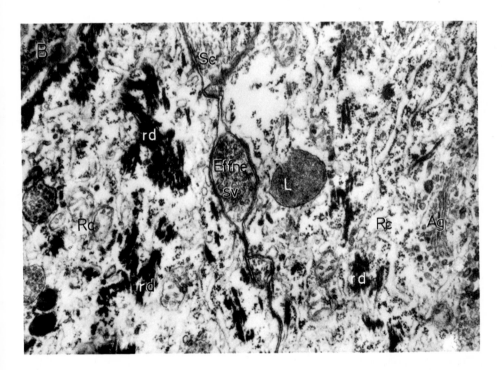

Fig. 114A and B. Receptor cells in cephalopods. A. Apex of receptor cell in the macula of the octopus (×2,600). B. Section through two neighbouring receptor cells in the crista of the squid (×31,500) (VINNIKOV *et al.*, 1971). *Rc* receptor cells; *bb* basal body; *St* stereocilia-like microvilli; *Sc* supporting cell; *F* phalanx; *mv* microvilli; *ot* otoconia; *r* rootlets; *Effne* efferent nerve endings; *sv* synaptic vesicles; *K* kinocilia; *L* lysosome; *rd* distal rootlet sectors; *Ag* Golgi apparatus sectors

are located adjacent to the central processes of receptor cells. As electron microscopic observations and cytochemical data have shown, some of these fibers are filled with synaptic vesicles and exhibit a high acetylcholinesterase activity (Fig. 115). Synaptic thickenings of membranes are often observed between these fibers, indicating a functional contact between them, and thus forcing us to consider the layer of nerve fibers as a neuropil. Moreover, fibers containing numerous synaptic vesicles and exhibiting high acetylcholinesterase activity may leave the layer of nerve fibers and terminate in synapses at the base and on the lateral surfaces of receptor cells (Fig. 115). Although we have no direct experimental proof, these facts lead us to believe that the fibers in question are efferent fibers. Thus, as we shall see below, it seems that the function of receptor cells in statocysts of cephalopods is regulated in the same way as in vertebrates by means of feedback, i.e. by an efferent innervation; this was evident from electrophysiological experiments (BUDELMANN and WOLFF, pers. comm.). Thus, the statocysts of cephalopod molluscs can be considered as quite effective devices, namely as equilibrium organs, which in many respects (including their connections with the central nervous system and other sense organs) are just as effective as the equilibrium organs of vertebrates.

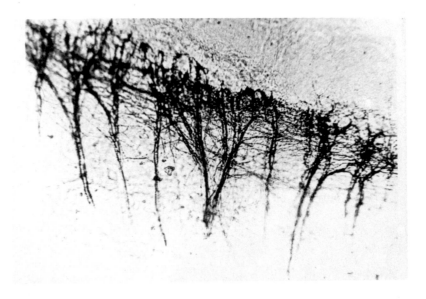

Fig. 115. Cholinesterase activity in efferent nerve fibers and nerve endings of the crista in the statocyst of the octopus (*Octopus* sp.) (VINNIKOV *et al.*, 1968). Treatment according to KOELLE (× 140)

We shall not here give special consideration to the statocysts of echinoderms and urochords, which unfortunately have not been studied to any great extent. Although these animals are representatives of the Deuterostomia, both species have, in addition to typical statocysts equipped with otoconia, primitive multicellular or unicellular gravireceptors of the lithocyte type found in coelenterates and ciliated worms (the spheridium of echinoderms, the lithocyte of ascidian larvae) (DILLY, 1962; EAKIN and KUDE, 1971; HYMAN, 1955).

Thus, an analysis of the evolution of the gravireceptor in invertebrates shows how natural selection has by "trial and error" finally achieved the most rational structure. For the gravireceptor in all independently arising phyla practically the same elements are utilized: a primary sensory cell, equipped with kinocilia (less frequently stereocilia) and a "standard mass" in the form of an otolith or otoconia. In Ctenophora, however, receptor cells seem to be secondary sensory cells. The mechanochemical mechanism responsible for the movement of kinocilia, i.e. of the flagellum, was already perfected on the molecular level in Protozoa; this involves the interaction of low-molecular-weight ATP, supplied by cellular mitochondria, with high-molecular-weight ATPase present in the $9 \times 2 + 2$ fibrils of the flagellum.

The processes that ensure the vital activity of cells, both in a state of relative rest and under conditions of stimulation, are made possible by the rich cytochemical and ultrastructural resources of the cell, apparently supplemented by neighboring supporting cells.

Our examples of the evolution of the gravireceptor in invertebrates have shown that, with the development of the motor activity in animals, this receptor was transformed from an organ that originated as an organ of strictly static equilibrium into an organ capable not only of regulating the behavior of an organism in the gravitational field, but also of coordinating its movements in space. This second function attains a special stage of development in vertebrates.

## 4. Evolution of the Structural and Functional Organization of the Gravireceptor in Vertebrates

The gravireceptor of vertebrates is located in what is called the membraneous labyrinth, which has a very complex structure and functional organization. At first glance, the membraneous labyrinth simply gives the impression of a complicated statocyst, as is typical for higher Protostomia. In reality, however, the labyrinth of vertebrates represents the peripheral portions of three sense organs: 1. maculae with otolith devices in the utricle, sacculus and lagena; 2. two (in the lamprey) or three (in all other vertebrates) semicircular canals with ampullae containing cristae or crests with cupulae; 3. Corti's organ (higher reptiles, birds, and mammals), located in the cochlea. As discussed, maculae and cristae were clearly represented in the statocysts of cephalopod molluscs. This is not only an external morphological similarity but is also a reflection of general functional relationships. Thus, the macula of the utricle can perceive the position of an organism with respect to the gravitational field, i.e. it is a gravireceptor (MAGNUS, 1924, 1962; ADRIAN, 1943; LOWENSTEIN and ROBERTS, 1949, 1951; GERNARD, 1949, 1950, 1959; SCHOEN, 1957; RUPPERT, MOUSHEGIAN, and CALAMBOS, 1962; GAZENKO et al., 1962; VINNIKOV, 1966a, 1966b; VINNIKOV et al., 1971). The maculae of the sacculus and lagena play an auxiliary role with respect to the utricle, while the macula of the sacculus is at the same time a receptor of vibration (LOWENSTEIN and ROBERTS, 1948, 1949, 1951; LOWENSTEIN and

SAND, 1940; ABRAMYAN, 1968). The cristae in the ampullae of the three semicircular canals located in three orthogonal cavities can perceive angular acceleratins (EWALD, 1892; MAGNUS, 1962) and, according to the latest data, linear accelerations (LOWENSTEIN, 1972). Corti's organ is an auditory organ. The sacculus, utricle and the lagena of the labyrinth together with the semicircular canals are designated as the vestibule or vestibular apparatus, in contrast to the auditory organ or Corti's organ.

The similarity between the statocysts of Protostomia and the labyrinth of vertebrates is particularly stricking in the embryonic stages. During embryonic development, the labyrinth originates as a thickening of the ectoderm or placode (KUPFER, 1891; MITROFANOV, 1892; VINNIKOV, 1946) on both sides of the still open neural tube, in the region which later becomes the afterbrain (medulla oblongata). The placode then descends into the appropriate mesenchyme, as a result of which a depression, known as the acoustic (auditory) fossa, is formed; this fossa becomes deeper and is transformed into the acoustic vesicle. During a certain period the fossa continues to communicate with the outer surface. This opening usually closes later, but in some lower vertebrates the connection of the vesicle with the outer environment may be preserved throughout life. The endolymphatic diverticulum or sac grows out from the dorsal wall of the acoustic vesicle (in the human embryo, at 6.3—6.7 mm length). Formation of the endolymphatic sac marks the beginning of the transformation of the vesicle into several sections communicating with each other, i.e. the labyrinth (BEST, ANSON, and GARDNER, 1947).

According to data obtained in our laboratory by TITOVA (1968), the embryonic development of the acoustic vesicle leads first to the appearance in this vesicle of a general precursor of future receptor organs, known as macula communis, under which the primordium of the eight ganglion is located. Then, simultaneously with the subdivision of the vesicle into the utricle, semicircular canals, and sacculus (adjacent to which, in birds and mammals, is the cochlear duct), the macula communis also divides into the corresponding receptor sectors, namely maculae, crests, and Corti's organ. Within receptor structures, the first symptom of cellular differentiation is the change in shape and dimensions of the nucleolus and the increased concentration of nucleic acids, total protein and its functional groups (—SS, —SH, —COOH). Once this differentiation is completed, a rearrangement of the above substances is observed, involving their localization in the nucleus, cuticle, etc. The specific differentiation of receptor cells is expressed in the' appearance on their apical surface of a single kinocilium, branching off from the basal body and containing $9 \times 2 + 2$ fibrils, and of a large number of microvilli, which are gradually transformed into stereocilia by the formation of numerous thin fibrils. Only then does the differentiation of synaptic structures start at the point of approach of nerve endings; this coincides with the appearance and rise of acetylcholinesterase activity. The differentiation of receptor cells and nerve endings is accompanied by the phenomenon of mitochondrial redistribution and increased activity of oxidizing enzymes (TITOVA, 1968). Thus, the same biologically active chemical compounds that are the main components of the structural organization of the receptor cell and determine its function are also responsible for its differentiation (TITOVA, 1968).

The embryonic development of the labyrinth in vertebrates allows us to draw an analogy between the acoustic vesicle and statocysts. This analogy refers to the ectodermal origin and vesicle-like shape, if only in the embryonic stages of vertebrates, of both structures. The principal difference, in all Protostomia except Ctenophora, is that the receptor cells of statocysts are primary sensory cells, whereas in the labyrinth of Deuterostomia vertebrates these cells are secondary sensory cells. Moreover, as was pointed out, such secondary sensory cells in vertebrates are present only in lateral-line organs, in the labyrinth, and in the gustatory organ. As we have seen, in the visual and olfactory organs of vertebrates, photoreceptors and olfactory cells are represented by primary sensory cells as in Protostomia.

In phylogenesis, the labyrinth of vertebrates arose on the basis of lateral-line mechanoreceptor organs, but by now these organs are consolidated into a single acoustico-lateral system; the receptor formations of this system are based on a secondary sensory hair cell (VINNIKOV, 1946). Secondary sensory cells appeared at the dawn of the evolution of vertebrates. As far as we can judge from sufficiently reliable paleontological data STENSIÖ, 1927; BYSTROV, 1957) the Agnatha, primitive vertebrates, which in the Silurian period had already adapted to living conditions in freshwater basins, had a well-developed system of lateral-line organs, which has persisted to the present in fishes and aquatic amphibians and in which secondary sensory cells are the receptor elements. In Agnatha, this system consisted of tubules or canals that, being embedded in the aspidin substance of the shell, has been preserved to our time. The tubules opened onto the external surface of the shell. Thus, this whole system of lateral-line organs communicated with the outer environment, i.e. water, whose vibrations represented the specific stumulus for this system, judging from present-day fish and amphibians. In recent fishes the canals of the lateral-line organs are filled with mucus and communicate with the outer environment either directly by means of pores or, in some species, indirectly, since these pores are closed by a membrane. In fishes, as well as in aquatic amphibians, the receptor elements of lateral-line organs may also be located on the surface of the skin. According to DISLER (1960), the structure and development of lateral-line organs is a reflection of the ecology of a given fish species. In certain amphibians, the lateral-line organs are subjected to rhythmic seasonal changes (KONZHUKOVA, 1938). According to the data of MALYUKINA (1955), lateral-line organs of fishes are capable of perceiving, as well as water vibrations, the entire range of subsonic frequencies and the lowest acoustic frequencies, right down to 25 cps. DIJKGRAAF (1954) denies that lateral-line organs are able to perceive acoustic frequencies.

According to electron microscopic and cytochemical data obtained in our laboratory by ARONOVA (1967, 1968), the lateral-line organs of the pike can respond to several stimuli. Thus, they exhibit shifts of their structural and cytochemical organization under the effect of a jet aimed in a cranio-caudal direction, at a pressure of about one atmosphere for a period of 10 minutes; they also respond by similar shifts to low-frequency oscillations (50 cps for 20 minutes) and to the effect of centrifugal forces involving 10 $g$ for 3 min in a dorso-ventral direction. These shifts are manifested in the exit of nucleolus ribosomes from the nucleus into the cytoplasm, where they build sectors of the endoplasmic reticulum, and in patterns exhibiting rearrangement, swelling and adherence of mitochondria. Further, an 8—13% fall in the protein content is observed in the case of a hydrodynamic stimulus, 30—33% under the effect of vibration, and 30—33% under the effect of centrifugal forces. Thus, receptor cells of lateral-line organs show a graduated response to each of the three stimuli applied. This fact indicates that lateral-line organs, endowed with a broader range of reception, could have been the source of the specialized and more precise function of reception that resulted in the formation during evolution of the labyrinth and, in particular, of that part of the labyrinth which can perceive gravitational forces and vibration. In certain fishes *(Mormiridae)*, the lateral-line organs are so modified *(Lorenzini ampullae)* as to be converted into electroreceptors (BULLOCK, 1961).

The system of lateral-line organs serves as the basis for the development of the labyrinth, i.e. the inner ear; it was originally in communication with the outer environment and can be found as early as the Silurian period in such Agnatha as Osteostraci. According to STENSIÖ (1927), the labyrinth in *Osteostraci kiaeraspus* had only two vertical semicircular canals—namely an anterior and posterior canal. Among present-day forms, such a characteristic is found only in the labyrinth of cyclostomes (RETZIUS, 1881; TRETYAKOV, 1916; DE BURLET, 1934).

Thus, the development of receptor structures of lateral-line organs and of the labyrinth during onto- and phylogenesis was associated with repeated alternation of functions; the appearance of sense organs with a wide variety of functions is essentially due to this fact. However, as was noted above, the same secondary sensory receptor cell lies at the basis of the structure of all labyrinth and lateral-line organs.

In lower vertebrates (fishes and amphibians), the organization of receptor structures in the labyrinth, including the semicircular canals, the utricle and sacculus, that perform the function of gravity reception, is based in type-II cells (Fig. 116); in addition, type-I cells are found in higher vertebrates, starting with reptiles and birds (Fig. 116). Individual buttonshaped nerve endings approach the cylindrical type-II cells; type-I cells, having a bowl-like shape, are enclosed in special, calyx-shaped nerve endings. Both types of cells are crowned with a bundle of hairs consisting of 60 to 70 stereocilia and a single kinocilium having a polar orientation with respect to the stereocilia and containing $9 \times 2 + 2$ fibrils. As we have seen, primary sensory receptor cells in the statocysts of Protostomia were crowned with a very large number (45—80 and more) of kinocilia, whereas in vertebrates the primary sensory cells of the labyrinth have only one kinocilium; on the other hand, 40 to 70 supplementary immobile hairs, the stereocilia, are found in vertebrates. These hairs have developed from microvilli (TITOVA and GRIBAKIN, 1967), are coated with an extension of the plasma membrane and contain up to 75 to 80 thin, densely packed fibrils. The diameter of each stereocilium does not exceed 30—40Å. The stereocilia branch off from a special cuticular plate of the receptor cell.

It is obvious that type-I cells, which appear for the first time in higher vertebrates, reflect not only a general improvement in orientation but also a change in the position of these animals in the gravitational field, which required a more universal and reliable method of transmitting the information received by receptor cells to the central nervous system. At the same time, the evolutionary transformations at the cellular level did not have any effect on the organization of the hairs and of their connections with the otolith membrane, which does not differ in any way in type-I cells from the phylogenetically original type-II cells. This is an illustration of the fact that primary physical transformations associated with reception of the Earth's gravitational field, were already resolved by natural selection at the dawn of evolution of multicellular animals in coelenterates and, in particular, in ctenophores. Later, when new models of the gravireceptor evolved in new animal phyla, including vertebrates, the same structure was inevitably produced again, because otherwise the effect of the gravitational field could not have been adequately perceived.

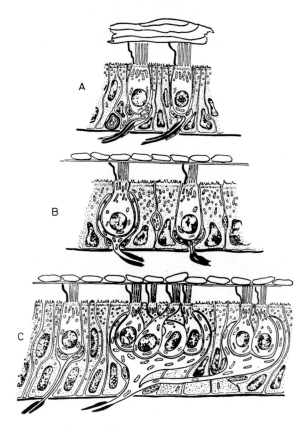

Fig. 116 A—C. Diagram showing the evolution of the structural organization of the utricle in (A) fish, (B) mammals and (C) birds (VINNIKOV, 1966a)

In receptor cells of vertebrates, the kinocilium always has a definite polar orientation with respect to the bundle of stereocilia and appears to be facing the stereocilia, being located in front of or behind them; they are arranged

in 7 parallel rows, each row consisting of 5—6—9 stereocilia. The length of
the stereocilia usually increases in the direction of the kinocilium from 0.5
to 5 μm. Modern electrophysiological methods have shown that the receptor
cells of lateral-line organs and of the labyrinth are stimulated only when the
stimulus is directed towards the stereocilia (Fig. 117). In this case, a depolarization

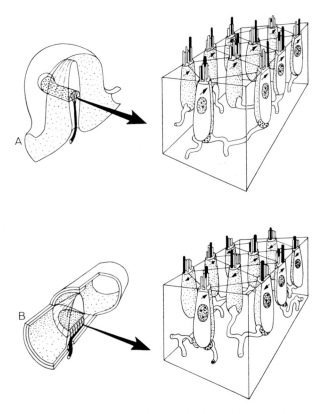

Fig. 117 A and B. Diagram of the polarization of kinocilia (A) in the crista of the semicircular
canal, and (B) in lateral-line organs (FLOCK and WERSÄLL, 1962 b)

of cellular membranes takes place and action currents can be detected in the
corresponding afferent nerves. If the stimulus is directed towards the opposite
side, i.e. to the kinocilium, hyperpolarization sets in and the cell is inhibited
(FLOCK, 1965; WERSÄLL, 1956; FLOCK et al., 1962 a, 1962 b). This circumstance
has given rise to the concept that the morphological polarization in receptor
cells of lateral-line organs and of the labyrinth coincides with the physiological
polarization. We have already been confronted with a somewhat similar phenomenon in the cnidoblasts of coelenterates, where the kinocilium is surrounded
on all sides by stereocilia, and also in the kinocilia (surrounded by stereocilia-like
microvilli) of primary sensory cells in the maculae and cristae of cephalopod

molluscs, as well as in Corti's organ. Apparently, in both coelenterates and cephalopod molluscs, the fact that a kinocilium is uniformly surrounded by stereocilia results in stimulation of the cell irrespective of the direction of the stimulus.

In lateral-line organs, the cells are divided into two groups in such a way that the kinocilia of adjacent cells are oriented in opposite directions: one cell is directed towards the head, and the other towards the tail end (FLOCK, 1965; ARONOVA, 1967), so that two neighboring cells appear to be mirror reflections of each other. It was, of course, on lateral-line organs of fishes that "spontaneous potentials", which have played such a significant role in our general understanding of nerve conduction, were first discovered (HOAGLAND, 1932). The spontaneous activity of lateral-line receptor cells represents the background against which responses to adequate stimuli are expressed. SAND (1937) found that the spontaneous activity of a nerve fiber increases when the canal is perfused with liquid in a head-to-tail direction, and decreases when the perfusion is carried out in the opposite direction. The rise of action currents in some nerve fibers and their decline in other fibers when the cupula of lateral-line organs is displaced, can thus be explained by the morphological polarization of receptor cells.

Very curious rules governing the polarization of receptor cells have also been detected in the cristae of semicircular canals in the labyrinth of vertebrates. In the crista of the horizontal canal the polarization of kinocilia with respect to stereocilia is always constant. In each receptor cell this polarization is oriented toward the utricle. Only centripetal stimulation, i.e. deflection of the cupula toward the utricle, is accompanied in the horizontal canal by the appearance of action currents and their inhibition during stimulation in the direction of the semicircular canals. The reserve relationships are found in the anterior and posterior ampullae of the semicircular canals. Thus, there is an obvious parallelism between the morphological structure and the bioelectrical function of the cell.

In the macula of the utricle, i.e. in the main gravireceptor of vertebrates, we are confronted with the fact that receptor cells having similar polarization assemble in groups that together form a mosaic, which in a general way reflects the planes of space. However, according to our data (VINNIKOV et al., 1971), the organization of this mosaic is slightly different in mammals as compared to birds, in birds as compared to reptiles, in reptiles as compared to amphibians, in amphibians as compared to fishes, and in fishes as compared to cyclostomes (Fig. 118). This mosaic ensures that only a certain group of cells is stimulated per unit time during the sliding of the otolith membrane. On the basis of physiological data obtained some time ago by MAGNUS (1924), and especially by SZENTÁGOTHAI and his associates (1967) [who also divided the utricle into 4 quadrants (Fig. 119)] it follows that every portion of this mosaic or quadrant may correspond to a definite group of muscles, which are involved in positioning the body and regulated by the function of the utricular and saccular maculae. The saccular macula, in turn, also has kinocilia polarization, which is characteristic only for this macula and differs in different classes of vertebrates, such as fishes (FLOCK, 1964), mammals (SPOENDLIN, 1966), and birds (ABRAMYAN, 1969); this polarization is particularly complex in birds. We once stated the view

(VINNIKOV, 1966a) that the difference in the pattern of distribution in the mosaic of receptor cells in the maculae of given vertebrate classes reflects the development and evolution of the musculature, in connection with the characteristic posture of these vertebrates in the gravitational field. We believe such a viewpoint receives confirmation when we compare the mosaic of the utricular macula in mammals and in birds. In birds, as we have seen, the mosaic is extremely complex, probably owing to characteristics in the development of their musculature connected with flight. In reptiles, however, and especially in the turtle, the mosaic is much

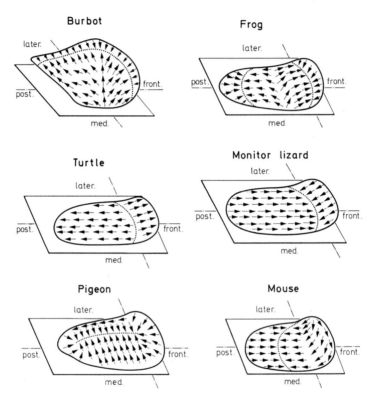

Fig. 118. Diagram of the morphological polarization of kinocilia (*arrows*) in relation to the stereocilia bundles in receptor cells of the utricle of vertebrates (fishes, amphibians, reptiles, birds, mammals) (VINNIKOV et al., 1971). The most distinct polarization areas are delimited by dotted lines

simpler, which should reflect the simpler nature of their body musculature. In amphibians, the mosaic, though somewhat similar to that of cyclostomes (LOWENSTEIN et al., 1968) and fishes (FLOCK, 1964), is more complex reflecting the appearance of extremities in these animals and the fact that they emerged from water onto dry land. Thus, the distribution pattern of receptor cells in maculae, depending as it does upon the polarization of kinocilia, is a reflection of ecological transformations associated with a change in the position of animals in the Earth's gravitational field (VINNIKOV, 1974).

Next, we must ask what happens to the receptor cell of the utricle during a stimulating deflection of stereocilia under the effect of the shearing forces that arise during sliding movements of the otolith membrane induced by the animal changing its position in the gravitational field.

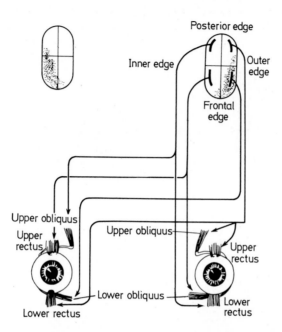

Fig. 119. Projection of eye muscles on the utricular macula (viewed from above) (SZENTAGOTHAI, 1967). The points indicate sectors of the macula where the thickest fibers terminate

Receptor cells in the labyrinth of vertebrates are characterized by an extraordinarily complex structural (Fig. 120) and cytochemical organization, which allows them to maintain their vital activity not only in a state of relative rest, but also under adequate stimulation conditions. Thus, we were able to establish that in all vertebrates during adequate stimulation with radial accelerations at $10\,g$ shifts take place in the subcellular and cytochemical organization of the nucleus and cytoplasm of the receptor cells of the utricle, and also of the sacculus and semicircular canal of the labyrinth (VINNIKOV et al., 1963a, 1963b; VINNIKOV et al., 1965a, 1966). These shifts manifest themselves in a reduction of the cytoplasmic RNA content, migration of the nucleolus towards the nuclear membrane, and the transfer of RNA (ribosomes) of the nucleolus from the nucleus to the cytoplasm, where at the same time a limited sector of rough endoplasmic reticulum is immediately induced; this sector appears under the light microscope as an escaped nucleolus (Fig. 121). These processes follow a particularly distinct course in guinea pigs, monkeys, and birds. It seems that in these animals a controlled exit of RNA of nucleoli from the nucleus into the cytoplasm can also take place spontaneously, without exposure to an experimental effect; it may thus reflect some sort of rhythmic passage of RNA from the nucleus into the cytoplasm (NEIFACH, 1965). We think the migration of nucleolar ribosomes across the nuclear membrane into the cytoplasm may ori-

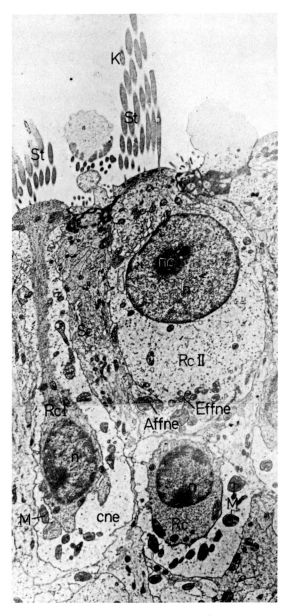

Fig. 120. Structural organization of receptor and supporting cells in the utricle of the mouse in a state of relative rest ( × 5,400) (VINNIKOV *et al.*, 1971). *Rc I, Rc II* receptor cells of type I and II; *Sc* supporting cell; *St* stereocilia; *K* kinocilium; *n* nucleus; *nc* nucleole; *M* mitochondria; *cne* cup-shaded nerve ending; *Effne* efferent nerve ending; *Affne* afferent nerve ending

ginally have been the result of a mechanical effect of the gravitational field during overloads. Gradually, during the course of evolution, this phenomenon became an adaptive factor, promoting protein repair in connection with the considerable expenditure of structural and functional proteins (enzymes) by stimulated receptor cells during intensive work under the effect of accelerations. Monkeys and birds are apparently highly sensitive to overloads, and in these species the endoplasmic reticulum with ribosomes, in the hair cells of the utricle, can be located in both the basal and apical portions of the receptor cell, so that the exit of nucleolar RNA can take place both in either direction. In mice, however, under analogous overloads such phenomena are practically absent.

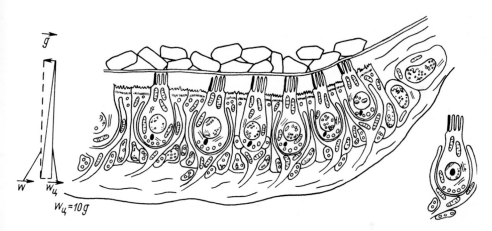

Fig. 121. Diagram of the utricle of the guinea pig, subjected to the action of a centripetal acceleration of 10 $g$ for 3 min (VINNIKOV et al., 1963a). Receptor cells shown in longitudinal section. Otoliths are located on the otolith membrane. The escape of nuclear RNA from the nucleus corresponds to the gravitational field vector. Right figure shows a receptor cell of the guinea pig utricle in a state of relative rest. Black dots indicate RNA in nucleoles and the cytoplasm. The diagram on the left shows the direction of the gravitational field vector

The observed phenomenon of the migration of ribosomes of the nucleolus from the nucleus to the cytoplasm, although experimentally induced, is of general biological significance. It demonstrates spatial regularities, associated with the exit of ribosomes from the nucleus into the cytoplasm, where they induce the formation of endoplasmic membranes, apparently, at the expense of a "priming" of the outer membrane of the nucleus. Formation of a rough endoplasmic reticulum sector indicates that the process of protein synthesis in the cell is being intensified, i.e. a feedback is present. The transfer of the nucleolus from the nucleus into the cytoplasm of the cell has been observed many times under the light microscope (KEDROVSKIY, 1959; TEWARI and BOURNE, 1962). in addition to our observations (VINNIKOV et al., 1963a, 1963b), the transport of ribosomes through pores of the nuclear membrane has been clearly demonstrated in cells of the *Chironomus* salivary gland by STEVEN and SWIFT (1966) using the electron microscope. This phenomenon represents a process of transport into the cytoplasm of large packets of RNA and, as was recently found, of a number of enzymes, too. The electron microscope shows (Fig. 8) how the ribosomes of the nucleolus, after leaving the nucleus, form around themselves in the cytoplasm a number of membranes of rough endoplasmic reticulum, i.e. begin to perform their function of protein synthesis. This assumption is confirmed by simultaneous cytophotometric investigations of the total protein content in such cells. Following the restoration of cytoplasmic RNA in the form of an escaped nucleolus, as seen in the light microscope (or as a local sector of rough endoplasmic reticulum, as seen in the electron microscope), a process of increased protein synthesis begins in the receptor cells of the utricle. Protein synthesis, after reaching a certain maximum value, drops almost to normal and then increases again, forming a multipeak curve with the highest peak observed 48 hours after exposure to a single effect (Fig. 122). Repeated overloads during this period (after 1, 2, 8 hours and 12 days) apparently exert an unfavorable effect, causing disruption or even cessation of protein synthesis. Thus, shifts in the subcellular organization of receptor cells in the utricle, induced by the action of overloads, can be interpreted with the aid of both qualitative and quantitative methods. We shall not examine here the distribution pattern of carboxylic, sulfhydryl, and thiol groups, nor the changes in the distribution of these groups during overloads, since these changes proceed more or less parallel to the overall content of the biologically active chemical compounds of the labyrinth, being high in fishes, reptiles, birds, and mammals, and lower in amphibians. The same applies to the activity of the dehydrogenase and cholinesterase studied.

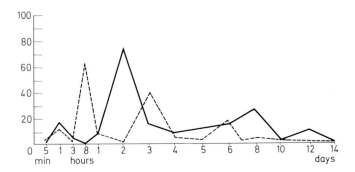

Fig. 122. Variation of the optical density of protein reaction products in the basal parts of receptor cells (based on cytophotometric data) after a single rotation (solid line) and repeated rotations (broken line) (VINNIKOV et al., 1963a). The abscissa shows the time elapsed after a single rotation. The ordinate shows relative units of optical density (arithmetical mean)

Studies of enzymes in receptor structures of the labyrinth, in particular of the utricle, have shown that, by using a combination of cytochemical and electron microscopic methods, it is possible to determine how the function of these enzymes, localized in mitochondria, is effected in receptor cells of the labyrinth. A study of the utricle of animals in a state of relative rest and exposed to overloads has shown that mitochondria of receptor cells can come into most intimate contact with the presynaptic membrane and abut tightly against this membrane. Owing to this contiguous position of mitochondria, a structure is formed, which consists of four membraneous layers: two mitochondrial and two synaptic layers, separated from each other by a very narrow cleft. Under the effect of overloads, the phenomenon of mitochondrial adjacency can be observed in the presynaptic region of both type-I and type-II receptor cells. This phenomenon can also be detected in calyx- and button-shaped nerve endings (Fig. 23—24). The phenomenon of mitochondrial adjacency is combined with a change in the activity of mitochondrial oxidative processes (Fig. 25). Prolonged and multiple overloads lead to a distinct drop in the activity of dehydrogenases (VINNIKOV et al., 1966; VINNIKOV, 1967a, 1967b; VINNIKOV and TITOVA, 1962a, 1962b).

In regard to the sacculus, data obtained in our laboratory by ABRAMYAN (1968, 1969) show this sector of the labyrinth to be mainly a receptor of vibrations. A pigeon was subjected to vibrations of 50 cps with an amplitude of 1 mm for 15 minutes or 2 hours, and the reaction of the receptor cells to such a functional load was noted. This reaction, which was investigated quantitatively, is characterized by bending of stereocilia and a change in the dimensions of nuclei. Characteristic changes were also observed in the distribution and content of nucleic acids, protein molecules, and functional groups (—SS, —SH, —COOH). The change in the dimensions of the nucleus is accompanied by migration of nucleolar ribosomes into the cytoplasm, where sectors of newly developed rough membranes, mitochondrial adjacency, etc. can be observed. Under overload conditions, the above shifts were less pronounced (ABRAMYAN, 1968).

Peculiar shifts were observed in nerve endings. As first established in Corti's organ, "dark" nerve endings filled with synaptic vesicles were found to be present in the vestibular part of the labyrinth, along with "light" nerve endings practically devoid of synaptic vesicles (SMITH and SJÖSTRAND, 1961; SMITH and RASMUSSEN, 1967). These "dark" nerve endings, as cutting tests have shown, are efferent endings (IURATO, 1962b; KIMURA and WERSÄLL, 1962). "Dark" nerve endings have been found on neural calyxes of type-I receptor cells and among boutons of type-II cells (WERSÄLL, 1956; ENGSTRÖM, 1958, 1961). Following sectioning of the vestibular nerve, degeneration of efferent myelinized fibers down to maculae and cristae is observed (RASMUSSEN and GAČEK, 1958; GAČEK, 1960). The number of afferent nerve fibers found in the vestibular nerve of the cat is 1,200; that of efferent fibers is about 200 (GAČEK, 1960). The nature of the cerebral nuclei, from which the efferent innervation of the vestibular part of the labyrinth originates, has not yet been clarified. According to some data, efferent fibers originate in Deiters' nuclei (RASMUSSEN and GAČEK, 1958; GAČEK, 1960); according to other data, they originate in the upper and medial vestibular nuclei (CARPENTER, 1960). Some investigators assume that efferent fibers, because of their acetylcholinesterase activity, originate in a special intercalary nucleus, located at a greater dorsal and medial distance from the cranial end of the lower vestibular nucleus and at a greater ventral distance from the lateral vestibular nucleus (ROSSI and CORTESINA, 1962a, 1962b; ROSSI et al., 1964). However, afferent fibers can also display enzymic activity (VINNIKOV and TITOVA, 1958b,

1961, 1964; DOHLMAN, FARKASHIDY, and SALONNA, 1958; VINNIKOV, TITOVA, and ARONOVA, 1965).

Electrophysiological data on the function of the efferent vestibular system are also contradictory (LEDOUX, 1956; SALA, 1963; BERTRAND and VEENHOF, 1964). We can agree with KISLYAKOV and ORLOV (1966) that all these studies still lack precise criteria for determining what constitutes efferent control of vestibular activity.

The localization of oxidative enzymes in the synapse region of receptor structures in the utricle, as well as in the sacculs, semicircular canals and Corti's organ, is combined here with the localization of enzymes of the cholinergic system. A diffuse activity of butyrylcholinesterase can be detected in all receptor structures of the labyrinth of vertebrates. An increased activity of this enzyme in receptor structures is observed only in cyclostomes and in birds. A very high butyrylcholinesterase activity is observed in protoplasmic cells of teleosts and in the semilunar plates of ampullae in the semicircular canals of birds and mammals. In view of this fact, we believe that this enzyme is involved in the secretory function. In the pigeon, upon introduction of $S^{35}$, an elevated metabolism in the region of semilunar plates was detected by the autoradiographic method (DOHLMAN, 1960a).

In contrast to butyrylcholinesterase, the localization of acetylcholinesterase was a constant factor in all vertebrate species studied by us. In the course of development of the labyrinth in vertebrates, in spite of a change in its function, this enzyme is always located in neurons of the eighth ganglion (TITOVA and VINNIKOV, 1964; VINNIKOV, TITOVA, and ARONOVA, 1965), in the synapse region of acoustic spots and crests in cyclostomes, birds and mammals, and also in Corti's organ in reptiles, birds and mammals (VINNIKOV and Titova, 1961; TITOVA and VINNIKOV, 1964; VINNIKOV, TITOVA, and ARONOVA, 1965). However, in Corti's organ this enzyme can be detected not only in synapses and in the cytoplasm, but also, as we have seen, in the hairs of receptor cells.

Pharmacological, biochemical and physiological data indicate that acetylcholinesterase is linked with acetylcholine, i.e. it represents a hydrolyzing enzyme of a cholinergic system. It should be noted that spontaneous potentials, which at the present time are linked with the quantum ejection of the acetylcholine (FATT and KATZ, 1951) present in synaptic vesicles (BREMEN, ANDERSON, and RESER, 1958; GRAY and WHITTAKER, 1962; WHITTAKER, 1965; DE ROBERTIS et al., 1960, 1962; KOELLE, 1967; NACHMANSON, 1967; and others), can be detected in animals both in a state of relative rest and under stimulation conditions (DE ROBERTIS, 1958). We have been able to detect synaptic vesicles in the synapse region in receptor cells of the utricle in all vertebrates we have investigated. These vesicles have also been described by other investigators (ROSSI, 1964; LOWENSTEIN, OSBORNE, and WERSÄLL, 1964) in the synapse region of the utricle of the ray, teleosts and amphibians, and also in the synapse region of cristae in rays and amphibians. A specific stimulation of the utricle by overloads modifies the activity of acetylcholinesterase: it first rises, then drops, parallel to the distribution of synaptic vesicles, which are particularly clearly visible in lower vertebrates. In the region of presynaptic membranes and synaptic rods one can observe the appearance of swollen or empty vesicles, or their "shadows", which apparently have already discharged their contents into the intersynaptic cleft. Isolated swollen or empty vesicles of irregular shape can also be detected in the cytoplasm of nerve endings. The above data clearly indicate that acetylcholinesterase of the labyrinth takes part in the transmission of afferent impulses from the receptor cells to the sensory nerve fiber of the neutron located in Scarp's ganglion. These neurons also exhibit the activity of acetylcholinesterase, which is especially high in teleosts (TITOVA and VINNIKOV, 1964; VINNIKOV, TITOVA, and ARONOVA, 1965). According to both our own and literature data, acetylcholinesterase activity can also be detected in efferent nerve endings, yielding "dark" endings at the base of receptor cells (DOHLMAN, FARKASHIDY, and SALONNA, 1958; DOHLMAN, 1960a, 1960b; IRELAND and FARKASHIDY, 1961; ROSSI and CORTESINA, 1962a, 1962b, 1963; ROSSI et al., 1964; and others). We do not agree with the statement that impulses can be transmitted with the aid of a cholinergic system only in efferent nerve endings; obviously, this system can also provide its service to transmit afferent impulses. Moreover, it is possible that adrenergic fibers can also take part in the transmission of a nerve impulse (SPOENDLIN, 1965, 1966). Thus, the transmission of impulses in the synapse region of receptor structures of the labyrinth in general, and of the utricle in particular, is achieved with the aid of a specific cholinergic system, and possibly of an adrenergic system, but apparently in all cases with the participation of energy processes associated with oxidative enzymes. According to FLOCK and LAM (1974) GABA seems to participate in this process.

We thus can discern a more or less orderly pattern in the structural, cytochemical and functional organization of the receptor cell in the vertebrate vestibular apparatus and of the shifts that take place in a cell on the cellular, subcellular, and sometimes even molecular level of organization. These shifts start from the moment when stereocilia are deflected towards the kinocilium under the influence of the shearing forces that develop when the otolith membrane slides in one direction or the other; these forces are themselves induced by a change in the position of the organism in the gravitational field. We believe that this mechanism constitutes the basis of the function of the gravireceptor.

# 5. Conclusion

A comparison of the structural, cytochemical and functional organization of the gravireceptors of invertebrates and vertebrates shows that the gravireceptor arose independently in different animal phyla, reaching its maximum development in the Protostomia in arthropods and molluscs, and in Deuterostomia in vertebrates. In representatives of these three phyla the gravireceptor is transformed into a complex equilibrium organ, which enables the animal not only to perceive its position with respect to the gravitational field and regulate the setting of its body accordingly, but also to perceive and regulate the characteristics of its movement in three-dimensional space. The realization of such complex regulation and coordination was made possible by connections with a correspondingly developing nervous system and other sense organs (vision, proprioception, tactile sense). Both the statocyst of invertebrates and the membraneous labyrinth of vertebrates arose during the course of evolution through slow transformations of mechanoreceptors until finally, by "trial and error", an instrument was created that was capable of adequately perceiving the position of the organism in the Earth's gravitational field. If we understand the general properties of gravity (which are also characteristic for the Earth's gravitational field), we can readily see why the gravireceptor in representatives of different phyla is always built to the same design. The design includes three basic elements: 1. the "standard mass" (lithocyte, otoconium, otolith), which is free to move when the position of the organism in the gravitational field undergoes a change; 2. the antenna (kinocilium, flagellum, chitin hair, stereocilia), which is deflected by the "standard mass" and which stimulates the receptor cell; 3. the receptor cell, which measures the magnitude and direction of the antenna deflection and transmits these parameters in encoded form to the central nervous system, either along its own nerve fiber (statocyst of invertebrates), or through a synapse to an afferent nerve fiber (membraneous labyrinth of vertebrates).

The first attempt to create such a model is seen in unicellular organisms, which are endowed with a statocyst-like organelle (DOGIEL, 1929). Among multicellular organisms, we can observe an attempt aimed at the realization of such a model in coelenterates, when there is a trend to immerse a primitive lithostyle with lithocytes into a newly formed cavity. Ctenophores are the first to have a gravireceptor (aboral organ) that contains on the cellular level of organization all the basic elements which where later adopted by all higher animals. Ciliated worms and nemerteans still utilize as a "standard mass" lithocytes, located in the statocyst cavity. In annelids, primary sensory cells with kinocilia appear for the first time, and the "standard mass" consists of otoconia or sand particles introduced from outside. The organization of their statocysts fits perfectly into the scheme outlined above.

The most clearcut correspondence between the above scheme and the statocyst can be observed in arthropods and molluscs, particularly in higher crustaceans and cephalopod molluscs. Not only gravireceptors but also receptors of angular accelerations are found in these two animal forms, which have developed independently of each other. Behavioral observations and electrophysiological studies show that the function of statocysts is exercised in combination with the function of other sense organs (vision, proprioreception, tactile sense) and regulated by the central nervous system. The organization of the gravireceptor in the labyrinth of vertebrates fits particularly well in the above scheme. The labyrinth of vertebrates, and in particular its utricular portion, is the homolog of the statocyst of invertebrates with the sole difference that its organization is based on secondary sensory cells. In addition, a distinct feature of the labyrinth is the presence of cristae in the semicircular canals, acting as receptors of angular and linear accelerations. In the labyrinth of higher vertebrates, the acoustic organ (Corti's organ) arises on the basis of the same receptor cells, just as receptor sectors, responsible for the perception of vibrations, arise on the basis of a statocyst in arthropods and cephalopods. In lower vertebrates, however, there is still no clearcut subdivision into an utricular and saccular macula (for example, in cyclostomes) and no horizontal semicircular canal. Nevertheless, in the labyrinth of lower vertebrates and in the vestibular part of higher vertebrates the "standard mass" is always represented by an otolith membrane with otoliths or otoconia. Displacement of the otolith membrane during a change of the body's position in the gravitational field is accompanied by the appearance of shearing forces, acting upon the antennae of receptor cells. Whereas in invertebrates, with the exception of coelenterates and cephalopod molluscs, these antennae normally consist only of flagella-kinocilia, containing 9 pairs of peripheral and two central fibrils, the receptor cell of vertebrates has only one kinocilium, which has a polar orientation with respect to the 50—60 stereocilia belonging to the same cell. There is reason to believe that the kinocilium is somehow attached to the otolith membrane, but the same cannot be reliably said of stereocilia; it is probable that the distal ends of stereocilia can freely "support" or "brush over" the otolith membrane. Receptor cells are stimulated by the deflection of stereocilia: if this deflection is directed towards kinocilia, the cell is excited, whereas, when the deflection occurs in the opposite direction, it is inhibited. In the first case, depolarization of the cellular membrane and an increase in the frequency of action currents take place, whereas in the second case, hyperpolarization and a drop in the frequency of biopotentials are observed (LOWENSTEIN, 1956; LOWENSTEIN, OSBORNE, and WERSÄLL, 1964).

Thus, in vertebrates, instead of a large number of kinocilia, another structural modification of an antenna, namely stereocilia, has arisen. The role of the single kinocilium is apparently reduced to regulating the degree of sliding and tension of the otolith membrane, and also of the accuracy with which the membrane returns to its original position in the area of each receptor cell. Receptor cells with a similar polarization of kinocilia form, as a rule, a rather complex two-, three-dimensional mosaic on the surface of the utricular macula of vertebrates. Details of this mosaic differ somewhat in representatives of different classes of vertebrates. There is reason to believe that these details reflect the appearance or reduction of certain groups of muscles, associated with the positioning of the body (SZENTAGOTHAI, 1967; MAGNUS, 1962; VINNIKOV, 1966a).

Evolutionary laws, associated with the increase in the general level of organization in vertebrates, never affect the first transformation of our scheme, i.e., the interaction between the "standard mass" and the hairs of the receptor cell, which indeed reflects the efficiency of this transformation. However, the second transformation, the way in which information is transmitted to the central nervous system, may undergo a change as their organization continues to rise. Thus, whereas the receptor cells in lower vertebrates (fishes and amphibians) are represented only by type-II cells, i.e., they transmit information to several button-shaped nerve endings, in higher vertebrates (reptiles, birds, mammals) type-I cells appear along with type-II cells. These cells are submerged, either alone or in groups, into calyx shaped nerve endings, so that practically any portion of their surface can perform a synaptic function. It is conceivable that greater reliability and possibly also greater sensitivity of the organ is achieved by the presence of these nerve calyxes, which sometimes service several cells (this is particularly well expressed in birds). Thus, evolutionary changes associated with the higher organization of vertebrates affect only the second transformation. Such data are still not available in regard to invertebrates. The vestibular and central connections in the labyrinth of vertebrates are well known, as well as the synergism of its activity with other analyzers of the organism. We have been able to detect certain cytochemical and ultrastructural changes that accompany the activity of the gravireceptor at the cellular and subcellular level, and in some cases even at the molecular level. We believe that analogous processes take place in the gravireceptors of invertebrates. In analyzing the function of antennae in the statocysts of invertebrates, we are confronted by a striking fact. These antennae, as a rule, are typical kinocilia containing $9 \times 2 + 2$ fibrils, in which at least $9 \times 2$ fibrils (peripheral) contain ATPase; the interaction of ATPase with ATP is responsible for the movement of the kinocilia. In the state of relative rest, the antennae of the primary sensory cells of the statocysts seem to possess spontaneous motility. It's quite possible that this motility is to some extent responsible for the spontaneous potentials recorded in the static nerve. The mechanical shearing forces that arise during a change of position of the otolith induce a sharp shift in the amplitude of movement of the antennae. This result in alteration of electrical activity in the static nerve. The molecular interaction between ATP and ATPase in a state of relative rest appears to be to some extent inhibited by a chemical substance, still unknown to us. This substance, however, must be easily modified or destroyed under the mechanical effect exerted on the kinocilium by the shearing forces of the moving otolith, when the organism changes its position in the gravitational field. Another possible assumption is that the interaction between low-molecular-weight ATP and high-molecular-weight ATPase requires, depending upon the nature of the latter, additional ions ($K^+$, $Na^+$, or $Mg^{++}$) to be liberated into the endolymph when the kinocilium is subjected to a mechanical effect. It is also not clear how the movement of the kinocilia brings about the stimulation of the receptor cell. This question concerns the nature of the mechanochemical processes of stimulation of the receptor cell associated with the movement of antennae. Can we accept the presence of some additional mechano-sensitive protein in plasma membrane which covers the antennae, or are these merely processes taking place within the flagellar fibrils and the system of powerful rootlets connected with them?

In vertebrates, stereocilia, i.e. complicated microvilli, replace kinocilia in the vestibular apparatus. This "replacement" can be considered as an example of the "economy" principle in evolution. For the kinocilia of invertebrates under relative rest conditions we have to assume the presence of some inhibiting factor which interferes with the molecular reaction between ATP and ATPase in the contractile fibrillar substrate, the effect of which is neutralized by the shearing motion of the otolith membrane transmitted to the tip of the kinocilium; stereocilia, however, require no such mechanism, being in effect immobile. Their movement are merely the result of the movement of the otolith membrane. However, there still remains the question of the presence of some protein localized in the plasma membrane of stereocilia, which, by changing its conformation during their bending, could conceivably serve as a trigger mechanism for enzymatic and ionic processes leading to excitation of the receptor cell. The suggestion that such a substance could be the ATPase in the plasma membrane (DUNCAN, 1967; and others) excludes a specific receptor protein, which, in our opinion, is always the basis of any kind of reception.

In this respect, the hypothesis of DOHLMAN (1960a, 1960b), further developed by CHRISTIANSEN (1964), is confronted by a number of difficulties. DOHLMAN'S hypothesis is that the polarization of stereocilia is connected with the deformation of polysaccharide molecules (hyaluronic complex), hypothetically located between the stereocilia; these molecules would be capable of generating potentials ranging from 10 to 100 mV. It is not clear with which enzymes this hyaluronidaseresistant polysaccharide should interact. How can it penetrate the otolith membrane if it is produced (as was pointed out) in another location? Finally, what purpose do the stereocilia serve if the potential is induced by polysaccharide molecules located deep between the stereocilia? We should not forget that mucopolysaccharides, to which the hyaluronic complex belongs, have been detected on the plasma membrane of microvilli in cells of the intestine and renal tubules, where they play a definite role in suction processes (ITO, 1965; BOYD and PORSONS, 1969). For this reason, the presence of mucopolysaccharides in the region of stereocilia, which are derivatives of microvilli, hardly argues in favor of their having a specific function in the gravireceptor of vertebrates. The hyaluronic complex would appear to be present in otolith membranes and cupulae in the same way as, for example, acetylcholine is present in the endolymph of the labyrinth. However, we have not been able to detect acetylcholinesterase in the stereocilia of maculae and cristae; as we have seen, it is localized in the hairs of receptor cells of Corti's organ, where the interaction of acetylcholine with a specific protein and then with an enzyme leads to stimulation of auditory cells during the movement of the basillar membrane (VINNIKOV and TITOVA, 1961). It looks as if the problem of the mechanism of the function of stereocilia in maculae and cristae at the molecular level will be resolved in the near future with advances in cytochemical and electron microscopic methods. Nevertheless, the functional significance of stereocilia is great. According to DOHLMAN'S calculations (DOHLMAN, 1960a, 1960b), the total area of stereocilia membranes in the utricle of vertebrates is equal to about 2,000—4,000 $\mu m^2$, whereas the remaining plasma membrane of the cells covers an area of only 200—300 $\mu m^2$. Thus, in the course of the evolution of invertebrates a universal model of organ emerged, capable of perceiving the position of the body in the gravitational field. In spite of the completely different origin and evolutionary course of, for example, higher crustaceans, cephalopod molluscs, and vertebrates, their statocysts and vestibular apparatus exhibit a striking similarity at the organic, cellular, subcellular levels and, we believe, molecular levels of organization. The differences observed are essentially only different variations of the solution to the problem, of gravitation reception, and are associated with differences in the environment of various animals.

# Chapter IX

# The Molecular Theory of Sensory Reception

In this final chapter we shall try to summarize the information presented in the preceding chapters. In each of these chapters we have set out and compared the main factual results of studies carried out with the aid of electron microscopic, cytochemical, biochemical and electrophysiological methods, on the photoreceptors of vertebrates, insects and cephalopod mollusks, the taste cells of vertebrates and insects, the auditory cells of vertebrates and insects, the receptor cells of the organ of gravitation of coelenterata, ctenophora, ciliated worms, annelids, arthropods, molluscs, and vertebrates.

A study of the structural organization of the receptor cells of vertebrates and invertebrates (see Chapters IV to VIII) has confirmed earlier beliefs that only two modifications of such cells exist: primary and secondary sensory cells (HANSTRÖM, 1928; ZAVARZIN, 1941; VINNIKOV, 1946; BUDDENBROCK, 1952). Primary sensory cells thought to appear for the first time in the process of evolution in ciliated worms and annelids, are characterized by the fact that they are equipped with specialized peripheral processes capable of receiving the energy of a stimulus and are crowned by a mobile flagella containing $9 \times 2 + 2$ or $9 \times 2 + 0$ fibrils, or microvilli (or their derivatives, stereocilia), or both (VINNIKOV, 1964, 1965a, 1965b, 1967a, 1967b; VINNIKOV, 1969, 1970b, 1974). Any stimulus they receive is transmitted as an impulse along the central process to the corresponding part of the central nervous system. Primary sensory cells in invertebrates constitute the basic universal type of specialized receptor elements with which all types of reception are associated. In vertebrates, these cells are represented by only two, essentially relict modifications, namely the photoreceptors in the retina of the eye, and the olfactory cells of the olfactory organ, which develop as part of the nervous system (VINNIKOV, 1946, 1947; VINNIKOV and TITOVA, 1957a).

In addition to primary sensory cells, a new receptor modification appeared as early as the Silurian period in the Agnata, ancestors of the vertebrates; this was the secondary sensory cells (STENSIÖ, 1927; BYSTROV, 1957). These cells also seem to appear in Ctenophora. Secondary sensory cells have neither a peripheral nor a central process but, as in primary sensory cells, reception is usually accomplished with the aid of mobile flagellum-like hairs containing $9 \times 2 + 2$ fibrils, kinocilia, microvilli and their derivatives, namely immobile stereocilia (VINNIKOV, 1964, 1965a, 1965b, 1966a, 1966b, 1967a, 1967b, 1969, 1970b, 1974). Stimulation is transmitted with the aid of a synaptic mechanism through the enveloping terminal ramifications of afferent nerve fibers that branch off from the corresponding afferent neurons. Secondary sensory cells include the receptor elements of lateral-line organs of lower vertebrates, hair cells of the inner ear, located both in the cristae and in the maculae acusticae of the vestibule, also found in the organ of Corti and, finally, the receptor cells of the taste buds. In embryogenesis, the secondary sensory receptor cells develop from the special thickenings of "placoids" and then become connected to appropriate parts of the nervous system (VINNIKOV, 1946; VINNIKOV and TITOVA, 1957a). The organization of receptor cells in coelenterata, and echinoderms is still not completely clear; it is possible that these cells as well as those in ctenophora are secondary sensory cells.

Consequently, the receptor cells of sense organs, in spite of the divergent ways (KHLOPIN, 1946) and periods of their development in the evolution of different phyla of multicellular animals, exhibit a distinct parallelism (ZAVARZIN, 1941) in that portion which is organized in the form of kinocilia or microvilli and their derivatives (stereocilia) and which interacts directly with the energy of a given stimulus. Thus, the evolution of all receptor cells of the sense organs is always based on a cell equipped with flagella and microvilli or their derivatives (Fig. 123). Perhaps such an organization of receptor cells reflects the origin of multicellular animals from flagellates (ERWIN and BLOCH, 1964; IVANOV, 1968). As described above, in some of these animals *(Diflagella)*, the flagella are functionally connected with the eyespot, which contains both carotenoids and chlorophyll and, depending upon the illumination, functions as either a receptor or synthesizer (WOLKEN, 1956). SEVERTSOV (1967) considered the gradual histological changes of indifferent receptor cells or their replacement by specialized cells in sense organs as an aromorphosis.

Whereas the microvilli and their derivatives, the immobile stereocilia, are characterized by the relatively simple structure of their fibrillar apparatus, the kinocilia, as described, contain $9 \times 2 + 2$ fibrils and are capable of undergoing automatic and continuous movement. This movement is already observed in Protozoa, again the *Diflagella* where the eye spot is functionally connected with the flagella, and the long-known retinomotor phenomena involving the shortening and lengthening of the rods and cones in photoreceptors (ANGELUCCI, 1878). Finally, the movement of kinocilia in the olfactory cells of vertebrates (BRONSHTEIN, 1964) and of hair cells in the labyrinth (VINNIKOV and TITOVA, 1961) was established in our laboratory.

A special study would be required to determine the significance of the movement of kinocilia in receptor cells for the physiology of the sense organs. We shall merely remark that this movement seems to represent an active search for a specific stimulus in the surrounding environment, and it corrects or measures this stimulus within the limits of threshold values by means of selfadjustment or automatic control, i. e. its function is to create optimum reception conditions. The macroscopically well-known processes of movement (for example in the eye, the function of oculomotor muscles and of the iris and ciliary body muscles) should now be extended to the receptor cell itself. We could give many more examples in this regard. Undoubtedly microvilli are also capable of movement (ITO, 1965; BOYD and PORSONS, 1969; THUNEBERG and POSTGAARD, 1969), forming rhabdomers (GRIBAKIN, 1967a, 1967b, 1969a, 1969b) and, under the effect of shearing forces, so are stereocilia (VINNIKOV et al., 1971). However, whereas the mechanism of the movement of kinocilia is associated with the interaction between low-molecular ATP and high-molecular ATPase (ENGEL-HARDT, 1957) present in the 9 pairs of peripheral fibrils, the mechanism of the movement of microvilli is still not completely clear, though their movement may well be caused by the same mechanochemical processes, as is proved by the presence in their fibrills of the specific contractile protein, tubuline.

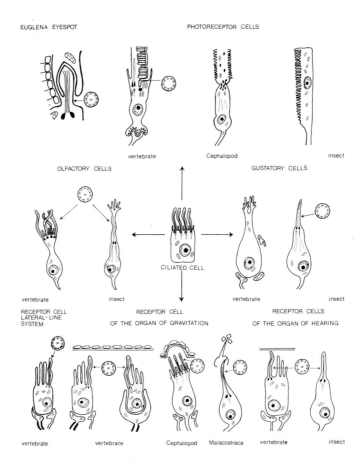

Fig. 123. Scheme of the evolution of receptor cells in the most highly developed representatives of animal phyletic lines

Taking into account the constant nature, special role and structure of the flagella (comprising kinocilia, microvilli and stereocilia) in the receptor cells of sense organs, we came to the conclusion that they should be considered as special mobile and universal antennae capable of automatically perceiving various forms of energy reaching them from the external environment (VINNIKOV, 1964, 1965a, 1965b, 1966a, 1966b, 1967a, 1967b, 1969, 1970a, 1970b, 1974). The antennae of receptor cells are the most ancient information transducers.

Thus, the receptor cells of sense organs, in contrast to neurons which receive and transmit information only through synapses, are stimulated directly by various forms of energy from the external environment, usually acting on the mobile antennae. If the receptor cell in the synapse region (see Chapter III) receives and transmits information with the aid of a mediator or ephaptic mechanism in the same way as nerve cells (NACHMANSON, 1959; ECCLES, 1964) the question is how does the cell effect the reception (or encoding) and conversion into information of the energy of an external stimulus in the antenna region? If the transmission and reception of information in the synapses takes place essentially in the region of the pre- and postsynaptic membranes, it is natural to assume that in the antenna this function is also performed by the plasma membrane coating the antenna. The anatomical relations in the sense organs are of such a nature as to leave no doubt that an interaction between an energy stimulus from the external environment and the receptor cell is possible only in the region of the plasma membrane of the antenna. What properties do cellular membranes in general and the plasma membrane in particular possess that allow them to effect such a transformation? In Chapter I we examined the characteristics of the structural and biochemical organization of biological membranes and showed that it is a supermolecular structure consisting of a bimolecular layer of lipids, bound on both sides by a double layer of protein molecules (ROBERTSON, 1967; SJÖSTRAND, 1967). During the transmission of nerve impulses, a change occurs in the permeability of synaptic membranes of neurons for $K^+$ and $Na^+$ ions; this is accompanied by depolarization of the postsynaptic membrane and the appearance of a biopotential along the neural fiber. The simplest assumption was thus (cf. DAVIS, 1958; GRUNDFEST, 1961, and many others) that in the sense organs too under the effect of the energy of an external stimulus the encoding, i.e. the primary transformation, consists in a depolarization of the plasma membrane of the antennae of the receptor cell.

Just as, for example, the cholinoreceptive protein is found in synapses with a cholinergic transmission, it is generally possible to detect in the plasma membrane of the antennae of the receptor cells, the localization of protein molecules that are specific for each of the sense organs (see Chapter IV—VIII) and are the first to interact with energy from the external environment (Fig. 124). It follows that the polarization of receptor cells of sense organs or the appearance of the receptor potential, i.e. the transmission of information, must always be preceded by a primary, specific interaction between a discrete energy unit of the stimulus and a specific protein molecule of the plasma membrane of the antenna, i.e. an encoding process. This encoding is thus the trigger mechanism for the overall stimulation of the receptor cell that accompanies the transmission of information.

The sensory perception and encoding of energy, i.e. the translation of the "language" of external stimuli (photons, molecules of gustatory and odoriferous substances, sound, gravitation, etc.) into the "language" of the receptor cell takes place at the molecular level of organization. There is in the plasma membrane of the antenna of a receptor cell a special molecule [rhodopsin (WALD, 1960), molecules of sweet- or bitter-sensitive proteins (DASTOLI and PRICE, 1966; DAS-

TOLI, LOPIEKES, and DOIG, 1968), molecules of olfactory proteins ASH, 1969;
RIDDIFORD, 1970) and a cholinoreceptive protein (VINNIKOV and TITOVA, 1961,
1963, 1964; VINNIKOV and KOICHEV, 1969)]. These molecules correspond to
discrete units of a definite form of energy, e. g. electromagnetic (photon) energy,
the chemical energy of "gustatory" or "olfactory" molecules, mechanical energy
("acoustic" vibrations of gas or liquid molecules) and so on.

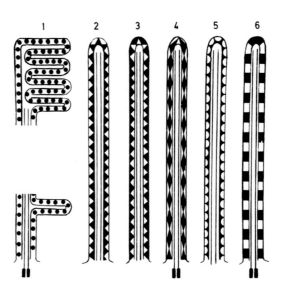

Fig. 124. Diagram showing how receptive protein molecules are mounted into the plasma membrane
of receptor cell antennae. *1* rhodopsin (photoreceptor); *2* and *3* sweet-sensitive and bitter-sensitive
protein (gustatory cell); *4* olfactive protein (olfactory cell); *5* cholinoreceptive protein (hair cell);
*6* hypothetical receptive protein (receptor cell of gravitation organ)

   We can agree with the statement that "in protein nature has found a unique
instrument, whose specificity it utilizes to achieve a tremendous selectivity and
multiplicity of effect" (CRICK, 1960). Reception, strictly speaking, involves two
stages: 1. encoding, i. e. the transformation of an external stimulus, and 2. transmission of the encoded information in the form of nerve impulses from the receptor
cell through synapses and numerous conductors to the central parts of the
relevant analyzer, where the decoding of the transmitted information takes place.
These processes, also are considered of present as molecular events (UNGAR,
1972).
   When the problem is formulated in this fashion, certain energy problems
arise. Thus, it has long been known that a single photon is sufficient for the
stimulation of a visual cell (VAVILOV, 1950). Beidler's equation (BEIDLER, 1964)
quoted in this book (Chapter V) shows how insignificant is the energy consumption
required for the stimulation of a gustatory cell. The role of the energy stimulus
is apparently not only to supply the energy required for the process of stimulation
of the receptor cell, but rather what we might call "closing the circuit". The

receptive protein molecule can be present in a state of either "rest" or "stimulation". These states are separated by a potential "barrier" which prevents spontaneous stimulation of the molecule under the effect of thermal movement. The external stimulus supplies the protein molecule with the energy required to cross this "barrier". This passage is accompanied by the change in the conformation of the molecule. The energy of the external stimulus, as we shall see below, must act upon a definite chemical bond of the receptive protein molecule; we think this is what determines the specificity of the interaction between a given molecule and a given stimulus.

However, although the coding, i.e. the direct conversion of the energy of external stimuli, does not require a large expenditure of energy, the transmission of the encoded information, i.e. a nerve impulse, needs from the very beginning a tremendous intensification of the energy of the excited receptor cell (ENGEL-HARDT, 1969). A rapid rise in the activity of ATPase is indeed observed in the plasma membrane of the antenna of every receptor cell in every sense organ (SCARPELLI and CRAIG, 1963; BRONSHTEIN and PYATKINA, 1969a; NAKAI and HILDING, 1967). Furthermore, complex mitochondrial aggregates are present for example, the ellipsoid of photoreceptors; these are suppliers of ATP and powerful energy boosters (LUKASHEVICH-TSIRULIS, 1964, 1966). During transmission of the nerve impulse, the mitochondria are seen to adhere to the membranes, particularly in the synapse region (VINNIKOV, 1967a, 1967c). This is a clear indication of local transmission of ATP.

Thus, the specific process of reception is determined both by the characteristics of the protein molecules located in the plasma membrane of the antennae of receptor cells and by the nature of the energy of the external stimulus; it is intensified by the universal nonspecific molecular interaction between low-molecular ATP and high-molecular ATPase which is also built into the same plasma membrane, and incidentally, into the other membrane structures of the receptor cell. This fact, however, does not justify the assumption that ATPase itself, through alterations in the distance between its active centers under the effect of various stimuli, plays the role of universal receptive protein and is capable of encoding the stimulus in the form of information, as postulated by DUNCAN (1967) and others.

The possibility of that there may be special bonds between the receptive protein molecules and ATPase, is, of course, not excluded, even if these bonds turn out to be of the myosin-ATPase type discovered by ENGELHARDT and LJUBIMOVA (1939), where, as is well known, the function is determined by the structure of the myosin molecules. The postulate that rhodopsin is an enzymic protein (OSTROVSKII and FEDOROVICH, 1965) has not yet been proved. The connections between the receptive protein molecules and some other proteins and lipids lead us to another problem—the problem of the structural and functional organization of the receptive membrane. The concept that receptive proteins may have an enzymic nature itself present a number of difficulties. The enzymatic theories of reception proposed, for example, for olfaction (KISTIAKOWSKY, 1950; BARADI and BOURNE, 1953) and for other senses have seldom been further developed or confirmed. Moreover, these theories contradict present concepts concerning the function and organization of enzymic protein molecules. Their active centers are known to be target-oriented only in respect to a definite chemical substrate (COSHLAND, 1964; PHILLIPS, 1968). In all sense organs which perform the most complex conversion of the energy of a stimulus, the interaction is always with a specific noncatalytic protein molecule. Of course, this fact should not be held to diminish the exclusive role of the wide variety of enzymes which regulate the function of receptive proteins and the further transmission of energy in the form of nerve impulses. The way in which enzymes participate in various types of conversion of a stimulus is described in detail in the appropriate sections of this book.

Thus, though reception demands the closest participation of enzymes, it does seem that receptive proteins are not themselves catalysts and hence should be classified in a special category. By the way, the concept of "receptive protein" was first introduced in 1906 by LANGLEY to describe the cholinoreceptor of synapses.

Returning to receptive proteins, we will give a brief description of what is known about each of them. The visual pigment, rhodopsin, is located in membranes of photoreceptor antennae and interacts with the energy of a photon (Chapter IV). The portion that reacts with a photon in this heterogenous lipoprotein molecule is retinal, which is a prosthetic group and a chromophore (WALD, 1968). The energy of one photon makes one molecule of retinal subject to *trans* isomerization; the protein portion of the molecule (opsin) undergoes a change in conformation at the moment of *trans* isomerization and simultaneous dissociation of retinal; at the same time, the chemical Schiff base linkages that united these molecules are liberated (HUBBARD et al., 1965). Although the function of retinal is universal, and isomerization takes place under the effect of any photon, only opsin is capable of effecting the specific encoding of the photon's quantum energy. Recent data indicate that in the dark retinal is linked by means of a Schiff base not directly to opsin, but rather to the lipid phosphatidylethanolamine that is present in rhodopsin (DAEMEN and BONTING, 1968). Like other proteins, rhodopsin can differ in size and molecular weight in different types of animals: 40,000 in vertebrates (DAEMEN et al., 1972) and 3,000 to 4,000 in insects (WOLKEN, MELLON, and CONTIS, 1957).

In the case of the sweet-sensitive (molecular weight 150,000) and bitter-sensitive receptive proteins (see Chapter V) localized in the plasma membrane of gustatory cell antennae, the molecular interaction with sweet and bitter food molecules is effected within the limits of London hydrogen bonds and is sufficient to cause a change in the conformation of the receptive molecule (DASTOLI and PRICE, 1966; DASTOLI, LOPIEKES, and DOIG, 1968).

Although the interaction between olfactory receptive protein molecules and molecules of odoriferous compounds appears to require the presence of ascorbic acid as a cofactor (ASH, 1969; see Chapter VI), it can presumably take place (by analogy with gustatory cells) with the participation of London hydrogen bonds or possibly Van der Waals forces (ASH, 1968, 1969).

In the case of antennae of auditory cells in Corti's organ (see Chapter VII), conformational shifts occur in the cholinoreceptive protein molecule when it interacts with an acetylcholine molecule, the quantum release of which we believe to be commensurate with the transformation of the mechanical energy of the molecules taking part in the transmission of a sound wave (VINNIKOV and TITOVA, 1961; VINNIKOV and KOICHEV, 1969). It is assumed that the active center of the cholinoreceptor contains an anionic group with which the cationic head of acetylcholine interacts, and also some kind of polarized group that reacts with the esterase portion of acetylcholine according to the dipole–dipole interaction principle (BARLOW, 1955, 1960; MIKHELSON and ZEIMAL, 1967, 1970). The qualitative difference between synapses and the cholinoreceptive protein in the plasma membrane of antennae in the hair cells of Corti's organ, which allows the conversion and encoding of an acoustic stimulus, may be associated with the special character of its structural organization and positioning, both of which can change in the course of evolution (MIKHELSON, 1967).

In the case of other mechanoreceptors, in particular the gravireceptor (see Chapter VIII), the presence of specific receptive protein in the plasma membrane of the antennae of their receptor cells is still hypothetical. However, as was recently shown for Vater-Pacini bodies, mechanochemical mechanisms form the basis for their stimulation (CHERNIGOVSKII et al., 1970). Even for receptive proteins which have been studied in greater detail, the alternating sequence of the amino acids is still unknown. Amino acid composition has been investigated only in opsin (HELLER, 1969) and the sweet-sensitive protein (DASTOLI, LOPIEKES, and DOIG, 1968), and their molecular weight has been determined. The primary, secondary, tertiary and quaternary structures of these proteins, i. e. their entire molecular organization, are still unknown. Such investigations of receptive proteins represent an exciting prospect for the future.

Using visual reception as our example, we have shown that the encoding of the energy of a photon is based on conformational shifts and breakdown of the heterogeneous rhodopsin molecule into retinal and opsin. Opsin may even continue to change its conformation after dissociation of retinal (MATTHEWS et al., 1963). Rhodopsin in the dark must possess a more or less stable conformation. The process that produces a change in the conformation of a protein molecule has two aspects, morphological and physical. Whereas the cooperative (morphological) aspect can be demonstrated best from an external viewpoint (VOLKENSHTEIN, 1965), the physical aspect of the change in molecular conformation has been studied only on individual proteins. This physical aspect is associated with changes that have to a lesser or greater extent been clarified, for example, in the case of hemoglobin (WEISSBLUTH, 1969). These changes affect absorption in the ultraviolet portion of the spectrum, magnetic properties, Mössbauer spectra, ligand field potentials, molecular orbitals, etc. We still have a very long way to go before the analogous properties of receptive proteins are fully known.

The action of a discrete unit of energy (stimulus) from the external environment upon a protein molecule, which is accompanied by the corresponding conformational transition, modifies the linkages of this molecule with neighboring lipids or other protein molecules; this process, according to present concepts, leads finally to a change in the permeability of the plasma membrane as a whole, which changes the ionic equilibrium, mainly for $Na^+$ and $K^+$, causing depolarization and the appearance of a receptor potential. By means of biochemical and cytochemical methods, it is possible to trace the change and distribution of $Na^+$ and $K^+$ ions when the receptor potential is generated during stimulation of receptor cells (ETINGOF, SHUKOLYUKOV, and LEONT'EV, 1964; HAGINS, ZONANA, and ADAMS, 1962; BONTING and BAGHAM, 1967; GOVARDOVSKII, 1969; KOICHEV, 1969b; VINNIKOV and KOICHEV, 1969).

Whereas $K^+$ ions are known to be localized in the cytoplasm of a cell, our work has shown that $Na^+$ ions are localized outside the receptor cell. For example, $Na^+$ ions can be produced in the olfactory organ by Bowman's glands and, together with the products of secretion, they enter the mucus which surrounds the antennae of the olfactory cells. In taste buds $Na^+$ ions are demonstrated on the outer surface of the microvilli membrane (PEVZNER, in press). $Na^+$ ions have been demonstrated in the cortilymph which surrounds the hair cells of Corti's organ. During embryonic development, if the disks are enclosed by an external environment contains $Na^+$ ions, as in the case of the rods of photoreceptors, $Na^+$ ions pass inside the disks, where they can be detected. The latest data show rhodopsin asymmetrically localized on the inner surface of the membranes of the disks (ABRAHAMSON, pers. comm.) which ought, in fact, to be considered as their outer surface. A similar asymmetrical (only on the outer protein layer) distribution in the plasma membrane can be assumed for the receptive protein molecules of taste cells (BEIDLER, pers. comm.). Thus, the ions which play an extremely important role in the transmission of the information encoded y receptive protein molecules are situated close at hand.

Thus, the action of a discrete stimulus upon a special receptive protein molecule, positioned apparently asymmetrically, i. e. only on the outer surface of the plasma membrane of the antenna of receptor cell, is the primary trigger mechanism and precedes the appearance of biopotentials, which are associated with the ultrastructural organization of the plasma membrane. The presence of potentials usually denotes a state of cellular excitation. However, the state of excitation of a receptor cell is by no means limited to depolarization of the plasma membrane. A complex process of molecular conversion has in fact preceded such a depolarization. Moreover, cytochemistry, biochemistry and electron microscopy reveal a pattern of extensive shifts, both in the ultrastructural organization and in the substrates and enzymes which have during the course of evolution moved to the sectors of the receptor cell that are most effective from a functional standpoint (VERZHBINSKAYA, 1954; KREPS and VERZHBINSKAYA, 1959). These shifts are manifested in the redislocation and swelling of the mitochondria, in changes and *de novo* formation of endoplasmic reticulum membranes, in modifications of the shape of the nucleus and of the position of the nucleolus, in the exit of ribosomes through the pores of the nuclear membrane into the cytoplasm, etc. (VINNIKOV, 1967). At the same time, substantial shifts are observed (and can be recorded with the aid of biochemical and cytochemical methods) in the substrates and enzymes involved in anaerobic and aerobic metabolism; these shifts occur in conjunction with oxidative phosphorylation. Changes are also observed in the biosynthesis of nucleic acids and proteins, which increases rapidly and sharply during brief stimulation (VINNIKOV and TITOVA, 1961). We do not yet know the sequence and association of the ultrastructural and cytochemical shifts that occur during stimulation. There is no doubt, however, that the excitation of a receptor cell is not limited merely to processes occurring on the plasma membrane of the cell. Excitation affects the entire cytoplasm of the receptor cell as a whole; this cytoplasm is characterized by a peculiar structure and stable character in every one of the sense organs. Excitation is ultimately resolved by the transmission of the encoded information through synapses to the central nervous system in the form of nerve impulses by ephaptic or mediator means, the general mechanisms of which have been discussed in the appropriate chapters of this book.

The specific character of the information was determined right from the start by the primary coding transformation that tooks place at the moment when the energy of the external stimulus acted upon the protein receptive molecule located in the plasma membrane of the antenna. The processes which can be observed on plasma membranes, in the cytoplasm, and in synapses of the receptor cell are secondary, noncoding processes; they are practically the same in all sense organs, and they do not alter the character of the information. Decoding, i. e. the final conversion of information, takes place in neurons of the central portions of analyzers, where the information undergoes a final analysis and synthesis.

In view of what has been stated above, it is difficult for us to agree with certain concepts advanced by DAVIS (1964) and presented in the preface to the English translation of our book (with TITOVA as co-author) entitled: "Organ of Corti" (1964). DAVIS suggests that the cytoplasm of the receptor cell is simply a peculiar "pool" which metabolically services the bioelectric processes taking place on its surface. We also find it difficult to agree that the process of depolarization of the membrane is the mechanism that triggers the stimulation of the receptor cell in general. Let us consider the hair cell of Corti's organ: it is hard to believe that this process is not preceded by an encoding process involving molecular interaction between acetylcholine and the cholinoreceptive protein as a result of the conversion of the acoustic stimulus in the middle and inner ear. The view that a deformation of the plasma membrane without any change in molecular conformation of the protein is sufficient to induce a receptor potential in the mechanoreceptors of vertebrates and insects in general (and in Corti's organ in particular) is apparently quite widely accepted (DAVIS, 1958; THURM, 1965a, 1965b; GOLDMAN, 1965). Indeed, it is frequently observed that the energy of a mechanical stimulus causes either a contraction of the mobile flagellum or a deflection of the immobile stereocilium; in this case a deformation of the plasma membrane actually takes place so that deformation must be considered as one of the possible ways of encoding a stimulus. Although there is no doubt that, as we have shown, other transformations take place in these receptors, for example in the Pacinian corpuscles (IL'INSKII, 1966; MIRKIN, 1966a—1966c; CHEREPNOV, 1968), these have not yet been studied to a sufficient extent. Nevertheless, the body of factual material presented above leads us to believe that every mechanical stimulus undergoes conversion into a mechanochemical stimulus and that the appearance of a biopotential is preceded by a process involving a change in the conformation of protein molecules, still unknown to us, which are specific for each mechanoreceptor. Naturally, this assumption would also apply to the gravireceptor (Chapter VIII).

This concept poses a number of evolutionary questions, but first and foremost: how did the receptor cell and its specific structures—the antennae and the receptive protein molecules—develop during phylo- and ontogenesis? The receptor cell alone is able to encode an energy stimulus and transmit it in the form of specific information. We know that energy stimuli, such as photons, acoustic vibrations, the energy of gustatory and odoriferous compounds, gravitation, etc., are capable of exerting a general, nonspecific effect upon any cell. We made a special demonstration of this on an example showing the effect of sound (VINNIKOV and TITOVA, 1961). The sorption of an intravital dye during acoustic stimulation, both *in vivo* and *in vitro*, has the same quantitative value for Corti's organ (cochlea) as for other tissues. Thus, sorption takes place within the limits of the audiogram, which means that Corti's organ and other tissues "hear" in the same way (NASONOV and RAVDONIK, 1947; VINNIKOV and TITOVA, 1961, 1964). Another example enabled us to demonstrate that cells and tissues show the same sensitivity toward molecules of odoriferous compounds. Odoriferous compounds were allowed to act directly upon the plasma membrane of the giant neuron of *Aplisia* into which a microelectrode had been inserted and were found to cause a slow change of the membrane potential; the depolarization was accompanied by a pulse discharge resembling an olfactogram (ARVANITAKI, TAKEUCHI, and CHALANOZITIS, 1967). Other similar examples can be cited. Clearly, the nonspecific reaction of a cell to the energy of a stimulus from the external environment is transformed into a specific reaction when it takes place in a receptor cell; if this were not so, reception would not reflect objective reality.

This raises yet another question: How can the receptor cell make such an adequate encoding from the energy of a stimulus when its "specific" reaction to this stimulus does not differ from the analogous nonspecific reaction of any other tissue cell? We think it is able to effect an equivalent encoding because of the creation, during the phyloembryogenesis of receptor cells, of a special molecular "extension". This takes the form of molecules of receptive protein, built into the plasma membrane of the antennae and capable of undergoing a specific reaction with a discrete unit of a particular form of energy from the external environment. The appearance of such protein molecules, which must have been the expression of mutations, requires the presence of appropriate genes to control the biosynthesis of proteins. These genes were created over many generations and were fixed by natural selection after further changes in the genetic stock had been induced by new random mutations (ANFINSEN, 1967).

A concrete study of the phylo- and ontogenesis of certain receptive proteins in the sense organs shows that Hekkel-Müller's theory of recapitulation is also applicable at the molecular level of evolution; this notion was advanced for the first time in biochemistry by KREPS (1967) for phospholipids of the brain. Thus, the rhodopsin molecule, in its origin, is a heterogeneous molecule. The vitamin A present in this molecule is a derivative of the $\beta$- and $\alpha$-carotenes that are found in the grains or more precisely the quantosomes, present in the chloroplast membranes of plants-Carotenoids, being light-sensitive, are localized in the vicinity of chlorophyll and play an auxiliary role in the processes of photosynthesis. The light sensitivity of carotenoids is preserved when these compounds enter into the organism of animals, where two molecules of vitamin

A are obtained from $\beta$-carotene by rupture of its chain and addition of water, and one molecule of vitamin A is from $\alpha$-carotene. Thus, retinal, the prosthetic group of opsin, has a long evolutionary history, being associated with the molecular organization of plant photosynthesis; after entering the animal organism it continues to perform its light-sensitive function by means of idioadaptation (SEVERTSOV, 1967).

The structural and functional evolution of the heterogeneous rhodopsin molecule can be compared with a such well-known Darwinian example as the matching development of the shape of the calyx of the red clover flower and the length of the stylet of the bumblebee. Obviously the calyx and the stylet, like carotenoids and opsin, developed independently. Yet by their structural and functional association the continuation of the plant species is assured in the one case and the realization of photoreception by animals in the other.

A knowledge of the phylogenesis of the rhodopsin molecule is helpful in understanding from a molecular standpoint the details of the embryogenesis of receptor cells. In our own and other laboratories it has been possible to observe how the disk membranes in outer segments of rods and cones of vertebrates develop at the expense of the plasma membrane of the flagellum (containing $9 \times 2 + 0$ fibrils) in the embryonic photoreceptor (NILSSON, 1964a, 1964b; GOVAR-DOVSKII and KHARKEEVICH, 1966a, 1966b). At all stages of ontogenesis, the development of these membranes is regorously controlled by the synthesis of opsin in the nucleus-containing portion of the cell. From here the opsin travels, together with other protein molecules, into the membrane region of the flagellum (DROZ, 1961, 1963; YOUNG and DROZ, 1968; YOUNG, 1968). This region also receives from the pigment layer of the retina oxidized vitamin A (retinal), stored in the liver of the embryo of the adult animal, which has acquired it with its food in the form of carotenoids from plants. The combination of opsin and retinal in the heterogeneous rhodopsin molecule leads in turn, as can be observed in the electron microscope, to the development of the disk membranes in which opsin and retinal are localized. Under experimental conditions, if the two parts of this heterogeneous molecule are not allowed to combine (for example, in tissue cultures or because of vitamin-A deficiency, the disks will fail to develop or will undergo atresia (GOVARDOVSKII and KHARKEEVICH, 1966a; DOWLING and GIBBONS, 1961; EAKIN, 1964). Addition of vitamin A to the animal's diet is accompanied by the development or restoration of the disk membranes. Thus, the organization of the heterogeneous molecule of rhodopsin during ontogenesis reflects the development and differentiation of disk membranes in the photoreceptors of vertebrates during phylogenesis.

Molecular organization constitutes the base on which cellular organization is built during phylo- and ontogenesis. Thus, representatives of the "younger" phyla, i.e. vertebrates, have cones with the same ultrastructural organization, regardless of the light perceived. The difference in color reception, which is associated with the characteristic features of opsin, must be attributed to the molecular level and has, in our opinion, not yet found morphological expression at the cellular level. In representatives of more "ancient" phyla, on the other hand, for example insects, molecular differences have led to the appearance of different types of cells, differing morphologically from each other and capable of perceiving three different colors. This discovery was made in our laboratory (GRIBAKIN, 1969a—1969d).

The molecular evolution of other sense organs has not yet been studied and only isolated, fragmentary data are available. We still do not know the exact location site of sweet- and bitter-sensitive proteins in gustatory receptor cells; the location of these proteins can be provisionally assigned to the plasma membrane of the microvilli where they seem to be asymmetrically localized in the outer protein layer of the cell membrane (BEIDLER, pers. comm.). However, we do know that, in man at least, molecules of sweet-sensitive protein are already synthesized in the taste buds of a 13-week-old fetus (DE SNOO, 1937; WINDLE, 1940).

Again, whereas in vertebrates molecular differences at the cellular level have not yet found morphological expression (i.e. sweet-sensitive and bitter-sensitive cells are indistinguishable) gustatory cells with a clearly distinguishable special function are found in certain insects (DETHIER and HANSON, 1965; ELIZAROV and SINITSYNA, 1969). Relationships resembling those of gustatory reception are also found in olfaction (ASH, 1969; ASH and SKOGEN, 1970; RIDDIFORD, 1970). In the organ of Corti of vertebrates, the activity of acetylcholinesterase (VINNIKOV and TITOVA, 1961; KANEKO and DALY, 1969) and presumably the cholinoreceptive protein coupled with it, can actually be observed; we have seen it in the antennae and synapses of hair cells in birds and mammals, however, during embryogenesis these compounds are present only in those coils of the cochlea in which the structural and functional differentiation of Corti's organ is completed. The activity of the enzyme can be seen first in the basal coils, then it gradually appears in the other coils of the cochlea (TITOVA, 1968; DEL BO and CONTI, 1961). In stereocilia of receptor cells of the vestibule, the activity of acetylcholinesterase is absent in embryogenesis as well as in definitive stages.

Thus, an extensive study of the onto- and phylogenesis of the molecular and cellular organization of sense organs needs to be undertaken. At present, we can only state that sense organs are indeed amazing biophysical instruments, and that their structure and functional evolution at all levels of organization (including the molecular level), are strictly determined. In the case of vision, they conform to the laws of the quantum theory of light; for hearing, to the laws of propagation and conversion of the energy of an acoustic wave; for organs of taste and smell, to the energy of gustatory and odoriferous compounds; for gravitation, to the laws of the Earth's gravitational field, and so on. This arrangement was the result of natural selection during many millions of years of evolution. The need to satisfy biophysical laws for the fulfillment of the same reception function is precisely what led to such a surprising parallelism of molecular, cellular and organ organization, either transmitted by heredity from some forms to others, or created *de novo* by parallel development. Years ago we pointed out that during the course of evolution reception is first determined qualitatively and its increasing complexity is then achieved by means of extensions in appropriate centers (VINNIKOV, 1947). Such conservatism relative to the cellular and molecular organization of receptor cells, already laid down by natural selection during the early stages of phylogenesis, is combined with complex evolutionary transformations in the central nervous system. According to the data of KARAMYAN (1965, 1970), obtained from representatives of all classes of vertebrates, the evolution of the central nervous system takes place according to the principle of stage-by-stage development or function exchange in an ascending direction. During this process a definite correlation is established between the level of organization of the nervous substrate and its function, and a general trend is noted to development from diffuse, nonspecialized forms of existence towards discrete, more specialized forms of nervous activity. Progressive development of the central nervous system, in turn, is accompanied by the appearance of the efferent innervation of receptor cells which allows the central regulation of the sensory organs by means of feedback mechanisms (VINNIKOV, 1967b).

The author is well aware that there are still a great many "blank spots" in the answer to the problem raised here. However, he believes that an investigation of this problem from an evolutionary standpoint presents the most promise and may enable the foundations of a molecular theory of reception to be laid.

## Note Added in Proof

This monograph was written in 1970, and the translation took rather a long time; it is therefore only natural that the contents are somewhat out of date. The author regrets that he could not discuss such topical points as the absence of ATP-ase activity in the outer segments of retine, the localization of ERP generators in rods and cones, the filter mechanism of PL perception in arthropods and so on. Nevertheless, the author feels that his general approach to the problem of sensory reception has not been modified by recent findings, and he hopes that his mistakes, if any, will serve to stimulate further study in this field.

# References

ABRAHAMSON, E. W., OSTROY, S. E.: The photochemical and macromolecular aspects of vision. In: Progress in Biophys. Molec. Biol. **17**, 181 (1967).

ABRAHAMSON, E. W., WIESENFELD, J.: The structure spectra and photochemistry of visual pigments. Exp. Eye Res. **8**, 242 (1969).

ABRAMYAN, R. A.: Histochemical study of the sacculus of birds under conditions of relative rest and adequate stimulation. Zh. evolyuts. biokhim. fiziol., **4**, 376 (1968).

ABRAMYAN, R. A.: Cytochemical and electron microscopic study of the sacculus of birds. Author's abstract of dissertation, Leningrad 1969.

ADRIAN, E. D.: Discharges from vestibular receptors in the cat. J. Physiol. (Lond.) **101**, 389 (1943).

ADRIAN, E. D.: The role of air movement in olfactory stimulation. J. Physiol. (Lond.) **114**, 4 (1951a).

ADRIAN, E. D.: Olfactory discrimination. Ann. Psychol. **50**, 107 (1951b).

AI, N., TAKAGI, S. F.: The effects of ether and chloroform in the olfactory epithelium. Jap. J. Physiol. **13**, 454 (1963).

AKERT, K.: Dynamic aspects of synaptic ultrastructure. Brain Res. **49**, 511 (1973).

AKHTAR, M., BLOSSER, F. T., DEWHURST, P. B.: The reduction of rhodopsin derivative. Life Sci. **4**, 1221 (1965).

AKIMUSHKIN, I. I.: Golovonogie mollyuski morei SSSR (Cephalopod Mollusks of U.S.S.R. Seas). Izd. Akad. Nauk SSSR, Moscow 1963a.

AKIMUSHKIN, I. I.: Primaty moryai (Primates of the Sea). Gos. Izd. Geograf. Liter, Moscow 1963b.

ALEKSANDROV, V. Ya., ARRONET, N. I.: Adenosine triphosphate causes movement of the cilia of the ciliated epithelium destroyed by glycerine extraction (cellular model), Dokl. Akad. Nauk SSSR *110*, **457** (1956).

ALEXANDER, G.: Entwicklungsgeschichte, Anthropologie, Varietalen. In: Denker, A., Kahler, O.: Handbuch der Hals-, Nasen- und Ohren-Heilkunde. Berlin: Springer 1926.

AMOORE, J. E.: The stereochemical theory of olfaction. I. Identification of the seven primary odours. Proc. Sci. Sect., Toilet Goods Ass., Special supplement **37**, 1 (1962a).

AMOORE, J. E.: The stereochemical theory of olfaction. 2. Elucidation of the stereochemical properties of the olfactory receptor sites. Proc. Sci. Sect., Toilet Goods Ass., Special Supplement **37**, 13 (1962b).

AMOORE, J. E.: Psychophysics of odor. In: Cold Spr. Harb. Symp. quant. Biol. **30**, 623 (1965).

AMOORE, J. E.: Computer correlation of molecular shape with odour: a model for structure–activity relationships. In: Taste and Smell in Vertebrates, p. 293. A Ciba Foundat. Symp. London: Churchill 1970.

ANDERSEN, H. T., FUNAKOSHI, M., ZOTTERMAN, Y.: Electrophysiological investigation of gustatory effect of various biological sugars. Acta physiol. scand. **56**, 462 (1962).

ANDRÉ, J., THIÉREY, J. P.: Mise en évidence d'une sous-structure fibrillaire dans les filaments axonématiques des flagelles. J. Microscop. **2**, 71 (1963).

ANDREEV, L. A.: The resonance theory of Helmholtz in the light of new data determining the action of the peripheral end of the acoustic analyzer of the dog. In: Collection of Works (Sbornik) on the Occasion of the Seventy-Fifth Birthday of I. P. Pavlov, p. 339. Leningrad 1924.

ANDRES, K. H.: Der Feinbau des Bulbus Olfactorius der Ratte unter besonderer Berücksichtigung der synaptischen Verbindungen. Z. Zellforsch. **65**, 530 (1965).

ANFINSEN, C. B.: The distribution of cholinesterase in the bovine retina. J. biol. Chem. **152**, 267 (1944).

ANFINSEN, C. B.: Molekulyarnye Osnovy Evolyutsii (Molecular foundations of Evolution), Inostr. literatura Moscow 1962.

ANFINSEN, C. B.: The formation of the tertiary structure of proteins. Harvey Lectures Ser. **61**, 95 (1967).

ANGELUCCI, A.: Histologische Untersuchungen über das retinale Pigmentepithel der Wirbelthiere. Arch. Anat. Physiol. 353 (1878).

ANICHIN, V. F.: The location and activity of acetylcholinesterase in the organ of Corti of animals under the effect of powerful high-frequency and medium-frequency sounds. Vestn. Oto-rino-laring. **6**, 9 (1964).

ANICHIN, V. F.: The distribution of nucleic acids and the change in the size of nuclei in hair cells of the organ of Corti under the effect of sound. Dokl. Akad. Nauk SSSR **163**, 1495 (1965).

ANICHIN, V. F.: Variation in the content of nucleic acids and the reaction of nuclei in hair cells of the organ of Corti in response to the effect of sound. Vest. Oto-rino-laring. **3**, 3 (1968).

ARDEN, G. B.: The dark reaction in visual cell suspension. J. Physiol. (Lond.) **123**, 386 (1954).

ARDEN, G. B., ERNST, W.: Mechanism of current production found in pigeon cones but not in pigeon or rat rods. Nature **222**, 528 (1969).

ARNSHTEIN, K. A.: Kontsevye apparaty vkusovogo nerva (Terminal Apparatus of the Gustatory Nerve), p. 22. Kazan 1893.

ARONOVA, M. Z.: Electron microscopic study of the lateral line organs of the pike *(Esox lucius)*. Arkh. Anat. Gistol. Embriol. **53**, 30 (1967).

ARONOVA, M. Z.: Electron microscopic and cytochemical study of the lateral line organs of the pike *(Esox lucius)*, Author's abstract of dissertation, Leningrad 1968.

ARVANITAKI, A.: Effects evoked in an axon by the electric activity of a contiguous one. J. Neurophysiol. **5**, 89 (1942).

ARVANITAKI, A., CHALANOZITIS, N.: Prototypes d'interactions neuroniques et transmission synaptiques, Données bioélectriques de préparations cellulaires. Arch. Sci. Physiol. **3**, 547 (1949).

ARVANITAKI, A., TAKEUCHI, H., CHALANOZITIS, N.: Specific unitary osmotic receptor potentials and spiking patterns from giant nerve cells. In: Olfaction and Taste, II, p. 573. Proc. 2d Int. Sympos. Oxford: Pergamon Press 1967.

ARVY, L.: Contribution à l'histoenzymologie des chémorécepteurs linguaux chez le mouton domestique. C. R. Acad. Sci. (Paris) **248**, 21 (1959).

ARVY, L.: Enzymes et appareil gustatif lingual chez le lapin domestique. Ann. Biol. anim. **1**, 145 (1961).

ASAKURA, S., EGUCHI, G., YINO, T.: Self-assembly of *Salmonella* flagellins. In: Seventh International Congress of Biochem., Abstr. II, p. 229 (1967).

ASH, K. O.: Chemical sensing: an approach to biological molecular mechanisms using difference spectroscopy. Science **162**, 452 (1968).

ASH, K. O.: Ascorbic acid; cofactor in rabbit olfactory preparations. Science **165**, 901 (1969).

ASH, K. O., SKOGEN, T. D.: Chemosensing: selectivity, sensitivity and additive effects on a stimulant-induced activity of olfactory preparations. J. Neurochem. **17**, 1143 (1970).

ASTBURY, W. T., BEIGHTON, E., WEIBULL, C.: The structure of bacterial flagella. Symp. Soc. exp. Biol. **9**, 282 (1955).

AUSTIN, L., MORGAN, J. G.: Incorporation of $^{14}$C-labelled leucine into synaptosomes from rat cerebral cortex in vitro. J. Neurochem. **14**, 374 (1967).

AUSTIN, L., MORGAN, J. G.: Synaptosomal protein synthesis in cell-free system. J. Neurochem. **15**, 41 (1968).

AUTRUM, H.: Über Gehör und Erschütterungssinn bei Locustiden. Z. vergl. Physiol. **28**, 580 (1941).

AUTRUM, H.: The physiological basis of colour vision in honeybees. In: Ciba Foundation Symposium on physiology and experimental psychology of colour vision (De Reuck, A.V.S., Knight, I., Eds.), p. 286. London: Churchill 1965.

AUTRUM, H.: Colour vision in man and animals. Naturwissenschaften **55**, 10 (1968).

AUTRUM, H., AUTRUM, T., HOFFMANN, CH.: Komponent und Retinogramm von *Calliphora* und ihre Abhängigkeit von der Spektralfarbe. Biol. Zbl. **80**, 513 (1961).

AUTRUM, H., SCHNEIDER, W.: Vergleichende Untersuchungen über den Erschütterungssinn der Insekten. Z. vergl. Physiol. **31**, 74 (1948).

AUTRUM, H., STUMPF, H.: Das Bienenauge als Analysator für polarisiertes Licht. Z. Naturforsch. **5**, 116 (1950).

AUTRUM, H., ZWEHL, V.: Die Sehzellen der Insekten als Analysatoren für polarisiertes Licht. Z. vergl. Physiol. **46**, 1 (1962a).

AUTRUM, H., ZWEHL, V.: Zur spektralen Empfindlichkeit einzelner Sehzellen der Drohne *(Apis mellifera)*. Z. vergl. Physiol. **46**, 8 (1962b).

AUTRUM, H., ZWEHL, V.: Ein Grünrezeptor im Drohnenauge *(Apis mellifera)*. Naturwissenschaften **50**, 698 (1963).

AUTRUM, H., ZWEHL, V.: Spektrale Empfindlichkeit einzelner Sehzellen des Bienenauges. Z. vergl. Physiol. **48**, 357 (1964).

BABUCHIN, A. I.: Beiträge zur Entwicklungsgeschichte des Auges, besonders der Retina. Würzburger Naturw. Z. **4**, 1 (1863).

BABUCHIN, A. I.: Über den Bau der Cephalopodenretina. Würzburger Naturw. Z. **5**, 127 (1864).

BABUCHIN, A. I.: Das Geruchsorgan. In: Stricker's Handb., Lehre v. d. Gewebe d. Menschen u. d. Thiere, p. 964 (1872).

BAIRATI, A., IURATO, S., PERNIS, B.: Biophysical properties of the tectorial membrane of Corti. Exp. Cell. Res. **13**, 207 (1957).

BAKER, C. L.: Spermatozoa of *Ampiuma tridactilum:* morphology, helical motility and reversibility. Amer. Zool. **1**, 340 (1961).

BARADI, A. F.: A note on morphology and phosphatase histochemistry of cat lingual papillae. J. Histochem. Cytochem. **2**, 448 (1963).

BARADI, A. F., BOURNE, G. H.: Localization of gustatory and olfactory enzymes in the rabbit and the problems of taste and smell. Nature **168**, 977 (1951a).

BARADI, A. F., BOURNE, G. H.: Theory of tastes and odors. Science **113**, 660 (1951b).

BARADI, A. F., BOURNE, G. H.: Gustatory and olfactory epithelia. Internat. Rev. Cytol. **2**, 289 (1953).

BARADI, A. F., BOURNE, G. H.: Histochemical demonstration of cholinesterase in gustatory and olfactory epithelia. J. Histochem. Cytochem. **7**, 1 (1959a).

BARADI, A. F., BOURNE, G. H.: New observations on the alkaline glycerophosphatase reaction in the papilla foliata. J. biophys. biochem. Cytol. **5**, 173 (1959b).

BARBER, V. C.: Preliminary observations on the fine structure of the octopus statocyst. J. Microscop. **4**, 547 (1965).

BARBER, V. C.: The fine structure of the statocyst of *Octopus vulgaris*. Z. Zellforsch. **70**, 91 (1966).

BARBER, V. C.: The structure of mollusc statocysts, with particular reference to Cephalopods. Symp. zool. Soc. (Lond.) **23**, 37 (1968).

BARBER, V. C., BOYDE, A.: Scanning electron microscopic studies of cilia. Z. Zellforsch. **84**, 269 (1968).

BARBER, V. C., DILLY, P. N.: Some aspects of the fine structure of the statocysts of the molluscs *Pecten* and *Pterotrachea*. Z. Zellforsch. **94**, 462 (1969).

BARBER, V. C., WRIGHT, D. E.: The fine structure of the sense organs of the cephalopod mollusc *Nautilus*. Z. Zellforsch. **102**, 293 (1969).

BARBER, V. C., EVANS, E. M., LAND, M. F.: The fine structure of the eye of mollusc *Pecten maximus*. Z. Zellforsch. **76**, 295 (1967).

BARER, R., JOSEPH, S., MEEK, G. A.: Membrane interrelationships during meiosis. In: Proc. Fourth International Conference on Electron Microscopy, Part II, p. 233. Berlin—Göttingen—Heidelberg: Springer 1960.

BARETS, A., SZABO, T.: Appareil synaptique des cellules sensorielles de l'ampoule de Lorenzini chez la torpille, *Torpedo marmorata*. J. Microscop. **1**, 47 (1962).

BARLOW, R. B.: Introduction to Chemical Pharmacology. London 1955.

BARLOW, R. B.: Steric aspects of drug action. Biochem. Soc. Sympos. **19**, 46 (1960).

BAUER, V.: Über die anscheinend nervöse Regulierung der Flimmerbewegung bei den Pippenquallen. Z. allg. Physiol. **10**, 230 (1910).

BAUMANN, CH.: Receptorpotentiale der Wirbeltiernetzhaut. Pflügers. Arch. ges. Physiol. **282**, 92 (1965).

BECK, C.: Kernveränderungen der Haarzellen nach Beschallung. Arch. Ohr.-, Nas.- u. Kehlk.-Heilk. **167**, 262 (1955).

BECK, C.: Feinere Stoffwechselreaktionen an den Sinneszellen des cortischen Organs nach Reintonbeschallung. Arch. Ohr.-, Nas.- u. Kehlk.-Heilk. **175**, 374 (1959).

BECK, C.: Biochemie des Ohres. Arch. Ohr.-, Nas.- u. Kehlk.-Heilk. **3**, 115 (1965).

BECK, C., MICHLER, H.: Feinstrukturelle und histochemische Veränderungen an den Strukturen der Cochlea beim Meerschweinchen nach dosierter Reintonbeschallung. Arch. Ohr.-, Nas.- u. Kehlk.-Heilk. **174**, 496 (1960).

BEETS, M. G.: Structure and odour. In Monograph: Molecular structure and organoleptic quality. Society of Chemical Industry, p. 54. London 1957.

BEIDLER, L. M.: A theory of taste stimulation. J. gen. Physiol. **38**, 133 (1954).

BEIDLER, L. M.: Physiology of olfaction and gustation. Ann. Otol. (St. Louis) **69**, 398 (1960).

BEIDLER, L. M.: The chemical senses. Ann. Rev. Psychol. **12**, 363 (1961a).

BEIDLER, L. M.: Taste receptor stimulation. In: Progress in Bioph. bioph. Chem., p. 107 (1961b).

BEIDLER, L. M.: Dynamics of taste cells. In: Olfaction and Taste, I, p. 133. Oxford, Paris: Pergamon Press 1963.

BEIDLER, L. M.: The mechanism of the stimulation of gustatory and olfactory receptors. In: Teoriya svyazi v sensornykh sistemakh (Theory of Communication in Sensory Systems), p. 114. Moscow: Izd. Mir. 1964.

BEIDLER, L. M.: Comparison of gustatory receptors, olfactory receptors and free nerve endings. In: Cold Spr. Harb. Symp. quant. Biol. **30**, 191 (1965).

BEIDLER, L. M.: A physiological basis of taste sensation. J. Food Sci. **31**, 275 (1965).

BEIDLER, L. M.: Anion influences on taste receptor response. In: Olfaction and Taste, II, p. 509. Procced. Sec. Int. Sympos., Tokio 1965. Oxford: Pergamon Press 1965.

VON BÉKÉSY, G.: Variation of phase along the basilar membrane with sinusoidal variations. J. acoust. Soc. Amer. **19**, 452 (1947).

VON BÉKÉSY, G.: Elasticity of the cochlear partition. J. acoust. Soc. Amer. **20**, 227 (1948).

VON BÉKÉSY, G.: Resonance curve and decay period at various points on the cochlear partition. J. acoust. Soc. Amer. **21**, 245 (1949a).

VON BÉKÉSY, G.: Vibration of the cochlear partition in anatomical preparation and in models of the inner ear. J. acoust. Soc. Amer. **21**, 233 (1949b).

VON BÉKÉSY, G.: Coarse pattern of electrical resistance in the cochlea of the guinea pig. J. acoust. Soc. Amer. **23**, 18 (1951a).

VON BÉKÉSY, G.: Microphonics produced by touching the cochlear partition with a vibrating electrode. J. acoust. Soc. Amer. **23**, 29 (1951b).

VON BÉKÉSY, G.: DC potentials and energy balance of the cochlear partition. J. acoust. Soc. Amer. **23**, 576 (1951c).

VON BÉKÉSY, G.: Gross localization of place of origin of the cochlear microphonics. J. acoust. Soc. Amer. **24**, 399 (1952a).

VON BÉKÉSY, G.: DC resting potentials inside the cochlear partition. J. acoust. Soc. Amer. **25**, 770 (1952b).

VON BÉKÉSY, G.: Direct observation of the vibrations of the cochlear partition under the microscope. Acta oto-laryng. (Stockh.) **43**, 197 (1952c).

VON BÉKÉSY, G.: Description of some mechanical properties of the organ of Corti. J. acoust. Soc. Amer. **25**, 770 (1953a).

VON BÉKÉSY, G.: Shearing microphonics produced by vibrations near the inner and outer hair cells. J. acoust. Soc. Amer. **25**, 786 (1953b).

VON BÉKÉSY, G.: Some electromechanical properties of the organ of Corti. Ann. Otol. (St. Louis) **13** (2), 448 (1954).

VON BÉKÉSY, G.: Current status of theories of hearing. Science **123**, 779 (1956).

VON BÉKÉSY, G.: Pendulums, travelling waves and the cochlea. Laryngoscope (St. Louis) **68** (3), 317 (1958a).

VON BÉKÉSY, G.: Funnelling in the nervous system and its role in loudness and sensation intensity on the skin. J. acoust. Soc. Amer. **30**, 399 (1958b).

VON BÉKÉSY, G.: Neural funnelling along the skin and between the inner and outer hair cells of the cochlea. J. acoust. Soc. Amer. **31** (9), 1236 (1959).

VON BÉKÉSY, G.: Experiments in Hearing. New York—Toronto—London 1960a.

VON BÉKÉSY, G.: Experimental models of the cochlea with and without nerve supply. In: Neural. Mechanisms of Auditory and Vestibular Systems (Eds. G. L. Rasmussen, W. F. Windle), p. 3. Springfield/Ill.: Ch. C. Thomas 1960b.

VON BÉKÉSY, G.: Sweetness produced electrically on the tongue and its relation to taste theories. J. appl. Physiol. **19**, 1105 (1964).

VON BÉKÉSY, G.: Temperature coefficients of the electrical thresholds of taste sensations. J. gen. Physiol. **49**, 27 (1965).

VON BÉKÉSY, G.: Taste theories and the chemical stimulation of single papillae. J. appl. Physiol. **21**, 1 (1966).

BELANGER, L. F.: Autoradiographic detection of $^{35}$S in the membranes of the inner ear of rat. Science **118**, 520 (1953).

BELANGER, L. F.: Observation on the development, structure and composition of the cochlea of the rat. Ann. Otol. (St. Louis) **65**, 1060 (1956).

BENEDETTI, E. L., EMMELOT, P.: Electron microscopic observations on negatively stained plasma membranes isolated from rat liver. J. Cell Biol. **26**, 299 (1967).

BENEDETTI, E. L., EMMELOT, P.: Hexanol array of subunits in tight junctions separated from isolated rat liver plasma membranes. J. Cell Biol **28**, 15 (1968).

BENJAMIN, R. M., HALPERN, B. P., MOULTON, D. G., MOZELL, M. M.: The chemical senses. Ann. Rev. Psychol. **16**, 381 (1965).

BENNET, M. V. L.: Nervous function at the cellular level. Physiol. Rev. **26**, 289 (1964).

BENNET, M. V. L., PAPPAS, G. D., ALJURE, E., NAKAJIMA, Y.: Physiology and ultrastructure of electrotonic junctions: II. Spinal and medullary electromotor nuclei in Mormyrid fish. J. Neurophysiol. **30**, 180 (1967).

BERGER, E. R.: Mitochondria genesis in the retinal photoreceptor inner segment. J. Ultrastruct. Res. **11**, 90 (1964).

BERNAL, G. D.: Molecular structure, biochemical function and evolution. In: Teoreticheskaya i matematicheskaya biologiya (Theoretical and Mathematical Biology), p. 110. Moscow: Izd. Mir 1968.

BERTRAND, R., VEENHOF, V.: Efferent vestibular potentials by canalicular and otolithic stimulations in the rabbit. Acta oto-laryng. (Stockh.) **58**, 515 (1964).

BEST, T. H., ANSON, B. J., GARDNER, W. G.: The developmental course of the human auditory vesicle. Anat. Rec. **99**, 55 (1947).

BETHE, A.: Versuche an Medusen als Beispiel eines primitiven neuromuskulären Reaktionssystems. Pflügers Arch. ges. Physiol. **235**, 288 (1935).

BIRKS, R., HUXLEY, N. E., KATZ, B.: The fine structure of the neuromuscular junction of the frog. J. Physiol. (Lond.) **150**, 134 (1960).

BIRYUZOVA, V. I., LUKOYANOVA, M. A., GEL'MAN, N. S., OPARIN, A. I.: Subunits in the cytoplasmic membranes of *Micrococcus lysodeicticus*. Dokl. Akad. Nauk SSSR **156**, 198 (1964).

BLASIE, J. K., DEWEY, M. M., BLAUROCK, A. E., WORTHINGTON, C. R.: Electron microscope and low-angle X-ray diffraction studies on outer segmentes membranes from the retina of the frog. J. molec. Biol. **14**, 143 (1965).

BLASIE, J. K., DEWEY, M. M., WORTHINGTON, C. R.: Molecular localization of the photopigment in the outer segment membranes of frog retinal receptors. J. Histochem. Cytochem. **14**, 769 (1966).

BLASIE, J. K., WORTHINGTON, C. R.: Molecular localization of frog retinal receptor photopigment by electron microscopy and low-angle X-ray diffraction. J. molec. Biol. **39**, 339 (1969).

BOCCA, E.: Le développement historique et l'état actuel de nos conaissances sur l'innervation cochléaire. J. franç. Oto-rhino-laryng. **3**, 165 (1954).

BODIAN, D.: Electron microscopy: two major synaptic types on spinal motoneurons. Science **151**, 1093 (1966a).

BODIAN, D.: Synaptic types of spinal motoneurons: an electron microscope study. Bull. Johns Hopk. Hosp. **119**, 16 (1966b).

BOECKH, J.: Elektrophysiologische Untersuchungen an einzelnen Geruchsrezeptoren auf den Antennen des Totengräbers (*Necrophorus*, Coleoptera). Z. vergl. Physiol. **46**, 212 (1962).

BOECKH, J.: Inhibition and excitation of single insect olfactory receptors and their role as a primary sensory code. In: Olfaction and Taste, II, p. 721. Proc. Intern. symp. 2nd., Tokyo 1967. Oxford: Pergamon Press 1967.

BOETTCHER, A.: Über Entwicklung und Bau des Gehörlabyrinths nach Untersuchungen an Säugetieren. Dresden 1869.

BOLL, F.: Zur Anatomie und Physiologie der Retina. Arch. Anat. Physiol. 4 (1877).

BOLL, F.: Thesen und Hypothesen zur Licht- und Farbenempfindung. Arch. Anat. Physiol. 1 (1881); Klin. Mbl. Augenheilk. **19**, 287 (1881).

BONTING, S. L., BANGHAM, A. D.: On the biochemical mechanism of the visual process. Exp. Eye Res. **6**, 400 (1967).

BONTING, S. L., CARAVAGGIO, L. L.: Rhodopsin: An enzyme? Invest. Ophthal. **2**, 520 (1963).

BONTING, S. L., CARAVAGGIO, L. L., CANNADY, M. R.: Studies on sodium-potassium activated adenosinetriphosphatases. Exp. Eye Res. **3**, 47 (1964).

BONTING, S. L., CARAVAGGIO, L. L., GOURAS, P.: The rhodopsin cycle in the developing vertebrate retina. I. Relation of rhodopsin content, electroretinogram and rod structure in the rat. Exp. Eye Res. **1**, 14 (1963).

BONTING, S. L., CARAVAGGIO, L. L., HAWKINS, N. M.: Studies on sodium-potassium activated adenosinetriphosphatase. IV. Correlation with cation transport sensitive to cardiac glycosides. Arch. Biochem. **98**, 413 (1962).

BONTING, S. L., DE PONT, J. J. H. H. M.: Schiff bases of retinaldehyde as a substrate for retinal dehydrogenase. Exp. Eye Res. **8**, 251 (1969).

BOORD, L.: The efferent cochlear bundle in the caiman and pigeon. Exp. Neurol. **3**, 225 (1961).

BOROVYAGIN, V. L.: Electron microscopic study of cones in the frog retina. Biofizika **7**, 154 (1962a).

BOROVYAGIN, V. L.: Submicroscopic structure of rods in the frog retina. Biofizika **7**, 734 (1962b).

BOROVYAGIN, V. L.: Submicroscopic morphology and structural relationship of receptor and horizontal cells of the retina. Biofizika **11**, 810 (1966).

BORTOFF, A., NORTON, A. L.: Positive and negative potential responses associated with vertebrate photoreceptor cells. Nature **206**, 626 (1965a).

BORTOFF, A., NORTON, A. L.: Simultaneous recording of photoreceptor potential and the PIII component of the ERG. Vision Res. **5**, 527 (1965b).

BOTEZAT, E.: Die sensiblen Nervenendapparate in den Hornpapillen der Vögel im Zusammenhang mit Studien zur vergleichenden Morphologie und Physiologie der Sinnesorgane. Anat. Anz. **34**, 449 (1909).

BOURNE, G. H.: Alkaline phosphatase in taste buds and nasal mucosa. Nature **161**, 445 (1948).

BOVEE, E. C., JAHN, T. L., FONSECA, J., LANDMAN, M.: Flagellar movements in some species of Mostigamebas. In: Abstr. 7th Ann. Meeting Biophys. Soc., MD 2.

BOWNDS, D., GAIDE-HUGUENIN, A. C.: Rhodopsin content of frog photoreceptor outer segments. Nature **225**, 870 (1970).

BOWNDS, D., WALD, G.: Reaction of the rhodopsin chromophore with sodium borohydrate. Nature **205**, 254 (1965).

BOYCOTT, B. B.: The functioning of the statocysts of *Octopus vulgaris*. Proc. roy. Soc. B **152**, 78 (1960).

BOYD, C. A. R., PORSONS, D. S.: The fine structure of the microvilli of isolated brush borders of intestinal epithelial cells. J. Cell Biol. **41**, 646 (1969).

BOZLER, E.: Sinnes- und nervenphysiologische Untersuchungen an Scyphomedusen. Z. vergl. Physiol. **4**, 37 (1926).

BRADLEY, R. M., STERN, J. B.: The development of the human taste bud during the fetal period. J. Anat. (Lond.) **101**, 743 (1967).

BRANTON, D.: Fracture faces of frozen membranes. Proc. nat. Acad. Sci. (Wash.) **55**, 1048 (1966).

BRANTON, D.: Fracture faces of frozen myelin. Exp. Cell. Res. **45**, 703 (1967).

BRAUN, J. V., KRÖPER, H., WIENHAUS, H.: Geruch und Konstitution. Ber. Dtsch. chem. Ges. **62**, 2880 (1929).

BREDBERG, G., LINDEMAN, H. H., ADES, H. W., WEST, R., ENGSTROM, H.: Scanning electron microscopy of the organ of Corti. Science **170**, 861 (1970).

VAN BREEMEN, V. L., ANDERSON, E., REGER, J. F.: An attempt to determine the origin of synaptic vesicles. Exp. Cell. Res., Suppl. **5**, 153 (1958).

BRESTKIN, M. P., LEBEDINSKII, A. V., ORBELI, L. A., STREL'TSOV, V. V.: On the mechanism of death of animals during electric trauma depending upon different directions through the organism. Fiziol. Zh. SSSR **15**, 542 (1932).

BRIDGES, C. D. B.: Study on the flash photolysis of visual pigments. 3. Interpretation of the slow thermal reactions following flash irradiation of frog rhodopsin solutions. Vision Res. **2**, 201 (1962).

BRIGGS, M. M.: Retinen-I in insect tissues. Nature **192**, 874 (1961).

BRIGGS, M. M., DUNCAN, R. B.: Odour receptors. Nature **191**, 1310 (1961).

BRIGGS, M. M., DUNCAN, R. B.: Pigment and the olfactory mechanism. Nature **195**, 1313 (1962).

BRODSKII, V. YA.: DNA and nuclear structures of ganglion cells of the retina during the synthesis of ribonucleic acid in the cytoplasm and nucleus. Dokl. Akad. Nauk SSSR **129**, 1409 (1959).

BRODSKII, V. YA.: Trofika kletki (The Trophic System of Cells). Moscow: Izd. Nauka 1966.

BRONSHTEIN, A. A.: Intra-vital observations of the movement of hairs of olfactory cells. Dokl. Akad. Nauk SSSR **156**, 715 (1964).

BRONSHTEIN, A. A.: Histochemistry of the olfactory organ. Arkh. Anat. Gistol. Embriol. **48**, 106 (1965).

BRONSHTEIN, A. A.: Some data on the fine structure and cytochemistry of olfactory receptors. In the collection of works (Sbornik): Pervichnye protsessy v retseptornykh elementakh organov chuvstv (Primary Processes in the Receptor Elements of Sense Organs), p. 65. Moscow—Leningrad: izd. Nauka 1966.

BRONSHTEIN, A. A., IVANOV, V. P.: Electron microscopic study of the olfactory organ of the lamprey. Zh. evolyuts. biokhim. fiziol. **1**, 251 (1965).

BRONSHTEIN, A. A., LEONT'EV, V. G.: The content of sodium and potassium in the mucus covering the olfactory mucose in vertebrates. Zh. evolyuts. biokhim. fiziol. **8**, 580 (1972).

BRONSHTEIN, A. A., PYATKINA, G. A.: Ultrastructural organization of the hairs of olfactory cells in bony fish. Tsitologiya **8**, 642 (1966).

BRONSHTEIN, A. A., PYATKINA, G. A.: Ultrastructural organization of the olfactory organ in the steppe turtle *Testudo horsfieldi*. Zh. evolyuts. biokhim. fiziol. **4**, 419 (1968).

BRONSHTEIN, A. A., PYATKINA, G. A.: Electron microscopic study of the location of sodium ions in the olfactory organ of the frog *Rana temporaria*. Zh. evolyuts. biokhim. fiziol. **5**, 274 (1969a).

BRONSHTEIN, A. A., PYATKINA, G. A.: Ultrastructural organization of the olfactory organ of birds. In: Tezisy VII Vsesoyuzn. konf. po elektronnoi mikroskopii (Reports of the VII All-Union Conference on Electron Microscopy), p. 130. Moscow 1969b.

BRONSHTEIN, A. I.: Vkus i obonyanie (Taste and Smell). Moscow—Leningrad: Izd. Akad. Nauk SSSR 1950.

BROWN, K. T., MURAKAMI, M.: A new receptor potential of the monkey retina with no detectable latency. Nature **201**, 626 (1964a).

BROWN, K. T., MURAKAMI, M.: Biphasic form of the early receptor potential of the monkey retina. Nature **204**, 739 (1964b).

BROWN, K. T., WATANABE, K., MURAKAMI, M.: The early and late receptor potential of monkey cones and rods. Cold. Spr. Harb. Symp. quant. Biol. **30**, 457 (1965).

BROWN, N. P.: On the structure and mechanics of protozoan flagellum. Ohio J. Sci. **34**, 247 (1945).

BROWN, P. K., GIBBONS, J. R., WALD, G.: The visual pigments of the mudpuppi, *Necturus*. J. Cell Biol. **19**, 79 (1963).

BROWN, P. K., WALD, G.: Visual pigments in human and monkey retinas. Nature **200**, 37 (1963).

BROWN, P. K., WALD, G.: Visual pigments in single rods and cones of the human retina. Science **144**, 45 (1964).

VON BRÜCKE, H., HELLAUER, H. F., UMRATH, K.: Sur la nature cholinergique des bourgeons gustatifs de la papille foliée du lapin. Arch. int. Physiol. **55**, 362 (1948).

VON BUDDENBROCK, W.: Über die Funktion der Statozysten im Sande grabender Meerestiere (*Arenicola* und *Synapta*). Biol. Zbl. **32**, 564 (1912).

VON BUDDENBROCK, W.: Die Statozysten von *Pecten*, ihre Histologie und Physiologie. Zool. Jahrb., Abt. allg. Zool. **35**, 301 (1915).

VON BUDDENBROCK, W.: Vergleichende Physiologie: I. Sinnesphysiologie. Basel: Birkhäuser 1952.

BUDELMANN, B.-U.: Die Arbeitsweise der Statolithenorgane von *Octopus vulgaris*. Z. vergl. Physiol. **70**, 278 (1970a).

BUDELMANN, B.-U.: Untersuchungen zur Funktion der Statolithenorgane von *Octopus vulgaris*. Ver. Dtsch. Zool. Ges. (Köln) **65**, 256 (1970b).

BULLOCK, T. H.: Functional organizations of the giant fiber system of *Lumbriculus*. J. Neurophysiol. **8**, 55 (1945).

BULLOCK, T. H.: Formation of nerve impulses in receptor and central neurons. Sovr. Probl. Biofiziki (Contemporary Problems in Biophysics) **2**, 248 (1961).

BULLOCK, T. H., HORRIDGE, G. A.: Structure and Function of the Nervous Systems of Invertebrates, Vol. I and II. San Francisco and London: Freeman 1965.

BURGEN, A. S. V., SHIPMAN, L. M.: Cholinesterase and succinic dehydrogenase in the central nervous system of the dog. J. Physiol. (Lond.) **114**, 296 (1951).

BÜRGER, O.: Fauna und Flora des Golfes von Neapel und der angrenzenden Meeres Abschnitte. Herausgegeben von der Zoologischen Station zu Neapel. Berlin 1895.

BURKHARDT, D.: Spectral sensitivity and other response characteristics of single visual cells in the arthropod eye. Symp. Soc. exp. Biol. **16**, 86 (1962).

BURKHARDT, D., AUTRUM, H.: Die Belichtungspotentiale einzelner Sehzellen von *Calliphora erythrocephala* Meig. Z. Naturforsch. **156**, 612 (1960).

BURKHARDT, D., WENDLER, L.: Ein direkter Beweis für die Fähigkeit einzelner Sehzellen des Insektenauges, die Schwingungsrichtung polarisierten Lichtes zu analysieren. Z. vergl. Physiol. **43**, 687 (1960).

DE BURLET, H. M.: Vergleichende Anatomie des stato-akustischen Organs. a) Die innere Ohrsphäre. In: Handbuch der vergleichenden Anatomie der Wirbeltiere (Bolk, Göppert, Kallius), S. 1293. Berlin: Springer 1934.

BURNASHEVA, S. A., EFREMENKO, M. V., LYUBIMOVA, M. I.: Study of adenosine triphosphatases or of the activity of isolated cilia in *Tetrahymena pyriformis* infusorians and the secretion of adenosine triphosphatase from these cilia. Biokhimiya **28**, 547 (1963).

BURNASHEVA, S. A., RASKIDNAYA, N. V.: Characteristics of ATPase in the cilia of *Tetrahymena pyriformis*. Dokl. Akad. Nauk SSSR **179**, 719 (1968).

BUVAT, R.: Electron microscopy of plant protoplasm. Internat. Rev. Cytol. **14**, 41 (1963).

BYSTROV, A. P.: The Past, Present and Future of Man. (Proshedshee, nastoyashchee i budushchee cheloveka) Leningrad: Medgiz 1957.

BYZOV, A. L.: Elektrofiziologicheskie issledovaniya setchatki (Electrophysiological Studies of the Retina). Moscow: Izd. Nauka 1966.

BYZOV, A. L., ORLOV, O. Yu.: Sources of the electroretinogram of cephalopods. Fiziol. Zh. SSSR **48**, 16 (1962).

CAGAN, R. H.: Biochemical studies of taste sensation. I Binding of C-labeled sugars to bovine taste papillae. Biochim. biophys. Acta (Amst.) **252**, 199 (1971).

CARASSO, N.: Etude au microscope électronique de la morphogénèse du segment externe des cellules visuelles chez le Pleurodèle. C. R. Acad. Sci. (Paris) **248**, 3058 (1959).

CARASSO, N.: Rôle de l'ergastoplasme dans l'élaboration du glycogène au cours de la formation du "paraboloïde" des cellules visuelles. C. R. Acad. Sci. (Paris) **250**, 600 (1960).

CARLSON, S. D., GEMNE, G., VAN DE BERG, J. S., ROBBINS, W. E.: Ultrastructure of retinular cells in normal and vitamin-A deficient tobacco moth *(Manduca sexta)*. In: XIII Int. Congress of Entomology, Moscow 1968.

CARLSON, S. D., STEEVES, H. R., VAN DE BERG, J. S., ROBBINS, W. E.: Vitamin-A deficiency: effect on retinal structure of the moth *Manduca sexta*. Science **158**, 268 (1967).

CARPENTER, M. B.: Experimental anatomical-physiological studies of the vestibular nerve and cerebellar connections. In: Neural Mechanisms of Auditory and Vestibular Systems (Eds. G. L. Rasmussen, W. F. Windle), p. 297. Springfield/Ill.: Ch. C. Thomas 1960.

DEL CASTILLO, J., KATZ, B.: Localization of active spots within the neuromuscular junction of the frog. J. Physiol. (London) **132**, 630 (1956).

CAVALLITO, C. J.: Structure-action relations throwing light on the receptor. In: Curare and Curare-like Agents (De Reuck, A. V. S., Ed.), p. 55. London: Churchill 1962.

CHAMBERS, L. A., FLOSDORF, H. V.: The denaturation of protein of sound nerves by audible frequencies. J. biol. Chem. **114**, 75 (1936).

CHEREPNOV, V. L.: The ultrastructure of the inner bulb of Pacinian bodies. Zh. evolyuts. biokhim. fiziol. **4**, 91 (1968).

CHERNIGOVSKII, V. N.: Interoretseptory (Interoreceptors). Leningrad: Medgiz 1960.

CHERNIGOVSKII, V. N.: Neirofiziologicheskii analiz kortikovistseral'noi reflektornoi dugi (Predstavitel'stvo vnutrennikh organov v kore golovnogo mozga) (Neurophysiological Analysis of the Corticovisceral Reflex Arc: Representation of Inner Organs in the Brain Cortex). Leningrad: Izd. Nauka 1967.

CHERNIGOVSKII, V. N., MASHANSKII, V. F., MIRKIN, A. S.: On the possible mechanism of Pacinian bodies excitation. Izv. Akad. Nauk SSSR (ser. biol.) **2**, 214 (1970).

CHILD, C. M.: Beiträge zur Kenntnis der antennalen Sinnesorgane der Insekten. Z. wiss. Zool. **58**, 475 (1894).

CHILD, C. M.: The swimming plate rows of the ctenophore, *Pleurobrachia*, as gradients: with comparative data on the other forms. J. comp. Neurol. **57**, 199 (1933).

CHRISTIANSEN, J. A.: Verschiebungspotentiale als Biegungspotentiale fadenartiger Polyelectrolyte aufgefaßt. Z. Elektrochem. **66**, 2 (1962).

CHRISTIANSEN, J. A.: On hyaluronate molecules in the labyrinth as mechanoelectrical transducers, and as molecular motors acting as resonators. Acta oto-laryng. (Stockh.) **57**, 33 (1964).

CHUN, C.: Die Ctenophoren des Golfes von Neapel und der angrenzenden Meer-Abschnitte. Leipzig: Engelmann 1880.

CHUN, C.: Die Cephalopoden, Oegopsida. Wiss. Ergebn. Valdivia, p. 18 (1910).

CHURCHILL, J. A., SCHUKNECHT, H. E., DORAN, R.: Acetylcholinesterase activity in the cochlea. Laryngoscope (St. Louis), **66**, 1 (1956).

CLAUDIUS, M.: Bemerkungen über den Bau der häutigen Spiralleiste der Schnecke. Z. wiss. Zool. **8**, 154 (1885).

COGAN, D., KUWABARA, T.: Tetrazolium studies on the retina. II. Substrate dependent patterns. J. Histochem. Cytochem. **7**, 334 (1959).

COGGESHALL, R. E.: A fine structural analysis of the statocyst in *Aplysia californica*. J. Morph. **127**, 113 (1969).

COHEN, M. J.: Oscillographic analysis of an invertebrate equilibrium organ. Biol. Bull. **105**, 363 (1953).

COHEN, M. J.: The function of receptors in the statocyst of the lobster *Homarus americanus*. J. Physiol. (Lond.) **130**, 9 (1955).

COHEN, M. J.: The response patterns of single receptors in the crustacean statocyst. Proc. roy. Soc. B **152**, 30 (1960).

COHEN, M. J.: The peripheral organization of sensory systems. In: R. F. Reiss (Ed.): Neural Theory and Modelling, p. 273. Stanford: Univ. Press 1964.

COHEN, M. J., DIJKGRAAF, S.: Mechanoreception. In: The Physiology of Crustacea (Ed. T. H. Waterman), Vol. 2, p. 65. New York: Academic Press 1961.

COHEN, M. J., KATSUKI, Y., BULLOCK, T.: Oscillographic analysis of equilibrium receptors in crustacea. Experientia (Basel) **9**, 434 (1953).

COHEN, A. I.: The ultrastructure of rods of the mouse retina. Amer. J. Anat. **107**, 23 (1960).

COHEN, A. I.: Some preliminary electron microscopic observations of the receptor outer segments of the retina of *Macaca rhesus*. In: Structure of the Eye, p. 151. New York: Academic Press 1961a.

COHEN, A. I.: The fine structure of extrafoveal receptors of the rhesus monkey. Exp. Eye Res. **1**, 128 (1961b).

COHEN, A. I.: The fine structure of the visual receptors of the pigeon. Exp. Eye Res. **2**, 88 (1963a).

COHEN, A. I.: Vertebrate retinal cells and their organization. Biol. Rev. **38**, 427 (1963b).

COLLINS, F. D.: Rhodopsin and indicator yellow. Nature **171**, 469 (1953).

COLLINS, F. D., LOVE, R. M., MORTON, R. A.: Studies in rhodopsin. 5. Chemical analysis of retinal material. Biochem. J. **51**, 669 (1952).

COLWIN, A. L., COLWIN, L. H.: Role of the gamete membranes in fertilization. In: Cellular Membranes in Development (Ed. M. Looke), p. 233. New York: Academic Press 1964.

CONE, R. A.: Early receptor potential of the vertebrate retina. Nature **204**, 736 (1964).

CONE, R. A.: The early receptor potential of the vertebrate eye. Cold Spr. Harb. Symp. quant. Biol. **30**, 483 (1965).

CORNFIELD, B. R.: Coordination and movement of the swimming plates of *Mnemiopsis leidyi* Aggasiz. Biol. Bull. Woods Hole **66**, 10 (1934).

CONGER, A. D., WELLS, M. A.: Radiation and aging: effect on taste structure and function. Radiat. Res. **37**, 31 (1969).

CORDIER, R.: Sur la double innervation des cellules sensorielles dans l'organe de Corti du pigeon. C. R. Acad. Sci. (Paris) **258**, 6238 (1964).

CORTI, A.: Recherches sur l'organe de l'ouie des mammifères. I Partie. Limaçon. Z. wiss. Zool. **3**, 106 (1851).

COSHLAND, D.: Catalysis in living nature and in the test tube. In the collection of works (Sbornik): Gorizonty biokhimii (Horizons of Biochemistry), p. 202. Moscow: Izd. Mir 1964.

COULOMBRE, A.: Cytology of the developing eye. Internat. Rev. Cytol. **4**, 161 (1961).

COUTEAUX, R.: Morphological and cytochemical observations on the postsynaptic membrane of motor endplates and ganglionic synapses. Exp. Cell Res. Suppl. **5**, 294 (1958).

COUTEAUX, R., TAXI, J.: Recherches sur la distribution des activités cholinestérasiques au niveau de la synapse myonévrale. Arch. Anat. micr. Morph. exp. **41**, 352 (1952).

CRICK, F.: Protein synthesis. In: Biological Reproduction of Molecules (V. L. Ryzhkov, Ed.), p. 209. Inostrannaya Literatura 1960.

CUNNINGHAM, W. R., CRANE, F.: Variation in membrane structure as revealed by negative staining technique. Exp. Cell. Res. **44**, 31 (1966).

DACHA, U., MARTINI, R.: Il riflesso di Tullio nei piccioni constimolazioni sonara di diversa altessa. Boll. Soc. ital. Biol. sper. **17**, 331 (1942).

DAEMEN, F. J. M., BONTING, S. L.: Biochemical aspects of the visual process. III. Specificity of the retinaldehyde effect on cation movements in rod outer segment. Biochim. biophys. Acta (Amst.) **163**, 212 (1968).

DALTON, A.: Golgi apparatus and secretion granules. In: The Cell, Vol. 2 (Eds. J. Brachet, A. Mirsky), p. 603. New York: Academic Press 1961.

DANEEL, R., ZEUTZSCHEL, B.: Über den Feinbau der Retina bei Drosophila melanogaster. Z. Naturforsch. **12**, B, 580 (1957).

DANIELLI, J. F., DAVSON, H. A.: A contribution to the theory of permeability of thin films. J. cell. comp. Physiol. **5**, 495 (1935).

DARTNALL, H. J. A.: The interpretation of spectral sensitivity curves. Brit. med. Bull. **9**, 24 (1953).

DARTNALL, H. J. A.: The Visual Pigments. New York: Wiley 1957.

DARTNALL, H. J. A., LYTHGOE, J. H.: The spectral clustering of visual pigments. Vision Res. **5**, 81 (1964).

DASTOLI, F. R., LOPIEKES, D., DOIG, A.: Bitter-sensitive protein from porcine taste buds. Nature **218**, 884 (1968).

DASTOLI, F. R., LOPIEKES, D., PRICE, S.: A sweet-sensitive protein from bovine taste buds. Purification and partial characterization. Biochemistry **7**, 1160 (1968).

DASTOLI, F. R., PRICE, S.: Sweet-sensitive protein from bovine taste buds: isolation and assay. Science **154**, 905 (1966).

DAVIES, J. T.: The mechanism of olfaction. In: Biological Receptor Mechanisms, p. 170. Cambridge: Univ. Press 1962.

DAVIES, J. T.: A theory of the quality of odours. J. theor. Biol. **1**, 7 (1962).

DAVIES, J. T., TAYLOR, F. H.: Molecular shape, size and adsorption in olfaction. In: Proc. 2nd Internat. Congr. Surface Activity, p. 329. London 4, 1957.

DAVIES, J. T., TAYLOR, F. H.: The role of adsorption and molecular morphology in olfaction: the calculation of olfactory threshold. Biol. Bull. **117**, 222 (1959).

DAVIES, D. D., GIOVANELLI, I., REES, T. A. P.: Plant Biochemistry. Oxford: Blackwell 1964.

DAVIS, H.: Energy into nerve impulses: hearing. Med. Bull. St. Louis. Univ. **5**, 43 (1953).

DAVIS, H.: The excitation of nerve impulses in the cochlea. Ann. Otol. (St. Louis) **63**, 469 (1954).

DAVIS, H.: Biophysics and physiology of the inner ear. Physiol. Rev. **37**, 1 (1957).

DAVIS, H.: A mechano-electrical theory of cochlear action. Ann. Otol. (St. Louis) **67**, 3 (1958).

DAVIS, H.: Mechanism of excitation of auditory nerve impulses. In: Neural Mechanisms of Auditory and Vestibular Systems (Eds. G. L. Rasmussen, W. F. Windle), p. 21. Springfield/Ill.: Ch. C. Thomas 1960.

DAVIS, H.: Some principles of sensory receptor action. Physiol. Rev. **41**, 391 (1961).

DAVIS, H.: Foreword to the English edition of the book: Organ of Corti, its Histophysiology and Histochemistry by Ya. A. Vinnikov and L. K. Titova. New York: Consultants Bureau 1964.

DAVIS, H.: A model for transducer action in the cochlea. Cold Spr. Harb. Symp. quant. Biol. **30**, 181 (1965).

DAVIS, H.: Biochemical mechanisms in hearing and deafness. Res. Otol. Internat. Symp. (Ed. M. M. Paparella), p. 361. Springfield/Ill.: Ch. C. Thomas 1970.

DAVIS, H., DEATHERAGE, B. H., ELDREDGE, D. H., SMITH, C. A.: Summating potentials of the cochlea. Amer. J. Physiol. **195**, 251 (1958).

DAVIS, H., DERBYSHIRE, A. J., LURIE, M. H., SAUL, L. J.: The electric response of the cochlea. Amer. J. Physiol. **107**, 311 (1934).

DAVIS, H., ELDREDGE, D. H.: An interpretation of the mechanical detector action of the cochlea. Ann. Otol. (St. Louis) **68**, 665 (1959).

DAVIS, H., FERNANDEZ, C., MCAULIFFE, D. R.: The excitatory process in the cochlea. Proc. nat. Acad. Sci. (Wash.) **36**, 580 (1950).

DAVIS, H., TASAKI, J., GOLDSTEIN, R.: The peripheral origin of activity with reference to the ear. Cold Spr. Harb. Symp. quant. Biol. **17**, 143 (1952).

DAVIS, H., TASAKI, J., SMITH, C. A., DEATHERAGE, G. H.: Cochlear potentials after intracochlear injection and anoxia. Fed. Proc. **14**, 112 (A) (1955).

DAVIS, M. E., POTTER, E. L.: Intrauterine respiration of the human fetus. J. Amer. med. Ass. **131**, 1194 (1946).

DAVSON, H., DANIELLI, I. F.: Permeability of Natural Membranes. New York: Macmillan 1943.

DEL BO, M., CONTI, A.: Distributione dell' acetilcolinesterasi nella lamina spirale della coclea di cavia. Arch. ital. Otol. **72**, 44 (1961).

DERBYSHIRE, A. J., DAVIS, H.: Probable mechanism for stimulation of the auditory nerve by the organ of Corti. Amer. J. Physiol. **113**, 35 (1935a).

DERBYSHIRE, A. J., DAVIS, H.: Action potential of the auditory nerve. Amer. J. Physiol. **113**, 476 (1935b).

DESMEDT, J. E.: Neurophysiological mechanisms controlling acoustic input. In: Neural Mechanisms of Auditory and Vestibular Systems (Eds. G. L. Rasmussen, W. F. Windle), p. 152. Springfield/Ill.: Ch. C. Thomas 1960.

DETHIER, V. G.: The physiology and histology of the contact chemoreceptors of the blowfly. Quart. Rev. Biol. **30**, 348 (1960).

DETHIER, V. G.: The Physiology of Insect Senses. London and New York 1963.

DETHIER, V. G., HANSON, F. E.: Taste papillae of the blowfly. J. cell. comp. Physiol. **65**, 93 (1965).

DETHIER, V. G., LARSEN, J. R., ADAMS, J. R.: The fine structure of the olfactory receptors of the blowfly. In: Olfaction and Taste, I, p. 105. Oxford, Stockholm: Pergamon Press 1963.

DETHIER, V. G., WOLBARSHT, M. L.: The electron-microscopy of chemosensory hairs. Experientia (Basel) **12**, 335 (1956).

DETWILLER, S. R.: Vertebrate Photoreceptors. New York: Macmillan 1943.

DEWEY, M. M., DAVIS, P. K., BLASIE, J. K.: Immunofluorescent localization of rhodopsin in the retina of the frog. J. Histochem. Cytochem. **14**, 789 (1966).

DEWEY, M. M., DAVIS, P. K., BLASIE, J. K., BARR, L.: Localization of rhodopsin antibody in the retina of the frog. J. molec. Biol. **39**, 395 (1969).

DIAMANT, H., FUNAKOSHI, M., STRÖM, L., ZOTTERMAN, Y.: Electrophysiological studies on human taste nerves. In: Olfaction and Taste, I, p. 193. Oxford, New York, Paris: Pergamon Press 1963.

DIAMANT, H., OAKLEY, B., STRÖM, L., WELLS, C., ZOTTERMAN, Y.: A comparison of neural and psychophysical responses to taste stimuli in man. Acta physiol. scand. **64**, 67 (1965).

DIJKGRAAF, S.: The supposed use of the lateral line as an organ of hearing in fish. Experientia (Basel) **10**, 586 (1954).

DIJKGRAAF, S.: The statocyst of *Octopus vulgaris* as a rotation receptor. Publicazioni della stazione Zool. de Napoli, **32**, 64 (1961).

DIJKGRAAF, S.: Nystagmus and related phenomena in *Sepia officinalis*. Experientia (Basel) **19**, 29 (1963a).

DIJKGRAAF, S.: Versuche über Schallwahrnehmung bei Tintenfischen. Naturwissenschaften **50**, 50 (1963b).

DILLY, P.: Studies on the receptors in the cerebral vesicle of the ascidian tadpole. I. The otolith. Quart. J. micr. Sci. **103**, 393 (1962).

DINGLE, J. T., LUCY, J. A.: Vitamin A, carotenoids and cell function. Biol. Rev. **40**, 422 (1965).

DISLER, N. N.: Organy chuvstv sistemy bokovoi linii i ikh znachenie v povedenii ryb (Sense Organs of the Lateral-Line System and Their Significance in the Behavior of Fish), Moscow: Izd. Akad. Nauk SSSR 1960.

DOGIEL, A. S.: Structure of the retina in ganoids, p. 2. Kazansk. Univ.: Trudy Obshch. Estestvoispyt. 1883.

DOGIEL, A. S.: Structure of the olfactory organ in ganoids, teleosts and amphibians, p. 16. Kazansk. Univ.: Trudy Obshch. Estestvoispyt. 1886.

DOGIEL, A. S.: Über das Verhalten der nervösen Elemente in der Retina der Ganoiden, Reptilien, Vögel und Säugetiere. Anat. Anz. **3**, 133 (1888).

DOGIEL, A. S.: Nerve endings in terminal (taste) buds of fish belonging to the sturgeon family. Zap. Akad. Nauk **5**, 31 (1897).

DOGIEL, V. A.: Die sogenannte Konkrementen-Vacuole der Infusorien als eine Statozyste betrachtet. Arch. Protistenk. **58**, 319 (1929).

DOGIEL, V. A.: The Coelenterate Type. Rukovodstvo po zoologii (Zoology Handbook), p. 268. Moscow—Leningrad: Biomedgiz. 1937.

DOHLMAN, G. F.: Modern views of vestibular physiology. J. Laryng. **73**, 154 (1959a).

DOHLMAN, G. F.: Modern concept of vestibular physiology. Laryngoscope (St. Louis) **69**, 865 (1959b).

DOHLMAN, G. F.: Histochemical studies of vestibular mechanisms. In: Neural Mechanisms of Auditory and Vestibular Systems (Eds. G. H. Rasmussen, W. F. Windle), p. 258. Springfield/Ill.: Ch. C. Thomas 1960a.

DOHLMAN, G. F.: Some aspects of the mechanism of vestibular hair cell stimulation. Confin. neurol. (Basel) **20**, 169 (1960b).

DOHLMAN, G. F.: Mechanismus der Haarzellenerregung. Acta oto-laryng. (Stockh.) **51**, 439 (1960c).

DOHLMAN, G. F., FARKASHIDY, I., SALONNA, F.: Centrifugal nervefibers to the sensory epithelium of the vestibular labyrinth. J. Laryng. **72**, 984 (1958).

DOHLMAN, G. F., ORMEROD, F. C., McLAY, K.: The secretory epithelium of the internal ear. Acta oto-laryng. (Stockh.) **50**, 243 (1959).

DOHLMAN, G. F., ORMEROD, F. C.: The secretion and absorption of endolymph. Acta oto-laryng. (Stockh.) **51**, 435 (1960).

DOLL, W., BOURNOT, K.: The odour of optical antipodes. Pharmazie **4**, 224 (1949).

DOOLITTLE, R. E., BEROZA, M., KEISER, J., SCHNEIDER, E. L.: Deuterization of the melon fly attractant, cue-lure, and its effect on olfactory response and infrared adsorption. J. Insect Physiol. **14**, 1697 (1968).

DOWLING, J. E., BOYCOTT, B. B.: Organization of the primate retina: electron microscopy. Proc. roy. Soc. B **166**, 80 (1966).

DOWLING, J. E., GIBBONS, I. R.: The effect of vitamin A deficiency on the fine structure of the retina. In: The Structure of the Eye, p. 85. New York: Academic Press 1961.

DOWLING, J. E., WALD, G.: Vitamin A deficiency and night blindness. Proc. nat. Acad. Sci. (Wash.) **44**, 648 (1958).

DOWLING, J. E., WALD, G.: The biological function of vitamin A acid. Proc. nat. Acad. Sci. (Wash.) **46**, 587 (1960).

DRAVNIEKS, A.: Possible mechanisms of olfaction. Nature **194**, 245 (1962).

DRAVNIEKS, A.: Properties of receptors through molecular parameters of odorivectors. In: Olfaction and Taste. (Ed. T. Hayashi), II, p. 89. Oxford, New York: Pergamon Press 1967.

DROZ, B.: Synthesis and migration of proteins in the visual cells of rats and mice. Anat. Rec. **139**, 222 (1961).

DROZ, B.: Dynamic condition of proteins in the visual cells of rats and mice as shown by radioautography with labelled amino acids. Anat. Rec. **154**, 157 (1963).

DUNCAN, C. J.: The molecular properties and evolution of excitable cells. Oxford: Pergamon Press 1967.

DUNCAN, R. B., BRIGGS, M. H.: Treatment of uncomplicated anosmia by vitamin A. Arch. Otolaryng. **75**, 116 (1962).

DUVAL, A., FLOCK, A., WERSÄLL, J.: The ultrastructure of the sensory hairs and associated organelles of the cochlear inner hair cell, with reference to directional sensitivity. J. Cell Biol. **29**, 497 (1966).

DYACHKOVA, L. N., KHAMORI, A.: Electron microscopic study of the ontogenesis of synapses in the ciliary ganglion of the chick. Tsitologiya **9**, 21 (1967).

DYSON, G. M.: Influence of chemical constitution on the odour of the mustard oils. Perf. Essent. Oil Record **17**, 20 (1926).

DYSON, G. M.: Odour and constitution among the mustard oils. I. The influence of alkyl groups. Perf. Essent. Oil Record **19**, 3 (1928a).

DYSON, G. M.: Odour and constitution among the mustard oils. II. The effect of halogen substitutents. Perf. Essent. Oil Record. **19**, 88 (1928b).

DYSON, G. M.: Odour and constitution among the mustard oils. VI. Natural mustard oils. Perf. Essent. Oil Record. **20**, 42 (1929).

DYSON, G. M.: Odour and constitution among the mustard oils. VII. Reactivity and odour. Perf. Essent. Oil Record **22**, 278 (1931).

DYSON, G. M.: Scientific basis of odours. Chemistry and Industry **57**, 647 (1938).

EAKIN, R. M.: Lines of evolution of photoreceptors. J. gen. Physiol. **46**, 357 (1962).

EAKIN, R. M.: Lines of evolution of photoreceptors. In: General Physiology of Cell Spezialization, Vol. 21 (Eds. D. Mazia, A. Tyler), p. 393. New York: McGraw-Hill 1963.

EAKIN, R. M.: The effect of vitamin-A deficiency on photoreceptors in the lizard *Sceloporus occidentalis*. Vision Res. **4**, 17 (1964).

EAKIN, R. M.: Evolution of Photoreceptors. Cold Spr. Harb. Symp. quant. Biol. **30**, 363 (1965).

EAKIN, R. M.: Evolution of photoreceptors. In: Evolutionary Biology, Vol. 2 (Eds. Th. Dobzhansky, M. K. Heht, C. Steere), p. 194. New York: Appelton-Century Croft 1968.

EAKIN, R. M., BRANDENBURGER, J. L.: Localization of vitamin A in the eye of a pulmonate snail. Proc. nat. Acad. Sci. (Wash.) **60**, 140 (1968).

EAKIN, R. M., KUDA, A.: Ultrastructure of sensory receptors in ascidian tadpoles. Z. Zellf. **112**, 287 (1971).

EAKIN, R. M., WESTFALL, J. A.: Fine structure of photoreceptors in *Amphioxus*. J. Ultrastruct. Res. **6**, 531 (1962).

EAKIN, R. M., WESTFALL, J. A.: Fine structure of the eye of chaetognath. J. Cell Biol. **21**, 115 (1964).

ECCLES, J. C.: The physiology of synapses. Berlin—Göttingen—Heidelberg—New York: Springer 1964.

ECCLES, J. C.: Fiziologiya sinapsov (Physiology of Synapses) (Ed. P. K. Anokhin). Moscow: Izd. Mir 1966.

EGGERS, F.: Ergebnisse von Untersuchungen am Johnstonschen Organ der Insekten und ihre Bedeutung für die allgemeine Beurteilung der stiftführenden Sinnesorgane. Zool. Anz. **57**, 224 (1923).

EGGERS, F.: Die stiftführenden Sinnesorgane. Zool. Bausteine **2**, 1 (1928).

EGUCHI, E., NAKA, K., KUWABARA, M.: The development of the rhabdom and the appearance of the electrical response in the insect eye. J. gen. Physiol. **46**, 141 (1962).

EGUCHI, E., WATERMAN, T. H.: Changes in retinula fine structure induced in the crab *Libinia* by light and dark adaptation. Z. Zellforsch. **79**, 209 (1967).

EHRENPREIS, S.: Isolation and identification of the acetylcholine receptor protein from electric tissue. Biochim. biophys. Acta (Amst.) **44**, 561 (1960).

EICHNER, D.: Zur Histologie und Topochemie der Netzhaut des Menschen. Z. Zellforsch. **48**, 137 (1958).

EICHNER, D., THEMANN, H.: Zur Frage des Netzhautglykogens beim Meerschweinchen. Z. Zellforsch. **56**, 231 (1962).

EICHNER, D., THEMANN, H.: Zur Frage der Glykogenlokalisation in der Netzhaut der Retina des Huhnes und Goldfisches. Z. Zellforsch. **70**, 330 (1963).

EIMER, T.: Versuche über künstliche Teilbarkeit von *Beroe ovatus*. Angestellt zum Zweck der Kontrolle seiner morphologischen Befunde über das Nervensystem dieses Tieres. Arch. mikr. Anat. **17**, 213 (1880).

EINTHOVEN, W.: Über Vaggusströme. Nach gemeinschaftlich mit A. Flohil und P. J. T. A. Bottaerd angestellten Versuchen. Pflügers Arch. ges. Physiol. **123**, 246 (1908).

ELIZAROV, Yu. A., SINITSYNA, E. E.: Physiological characteristics of chemoreceptor organs of insects. Trudy Vsesoyuzn. entom. obshch., Izd. Nauka (Leningrad) **53**, 274 (1969).

ELLIS, P. A.: Cholinesterase in the mammalian tongue. J. Histochem. Cytochem. **7**, 156 (1959).

EL-RAKHAWY, M. T.: The histochemistry of the lymphatic tissue of the human tongue and its probable function in taste. Acta anat. (Basel) **51**, 259 (1962a).

EL-RAKHAWY, M. T.: Succinic dehydrogenase in the mammalian tongue with special reference to gustatory epithelia. Acta anat. (Basel) **48**, 122 (1962b).

EL-RAKHAWY, M. T.: Alkaline phosphatases in the epithelium of the human tongue and a possible mechanisms of taste. Acta anat. (Basel) **55**, 323 (1963).

EL-RAKHAWY, M. T., BOURNE, G. H.: Cholinesterases in the human tongue. Bibl. anat. (Basel) **2**, 243 (1961).

ENGELHARDT, V. A.: Chemical basis of the locomotor function of cells and tissues. Vestn. Akad. Nauk SSSR **11**, 58 (1957).

ENGELHARDT, V. A.: Transformation of energy in biological systems. Vestn. Akad. Nauk SSSR **5**, 25 (1969).

ENGELHARDT, V. A., LYUBIMOVA, M. N.: Myosin and adenosine triphosphatase. Nature **144**, 663 (1939).

ENGELHARDT, V. A., LYUBIMOVA, M. N.: On the mechanochemistry of muscles. Biokhimiya **7**, 205 (1942).

ENGSTRÖM, H.: Microscopic anatomy of the inner ear. Acta oto-laryng. (Stockh.) **40**, 1 (1951).

ENGSTRÖM, H.: The structure of the basilar membrane. Acta oto-rhino-laryng. belg. **9**, 531 (1955).

ENGSTRÖM, H.: On the double innervation of the sensory epithelia of the inner ear. Acta otolaryng. (Stockh.) **49**, 109 (1958).

ENGSTRÖM, H.: Electron micrographic studies of receptor cells of the organ of Corti. In: Neural Mechanisms in Auditory and Vestibular Systems (Eds. G. L. Rasmussen, W. F. Windle), p. 48. Springfield/Ill.: Ch. C. Thomas 1960a.

ENGSTRÖM, H.: The cortilymph—the third lymph of the inner ear. Acta morphol. neerl.-scand. **3**, 195 (1960b).

ENGSTRÖM, H.: The innervation of the vestibular sensory cells. Acta oto-laryng. (Stockh.), Suppl., **163**, 30 (1961).

ENGSTRÖM, H., ADES, H. W.: Effect of high intensity noise on inner ear sensory epithelia. Acta oto-laryng. (Stockh.), Suppl. **158**, 219 (1960).

ENGSTRÖM, H., ADES, H. W., ANDERSON, A.: Structure Pattern of the Organ of Corti. Uppsala: Almqvist and Wiksell 1966.

ENGSTRÖM, H., ADES, H. W., BREDBERG, G.: Normal structure of the organ of Corti and the effect of noise-induced cochlear damage. Ciba Foundat. Sympos. on Sensation. Hearing Loss (Eds. G. E. W. Wolstenhouse, J. Knight), p. 127. London: Churchill 1970.

ENGSTRÖM, H., ADES, H. W., HAWKINS, J. E., jr.: Structure and function of the sensory hairs of the inner ear. J. acoust. Soc. Amer. **34**, 1356 (1962).

ENGSTRÖM, H., WERSÄLL, J.: Supporting structures and their relations to sensory cells and nerve endings. Acta oto-laryng. (Stockh.) **43**, 325 (1953).

ENGSTRÖM, H., WERSÄLL, J.: Structure and innervation of the inner-ear sensory epithelia. Int. Rev. Cytol. **7**, 535 (1958a).

ENGSTRÖM, H., WERSÄLL, J.: The ultrastructural organization of the organ of Corti and of the vestibular sensory epithelia. Exp. Cell. Res. **5**, 460 (1958b).

ENOCH, J.: The use of tetrazolium to distinguish between retinal receptors exposed and not exposed to light. Invest. Ophthal. **2**, 16 (1963).

ENOCH, J.: Physical properties of the retinal receptor and response of retinal receptors. Psychol. Bull. **61**, 242 (1964).

ERÄNKÖ, O., NIEMI, M., MERENMIES, E.: Histochemical observation on esterase and oxidative enzymes of the retina. In: The Structure of the Eye, p. 159. New York: Academic Press 1961.

ERBENGI, T., FERNER, H.: Histochemische Untersuchungen der Geschmacksknospen des Kaninchens. Z. Zellforsch. **61**, 673 (1964).

ERNST, K. D.: Die Feinstruktur von Riechsensillen auf der Antenne des Aaskäfers *Necrophorus* (Coleoptera). Z. Zellforsch. **94**, 72 (1969).

ERWIN, T., BLOCH, K.: Biosynthesis of unsaturated fatty acids in microorganisms. Science **143**, 1006 (1964).

ESAKOV, A. I.: Some problems concerning the electrophysiology of gustatory receptors. In the collection of works (Sbornik): Pervichnye protsessy v retseptornykh elementakh organov chuvstv (Primary Processes in Receptor Elements of Sense Organs), p. 14. Moscow—Leningrad: Izd. Nauka 1966.

ETINGOF, R. N.: Some problems concerning the biochemistry of light reception. In the collection of works (Sbornik): Pervichnye protsessy v retseptornykh elementakh organov chuvstv (Primary Processes in Receptor Elements of Sense Organs), p. 33. Moscow—Leningrad: Izd. Nauka 1966.

ETINGOF, R. N.: The biochemical bases of light reception. Usp. sovrem. Biol. **64**, 425 (1967).

ETINGOF, R. N., SHUKOLYUKOV, S. A., ZHUCHIKHINA, A. A.: On the lactatedehydrogenase activity of outer segments of the retina and of digitonin extracts of rhodopsin. Dokl. Akad. Nauk SSSR **175**, 234 (1967).

ETINGOF, R. N., SHUKOLYUKOV, S. A., LEONTEV, V. G.: Escape of $Na^+$ and $K^+$ ions from the outer segments of retinal photoreceptors under the effect of illumination and vitamin A. Dokl. Akad. Nauk SSSR **156**, 979 (1964).

EVANS, D. R., MELLON, D. F.: Electrophysiological studies of the water receptor associated with the taste sensilla of the blowfly. J. gen. Physiol. **45**, 487 (1962).

EVANS, S. M.: On the ultrastructure of the synaptic region of visual receptors in certain vertebrates. Z. Zellforsch. **71**, 499 (1966).

EWALD, J. R.: Physiologische Untersuchungen über die Endorgane des Nervus octavus. Wiesbaden 1892.

EXNER, S.: Physiologie der facettieren Augen von Krebsen und Insekten. Leipzig und Wien: Fr. Deuticke 1891.

FÄHRMANN, W.: Licht- und elektronenmikroskopische Untersuchungen an der Geschmacksknospe des neotenen Axolotls (*Siredon mexicanum* Shae). Z. mikr.-anat. Forsch. **77**, 117 (1967).

FÄHRMANN, W., SCHUCHARDT, E.: Licht- und elektronenmikroskopische Befunde an den Geschmacksknospen der Axolotlzunge. Experientia (Basel) **23**, 657 (1967).

FÄHRMANN, W., HOFFMANN, G., SCHUCHARDT, E.: Die Zellen der Geschmacksknospen und der Zellersatz. Naturwissenschaften **52**, 438 (1965).

FÄNGE, R., SCHMIDT-NILSEN, K., ROBINSON, M.: Control of secretion from the avian salt gland. Amer. J. Physiol. **195**, 321 (1958).

FARBMAN, A. I.: Electron microscope study of the developing taste bud in rat fungiform papilla. Developm. Biol. **11**, 110 (1965a).

FARBMAN, A. I.: Fine structure of the taste bud. J. Ultrastruct. Res. **12**, 328 (1965b).

FARBMAN, A. I.: Structure of chemoreceptors. In: Chemistry and Physiology of Flavors (Eds. H. W. Schultz, E. A. Day, L. M. Libley). Westport/Conn. 1967.

FATT, P., KATZ, B.: Some observations on biological noise. Nature **169**, 597 (1950).

FATT, P., KATZ, B.: An analysis of the end-plate potential recorded with an intracellular electrode. J. Physiol. (London) **115**, 320 (1951).

FAURÉ-FREMIÉT, E.: Gils vibratés et flagelles. Biol. Rev. **36**, 464 (1961).

FAUVEL, P.: Recherches sur les otocystes des annelides polychètes. Ann. Sci. Nat. (Zool.) Ser. (9), **6**, 1 (1907).

FAWCETT, D.: Cilia and flagela. In: The Cell, Vol. 2 (Eds. J. Brachet, A. E. Mirsky), p. 217. New York: Academic Press 1961.

FEDELE, M.: Il problema della regolazione del' attitiva vibrotile nei metazoi. Riv. Biol. **8**, 360 (1926).

FERGUSON, L. N., LOWRENCE, A. R.: The physicochemical aspects of the sense of taste. J. chem. Educ. **35**, 436 (1958).

FERNÁNDEZ-MORÁN, H.: Fine structure of the insect retinula as revealed by electron microscopy. Nature **177**, 742 (1956).

FERNÁNDEZ-MORÁN, H.: Fine structure of the light receptors in the compound eye of insects. Exp. Cell. Res., Suppl. **5**, 586 (1958).

FERNÁNDEZ-MORÁN, H.: The fine structure of vertebrate and invertebrate photoreceptors as revealed by low-temperature electron microscopy. In: The Structure of the Eye, p. 521. New York: Academic Press 1961.

FERNÁNDEZ-MORÁN, H.: Subunit organisation of mitochondrial membranes. Science **140**, 380 (1963).

FERRERI, G., GRIFO, S.: Mucopolisaccaridi acidi dei tessutivi labirintici. Valsalva **32**, 79 (1956).

FEX, J.: Auditory activity in centrifugal and centripetal cochlear fibers in cat. Acta physiol. scand. **55**, 189 (1962).

FINZI, A.: Richerche istochimiche sull' organo del Corti, cellule sensoriali e cellule di Hensen. Arch. ital. Otol. **69**, 817 (1958).

FLEISCHER, S., FLEISCHER, B., STOECKENIUS, W.: Fine structure of lipid-depleted mitochondria. J. Cell Biol. **32**, 193 (1967).

FLOCK, A.: Structure of the macula utriculi with special reference to directional interplay of sensory responses as revealed by morphological polarization. J. Cell Biol. **22**, 413 (1964).

FLOCK, A.: Electron microscopic and electrophysiological studies on the lateral-line canal organ. Acta oto-laryng. (Stockh.), Suppl. **199**, 1 (1965).

FLOCK, A.: Transducing mechanisms in the lateral-line organ receptors. Cold Spr. Harb. Symp. quant. Biol. **30**, 133 (1958).

FLOCK, A., KIMURA, R., LUNDQUIST, P. G., WERSÄLL, J.: Morphological basis of directional sensitivity of the outer cells of the organ of Corti. J. acoust Soc. Amer. **34**, 1351 (1962).

FLOCK, A., WERSÄLL, J.: Synaptic structures in the lateral-line canal organ of the teleost fish *Lota vulgaris*, J. Cell Biol. **13**, 377 (1962a).

FLOCK, A., WERSÄLL, J.: A study of the orientation of the sensory hairs of the receptor cells in the lateral-line organ of fish, with special reference to the function of the receptors. J. Cell Biol. **15**, 19 (1962b).

FRANCIS, C.: Succinic dehydrogenase in the visual cells. J. Physiol. (Lond.) **119**, 38.

FRANCIS, C.: Cholinesterase in the retina. J. Physiol. (Lond.) **120**, 435 (1953b).

FRANK, R. N., GOLDSMITH, T. H.: Adenosine triphosphatase activity in the rod outer segments of the pig's retina. Arch. Biochem. **110**, 517 (1965).

FRÄNKEL, G.: Der statische Sinn der Medusen. Z. vergl. Physiol. **2**, 658 (1925).

FRENKEL, Y.: On the mechanism of light absorption in solid bodies. Physiol. Rev. **37**, 459 (1931a).

FRENKEL, Y.: On the transformation of light into heat in solids. Physiol. Rev. **37**, 1276 (1931b).

FREY-WYSSLING, A., MÜHLETHALER, K.: Ultrastructural Plant Cytology. With an Introduction to Molecular Biology. Amsterdam, London, New York: Elsevier 1965.

FUKUDA, T., KOELLE, G. B.: The cytological localization of intracellular neuronal acetylcholinesterase. J. biophys. biochem., Cytol. **5**, 433 (1959).

FURUKAWA, T., FURSHPAN, E. J.: Two inhibitory mechanisms in the Mautner neurons of goldfish. J. Neurophysiol. **26**, 140 (1963).

FUTTERMAN, S.: The role of reduced triphosphopyridine nucleotide in visual cycle. J. biol. Chem. **238**, 1145 (1963).

FUTTERMAN, S., KINOSHITA, J. H.: Metabolism of the retina. I. Respiration of cattle retina. J. biol. Chem. **234**, 723 (1959).

GAĆEK, R. R.: Efferent component of the vestibular nerve. In: Neural Mechanisms of Auditory and Vestibular Systems (Eds. G. L. Rasmussen, W. F. Windle), p. 276. Springfield/Ill.: Ch. C. Thomas 1960.

GALAMBOS, R.: Suppression of auditory nerve activity by stimulation of efferent fibres to cochlea. J. Neurophysiol. **19**, 424 (1956).

GALL, J. G.: Centriole replication. A study of spermatogenesis in the snail *Viviparus*. J. biophys. biochem. Cytol. **10**, 163 (1961).

GAUDA, T.: Sul rapporto fra proprietà chimicofisiche dei sali e soglia di densazione per il loro sapore. Arch. Fisiol. **10**, 175 (1912).

GAWRILENKO, A. W.: Die Entwicklung des Geruchsorgans bei *Salmo salar*. Anat. Anz. **35**, 411 (1910).

GAZENKO, O. G., LIMANSKII, YU. P., RAZUMEEV, A. M., IZOSIMOV, G. O., BARANOV, V. I., CHICHKIN, V. A., GAYDAMAKIN, N. A.: Method of recording the action potentials of neurons in vestibular nuclei during adequate stimulation of vestibular receptors in cats. Izv. Akad. Nauk SSSR (Ser. biol.) **6**, 925 (1962).

GEL'MAN, N. S.: Molecular organization of biological membranes. Usp. sovrem. Biol. **64**, 379 (1967).

GEL'MAN, N. S.: Study of the structure of biochemical membranes by means of fragmentation with detergents. Usp. sovrem. Biol. **68**, 3 (1969).

GEL'MAN, N. S., LUKOYANOVA, M. A., OSTROVSKII, D. N.: Dykhatel'nyi apparat bakteriy (Respiratory Apparatus of Bacteria). Moscow: Izd. Nauka 1966.

GEREBTZOFF, M. A.: Development of cholinesterase activity in the nervous system. In: Biochemistry of the Developing Nervous System. New York 1955.

GEREBTZOFF, M. A.: Cholinesterases. New York: Pergamon Press 1959.

GEREBTZOFF, M. A., PHILIPPOT, E.: Lipids and olfactory Pigment. Acta oto-rhino-laryng. belg. **11**, 297 (1957).

GERHARDT, H. J.: Zur Verteilung der Succinodehydrogenase in der Meerschweinchenschnecke. Arch. Ohr.-, Nas.- u. Kehlk.-Heilk. **179**, 283 (1961).

GERHARDT, H. J.: Zur Verteilung der DPN- und TPN-diaphorase in der Meerschweinchenschnecke. Arch. Ohr.-, Nas.- u. Kehlk.-Heilk. **181**, 16 (1962).

GEREN, B. B.: The formation from the Schwann cell surface of myelin in the peripheral nerves of chick embryos. Exp. Cell. Res. **7**, 558 (1954).

GERNANDT, B. E.: Response of mammalian vestibular neurons to horizontal and caloric stimulation. J. Neurophysiol. **12**, 173 (1949).

GERNANDT, B. E.: The effect of the centrifugal force upon the nerve discharge from the horizontal canal. Acta physiol. scand. **21**, 61 (1950).

GERNANDT, B. E.: Vestibular mechanisms. In: Handbook of Physiology, sec. I. Neurophysiology, vol. I (Eds. J. Field, H. Magoun, V. E. Hall). American Physiological Society, Washington 1959.

GERNER, L.: Nemertinen der Gattungen *Cephalothrix* und *Ototyphlonemertes* aus dem marinen Mesopsammal. Helgoländer Wiss. Meeresunters. **19**, 66 (1969).

GERSHUNI, G. V.: Study of subsensory reactions during the activity of sense organs. Fiziol. Zh. SSSR **33**, 393 (1947).

GEUZE, J. J.: Observation on the function and the structure of the statocysts of *Lymnaea stagnalis* L. Netherlands J. Zool. **18**, 155 (1968).

GIBBONS, J. R.: Studies on the protein components of cilia from *Tetrahymena pyriformis*. Proc. nat. Acad. Sci. (Wash.) **50**, 1002 (1963).

352 References

GIBBONS, J. R.: An effect of adenosine triphosphate on the light scattered by suspensions of cilia. J. Cell Biol. **23**, 35 (1964).
GIBBONS, J. R., GRIMSTONE, A. V.: On flagellar structure in certain flagellates. J. biophys. biochem. Cytol. **7**, 697 (1960).
GISSELSSON, L.: The passage of fluorescin sodium to the labyrinthine fluids. Acta oto-laryng. (Stockh.) **37**, 268 (1949).
GISSELSSON, L.: Experimental investigation into the problem of humoral transmission in the cochlea. Acta oto-laryng. (Stockh.), Suppl. **82**, 1 (1950).
GIULIO, L.: Elektroretinographische Beweisführung dichroitischer Eigenschaften des Komplexauges bei Zweiflüglern. Z. vergl. Physiol. **46**, 491 (1963).
GLEBOV, R. N.: Biochemical aspects of the functioning of synaptic membranes. Tezisy 5-i Vsesoyuzn. konf. po neirokhimii 1968 (Reports of the 5th All-Union Conference on Neurochemistry 1968), p. 28.
GOGNIASHVILI, O. SH.: Histochemical study of the organ of Corti of birds. Arkh. Anat. Gistol. Embriol. **55**, 14 (1967a).
GOGNIASHVILI, O. SH.: Histochemical studies of the organ of Corti of birds under the effect of sound. Zh. evolyuts. biokh. fiziol. **3**, 272 (1967b).
GOGNIASHVILI, O. SH.: Histochemical and electron microscopic study of the organ of Corti of birds under conditions of relative rest and exposure to sound, Author's abstract of dissertation, Leningrad 1967c.
GOLDMAN, D. E.: The transducer action of mechanoreceptor membranes. Cold Spr. Harb. Symp. quant. Biol. **30**, 59 (1965).
GOLDSMITH, T. H.: On the visual system of the bee *(Apis mellifera)*. Ann. N. Y. Acad. Sci. **74**, 223 (1958).
GOLDSMITH, T. H.: Fine structure of the retinulae in the compound eye of the honey-bee. J. Cell Biol. **14**, 489 (1962).
GOLDSMITH, T. H.: The visual systems of insects. In: The Physiology of Insecta (Ed. M. Rockstein), p. 397. New York–London 1964.
GOLDSMITH, T. H., BARKER, R. J., COHEN, C. F.: Sensitivity of visual receptor of carotenoid-depleted flies: A vitamin-A deficiency in invertebrates. Science **146**, 65 (1964).
GOLDSMITH, T., ELLIS, R. A.: Monoamine oxidase activity in the tongue. Anat. Rec. **139**, 303 (1961).
GOLDSMITH, T. H., PHILPOTT, D. E.: The microstructure of the compound eye of insects. J. biophys. biochem. Cytol. **3**, 429 (1957).
GOLDSMITH, T. H., WARNER, L. T.: Vitamin A in the vision of insects. J. gen. Physiol. **47**, 433 (1964).
GOMAZKOVA, V. S.: On the alkaline phosphatase in the olfactory epithelium of some freshwater fish. In the collection of works (Sbornik): Materialy po biol. i gidrol. Volzhskikh vodokhranilishch (Data on the Biology and Hydrology of Volga Water Reservoirs), p. 92. Moscow: Izd. Akad. Nauk SSSR 1963.
GÖRNER, P. A.: Proposed transducing mechanism for a multiply innervated mechanoreceptor *(Trichobotrium)* in spiders. Cold Spr. Harb. Symp. quant. Biol. **30**, 69 (1965).
GÖTHLIN, G. H.: Experimental studies on primary inhibition of the ciliary movement in *Beroe cucumis*. J. exp. Zool. **31**, 403 (1920).
GOUREVITCH, A.: Consommation du glycogène par la rétine à lumière et à l'obscurité. J. Physiol. (Paris) **43**, 255 (1951).
GOUREVITCH, A.: La localisation histologique du glycogène dans la retine des poissons et sa consommation à la lumière. J. Physiol. (Paris) **46**, 633 (1954).
GOVARDOVSKII, V. I.: Comparative electron microscopic study of the structure and development of photoreceptors. Author's abstract of dissertation, Leningrad 1967.
GOVARDOVSKII, V. I.: Electron microscopic detection of sodium in the outer segments of photoreceptors in the light and in darkness. Tsitologiya **11**, 622 (1969).
GOVARDOVSKII, V. I.: Sodium and potassium concentration gradient in the retinal rod outer segment. Nature **234**, 53 (1971a).
GOVARDOVSKII, V. I., KHARKEEVICH, T. A.: Histochemical and electron microscopic study of the development of photoreceptor cells in tissue culture. Arkh. anat., gistol. embriol. **49**, 50 (1965).

GOVARDOVSKII, V. I., KHARKEEVICH, T. A.: Electron microscopic study of the structural development of the outer photoreceptor segment in the chick *(Gallus domesticus)*. Zh. evolyuts. biokhim. fiziol. **2**, 37 (1966a).

GOVARDOVSKII, V. I., KHARKEEVICH, T. A.: Embryonic development of photoreceptors. In: Pervichnye protsessy v retseptornykh elementakh organov chuvtsv (Primary processes in Receptor Elements of Sense Organs), p. 3. Moscow—Leningrad: Izd. Nauka 1966b.

GOVARDOVSKII, V. I., KHARKEEVICH, T. A.: Electron microscopic study of the retina in the hen *(Gallus bankiva domestica)*. Arkh. Anat. Gistol. Embriol. **52**, 53 (1967).

GOVARDOVSKII, V. I., TSIRULIS, T. P.: Development of mitochondria in photoreceptor ellipsoids of the lamprey. Tsitologiya **11**, 499 (1969).

GRANIT, R.: Sensory Mechanism of the Retina. Oxford: Univ. Press 1947.

GRANIT, R.: Receptors and Sensory Reception. New Haven: Yale Univ. Press 1955.

GRAY, E. G.: The fine structure of insect ear. Phil. Trans. B **243**, 75 (1960).

GRAY, E. G.: Electron microscopy of presynaptic organelles of the spinal cord. J. Anat. (Lond.) **97**, 101 (1963).

GRAY, E. G.: Round and flat vesicles in the goldfish CNS (abstract). In: 3rd Conf. Anatomists and Histologists in Bulgaria. Plovdiv, Medical and Physical Culture Publishing House, Sofia 1967.

GRAY, E. G.: Central nervous system. In: Elektronnomikroskopicheskaya anatomiya (Electron Microscopic Anatomy). Moscow: Izd. Mir 1967.

GRAY, E. G., WHITTAKER, V. P.: The isolation of nerve endings from brain and electron microscopic study of cell fragments derived by homogenization and centrifugation. J. Anat. (Lond.) **96**, 79 (1962).

GRAY, F. G.: Axo-somatic and axo-dendritic synapses of the cerebral cortex: An electron microscope study. J. Anat. (Lond.) **93**, 420 (1959).

GRAY, F. G.: Electron microscopy of excitatory and inhibitory synapses: a brief review. In: Progress in Brain Research (Eds. K. Akert, P. Wasser), Vol. **31**, p. 141. Amsterdam: Elsevier 1969.

GRAY, F. G., GUYLLIERY, R. W.: Synaptic morphology in the normal and degenerating nervous system. Int. Rev. Cytol. **19**, 111 (1966).

GRAY, J.: The movement of sea-urchin spermatozoa. J. exp. Biol. **32**, 775 (1955).

GREEN, D. E.: Biological membranes. In: Molekulyarnaya biologiya, problemy i perspektivy (Molecular Biology, Problems and Perspectives), p. 260. Moscow: Izd. Nauka 1964.

GREEN, D. E., ALLMAN, D. W., BACHMAN, E., BAUM, H., KOPACZYK, K., KORMAN, E., LIPTON, S., MACLENNAN, D., MCCANUELL, D., PERDUE, J. F., BIESKE, J., TZAGOLOFF, A.: Formation of membranes by repeating units. Arch. Biochem. **19**, 312 (1967).

GREEN, D. E., TZAGOLOFF, A.: The mitochondrial electron transfer chain. Arch. Biochem. **16**, 293 (1966).

GRELLMAN, K. H., LIVINGSTON, R., PRATT, D.: A flash-photolytic investigation of rhodopsin at low temperatures. Nature **193**, 1258 (1962).

GRENACHER, H.: Abhandlungen zur vergleichenden Anatomie des Auges. I. Die Retina der Cephalopoden. Abh. naturf. Ges. **16**, 207 (1886).

GRIBAKIN, F. G.: Ultrastructural organization of photoreceptor cells in the compound eye of the honeybee. Zh. evolyuts. biokhim. fiziol. **3**, 66 (1967a).

GRIBAKIN, F. G.: Types of photoreceptor cells in the compound eye of the working bee *Apis mellifera*. Electron microscopic data. Tsitologiya **9**, 1276 (1967b).

GRIBAKIN, F. G.: Ultrastructural organization of insect photoreceptors. Trudy Vsesoyuzn. entom. obshch. **53**, 238 (1969a).

GRIBAKIN, F. G.: Ultrastructural basis of color vision in the bee. Author's abstract of dissertation, Leningrad 1969b.

GRIBAKIN, F. G.: Types of visual cells in the compound eye of the working bee in relation to their spectral sensitivity. Tsitologiya **11**, 3 (1969c).

GRIBAKIN, F. G.: Cellular basis of colour vision in the honeybee. Nature **223**, 639 (1969d).

GRIBAKIN, F. G., GOVARDOVSKII, V. I.: Structure, visual pigments and optical properties of photoreceptors. Usp. sovrem. biol. **62**, 120 (1966).

GROTH, W.: Der Ursprung der Labyrinthplakode und des Ganglion statoacusticus im Vergleich zur Genese des Riechorgans beim Kaninchen. Z. Mikr.-anat. Forsch. **45**, 426 (1939).

GRUNDFEST, G.: Evolution of electrophysiological changes in sensory receptors. In the collection of works (Sbornik): Problemy evolyutsii funktsii i enzimokhimii protsessov vozbuzhdeniya (Prob-

354 References

lems of Evolution of the Function and Enzyme Chemistry of Excitatory Processes), p. 103. Moscow: Izd. Akad. Nauk SSSR 1961.

GUTH, L.: The effects of glossopharyngeal nerve transection on the circumvallate papilla of the rat. Anat. Rec. **128**, 715 (1957).

GUTH, L.: Taste buds on the cat's circumvallate papilla after reinnervation by glossopharyngeal, vagus and hypoglossal nerves. Anat. Rec. **130**, 25 (1958).

GUTH, L.: Histological changes following partial denervation of the circumvallate papillae (tongue) of the rat. Exp. Neurol. **8**, 336 (1963).

HAGINS, W. A.: Electrical signs of information flow in photoreceptors. Cold Spr. Harb. Symp. quant. Biol. **30**, 403 (1965).

HAGINS, W. A., ZONANA, H. V., ADAMS, R. G.: Local membrane current in the outer segments of squid photoreceptors. Nature **194**, 84 (1962).

HAJOS, F., KERPEL-FRONIUS, S.: Electron histochemical observations of succinic dehydrogenase activity in various parts of neurons. Exp. Brain. Res. **8**, 66 (1969).

HALL, M. O., BOK, D., BACHARACH, A. D. E.: Visual pigment renewal in the mature frog retina. Science **161**, 787 (1968).

HALL, M. O., BOK, D., BACHARACH, A. D. E.: Biosynthesis and assembly of the rod outer segment membrane system. Formation and fate of visual pigment in the frog retina. J. molec. Biol. **45**, 397 (1969).

HAMA, K.: Some observations on the fine structure of the giant nerve fibers of the earthworm, *Eisenia foetida*. J. biophys. biochem. Cytol. **6**, 61 (1959).

HAMA, K.: Fine structure of the lateral-line organ of the Japanese sea eel. In: Electron Microscopy, Vol. **2**, N 4. New York: Acad. Press 1962.

HAMILTON, D. V.: The calyceal synapse of type 1 vestibular hair cells. J. Ultrastruct. Res. **23**, 98 (1968).

HANAWA, J.: Photo-metabolism of the isolated outer segments of rods. Japan. J. Physiol. **6**, 218 (1956).

HANAWA, J., KIMURA, E., HOSOYA, Y.: The respiration of the isolated outer segments of rods. Japan. J. Physiol. **5**, 322 (1955).

HANAWA, J., KUGE, K.: The effect of light intensity upon the oxygen consumption of the isolated outer segments of rods. Japan J. Physiol. **11**, 38 (1961).

HANSTRÖM, B.: Vergleichende Anatomie des Nervensystems der wirbellosen Tiere. Berlin: Springer 1928.

HARA, R.: Changes in electrical conductance of rhodopsin on photolysis. J. gen. Physiol. **47**, 241 (1963—64).

HARA, T., HARA, R.: New photosensitive pigment found in the retina of the squid *Ommastrephes*. Nature **206**, 1331 (1965).

HARA, T., HARA, R.: Rhodopsin and retinochrome in the squid retina. Nature **214**, 574 (1967).

HARA, T., HARA, R.: Regeneration of squid retinochrome. Nature **219**, 450 (1968).

HARA, T., HARA, R., TAKEUCHI, J.: Vision in octopus and squid. Nature **214**, 572 (1967).

VON HARNACK, V. M.: Über den Feinbau des Nervensystems des Seesterns *(Asterais rubens)*, III. Mitteilungen. Die Structur der Augenpolster. Z. Zellforsch. **60**, 432 (1963).

HASE, H.: De- and regeneration of chloroplasts in the cells of *Chlorella protothecoides* as included by controlling nutritional and light conditions. In: Seventh International Congr. of Biochem., Abstract II, p. 223. Tokyo: Science Council 1967.

HASKELL, P. T.: Hearing in certain Orthoptera. I. Physiology of sound receptors. J. exp. Biol. **33**, 756 (1956a).

HASKELL, P. T.: Hearing in certain Orthoptera. II. The nature of the response of certain receptors to natural and imitation stridulation. J. exp. Biol. **33**, 767 (1956b).

HAYASHI, T.: Reactivities of actin as contractile protein. J. gen. Physiol. **50**, 119 (1967).

HAYDON, R. A., TAYLOR, J.: The stability and properties of bimolecular lipid leaflets in aqueous solution. J. theor. Biol. **4**, 281 (1963).

HEBB, G. C., WAITES, G. M.: Choline acetylase in antero- and retrograde degeneration of cholinergic nerve. J. Physiol. (Lond.) **32**, 667 (1956).

HEBB, G. C., WHITTAKER, V. P.: Intracellular distribution of acetylcholine and choline acetylase. J. Physiol. (Lond.) **142**, 187 (1958).

HEIDENHEIN, M.: Über die Sinnesfelder und die Geschmacksknospen der Papilla foliata des Kaninchens. Arch. mikr. Anat. **85**, 365 (1914).

HELD, H.: Untersuchungen über den feineren Bau des Ohrlabyrinthes der Wirbeltiere. I. Zur Kenntnis der cortischen Organe und der übrigen Sinnesapparate der Säugetiere. Abh. sächs. Ges. Wiss. Math.-Physik. Kl., Bd. **28**, S. 1 (1902).

HELD, H.: Die Cochlea der Säuger und der Vögel, ihre Entwicklung und ihr Bau. In: Handbuch der norm. und pathol. Physiol., Vol. **11**, p. 467. Berlin: Springer 1926.

HELLER, J.: Structure of visual pigments. Purification, molecular weight and comparison of bovine visual pigment. Biochemistry **7**, 2906 (1968).

HELLER, J.: Comparative study of a membrane protein. Characterization of bovine, rat and frog visual pigment. Biochemistry **8**, 675 (1969).

HELLSTRÖM, B.: The histochemical localization of succinic dehydrogenase in the retina of normal and oxygen-exposed animals. Acta path. microbiol. scand. **39**, 8 (1956).

HELMHOLTZ, G.: Uchenie o slukhovykh oshchushchenyakh kak fiziologicheskaya osnova dlya teorii muzyki (Theory of Auditory Sensations as a Physiological Basis for the Theory of Music). St. Petersburg 1875.

HELMHOLTZ, G.: O zrenii (On Vision). St. Petersburg 1896.

HENDLER, R. W.: Biological membrane ultrastructure. Physiol. Rev. **51**, 66 (1971).

HENSEN, V.: Zur Morphologie der Schnecke des Menschen und der Säugetiere. Z. wiss. Zool. **13**, 481 (1863).

HENSEN, V.: Über das Auge einiger Cephalopoden. Z. wiss. Zool. **15**, 155 (1885).

HERING, E.: Wissenschaftliche Abhandlungen, I. u. II. Herausgegeben von der Sächsischen Acad. d. Wissensch. zu Leipzig. Leipzig: Thieme 1931.

HERRICK, C.: The Brain of the Tiger Salamander, p. 76. Chicago: Univ. Chicago Press 1948.

HICKMAN, C. P.: Biology of the Invertebrates. St. Louis: Mosby 1967.

HIJI, V., KOBAYASHI, N., SATO, M.: A sweet-sensitive protein from the tongue of the rat. Kumamoto Med. J. **21**, 137 (1968).

HIJI, V., KOBAYASHI, N., SATO, M.: Binding capacities of sugars with the "sweet-sensitive protein" from rat tongue. Kumamoto Med. J. **22**, 104 (1969).

HILD, W., CALLAS, G.: The behavior of retinal tissue in vitro. Light and electron microscopic observations. Z. Zellforsch. **80**, 1 (1967).

HILDING, A. C.: Studien über die Anatomie und Funktion der Tectorial membran. Trans. Amer. Acad. Ophthal. Otolaryng. **57**, 35 (1953a).

HILDING, A. C.: The tectorial membrane in the theory of hearing; the significance of the insertion of the tectorial membrane in the transmission of sound vibrations to the hair cells and a theory of the mechanism of tone location in the cochlea. Ann. Otol. (St. Louis) **62**, 757 (1953b).

HILDING, D., WERSÄLL, J.: Cholinesterase and its relation to the nerve endings in the inner ear. Acta oto-laryng. (Stockh.) **55**, 205 (1962).

HIS, W.: Die Formentwicklung des menschlichen Vorderhirns vom Ende des ersten bis zum Beginn des dritten Monats. Abhandl. math.-phys. Classe d. Königl. Sächs. Ges. d. Wiss. **15**, 673 (1889).

HOAGLAND, H.: Impulses from sensory nerves of catfish. Proc. nat. Acad. Sci. (Wash.) **18**, 701 (1932).

HODGKIN, A.: Nervnyi impul's (The Nervous Impulse). Moscow: Izd. Mir 1965.

HODGSON, E. S.: Chemoreception. In: The Physiology of Insecta, p. 363. New York and London 1964.

HODGSON, E. S.: The chemical senses and changing viewpoints in sensory physiology. In: Viewpoints in Biology, p. 81. London 1965.

HODOSH, M., MONTAGNA, W.: Cholinesterase in the tongue of the potto (Periodicteus potto). Anat. Rec. **146** (I), 715 (1963).

HOFFMAN, C.: Bau und Vorkommen von proprioceptiven Sinnesorganen bei den Arthropoden. Ergeb. Biol. **27**, 1 (1964).

HOFFMAN-BERLING, H.: Geisselmodelle und Adenosintryphosphat (ATP). Biochim. biophys. Acta (Amst.) **16**, 146 (1955).

HOLWILL, M. E. J.: The motion of Strigomonas oncopelti. J. exp. Biol. **42**, 125 (1965).

HOLWILL, M. E. J.: Physical aspect of flagellar movement. Physiol. Rev. **46**, 696 (1966).

HOLWILL, M. E. J., SILVESTER, N. R.: The thermal dependence of flagellar activity in Strigomonas oncopelti. J. exp. Biol. **42**, 587 (1965).

HOPKINS, A.: The olfactory receptors in vertebrates. J. comp. Neurol. **41**, 253 (1926).

HOPKINS, J. M., WATSON, M. R.: The cilia of Tetrahymena pyriformis: isolation of ciliary segments. Exp. Cell. Res. **32**, 187 (1964).

HORRIDGE, G. A.: Presumed photoreceptive cilia in a ctenophore. Quart. J. micr. Sci. **105**, 311 (1964).

HORRIDGE, G. A.: Relations between nerves and cilia in ctenophores. Amer. Zool. **5**, 357 (1965a).

HORRIDGE, G. A.: Non-motile sensory cilia and neuromuscular junctions in a ctenophora independent effector organ. Proc. roy. Soc. B **162**, 333 (1965b).

HORRIDGE, G. A.: Statocysts of medusae and evolution of stereocilia. Tissue Cell **1** (2), 341 (1969).

HORRIDGE, G. A., BARNARD, P. B. T.: Movement of palisade in locust retinula cells when illuminated. Quart. J. micr. Sci. **106**, 131 (1965).

HUBBARD, R.: The respiration of the isolated rod outer limb of the frog retina. J. gen. Physiol. **37**, 373 (1954a).

HUBBARD, R.: The molecular weight of rhodopsin and the nature of the rhodopsin digitonin complex. J. gen. Physiol. **37**, 381 (1954b).

HUBBARD, R.: Retinene isomerase. J. gen. Physiol. **39**, 935 (1955—56).

HUBBARD, R.: The thermal stability of rhodopsin and opsin. J. gen. Physiol. **42**, 259 (1958—1959).

HUBBARD, R., BOWNDS, D., YOSHIZAWA, T.: The chemistry of visual photoreception. Cold Spr. Harb. Symp. quant. Biol. **30**, 301 (1965).

HUBBARD, R., DOWLING, J.: Formation and utilization of 11-*cis* vitamin A by the eye tissues during light and dark adaptation. Nature **193**, 341 (1962).

HUBBARD, R., ST. GEORGE, R. C. C.: The rhodopsin system of the squid. J. gen. Physiol. **41**, 501 (1957—58).

HUBBARD, R., KROPF, A.: Chicken lumi- and metaiodopsin. Nature **183**, 448 (1959).

HYMAN, L. H.: Observations and experiments on the physiology of medusae. Biol. Bull. Woods Hole **79**, 282 (1940).

HYMAN, L. H.: The Invertebrates, 4. New York: McGraw-Hill 1955.

IL'INSKII, O. B.: Some problems concerning the physiology of reception. In: Nervnaya kletka (The Nerve Cell), p. 187. Leningrad: Izd. LGU 1966.

IRELAND, R., FARKASHIDY, Y.: Studies on the efferent innervation of the vestibular end-organs. Ann. Otol. (St. Louis) **70**, 490 (1961).

ISHIGAMI, M., MAEDA, I., MISHIMA, I.: A retinen-tryptophan complex. Biochim. biophys. Acta (Amst.) **112**, 372 (1966).

ISHII, T. X., MURAKAMI, Y., BALOGH, K.: Acetylcholinesterase activity in the efferent nerve fibres of the human inner ear. Ann. Otol. (St. Louis) **76**, 69 (1967).

ISHIKAWA, H., BISCHOFF, R., HOLTZER, H.: Formation of arrow-head complexes with heavy meromyosin in a variety of cell types. J. Cell Biol. **43**, 312 (1969).

ISHIKAWA, T., YEN FEN REI: Intramitochondrial glycogen particles in rat retinal receptor cells. J. Cell Biol. **25**, 402 (1965).

ITO, S.: The lamellar systems of cytoplasmic membranes in dividing spermatogenic cells of *Drosophila vivilis*. J. biophys. biochem. Cytol. **7**, 433 (1960).

ITO, S.: The enteric surface coat on intestinal microvilli. J. Cell Biol. **27**, 475 (1965).

ITOIZ, M. E., CARRANZA, F. A., CABRINI, R. L.: Histoenzymatic study of the tongue mucosa in different species. Acta histochem. (Jena) **25**, 183 (1966).

IURATO, S.: Submicroscopic structure of the membranous labyrinth. I. The tectorial membrane. Z. Zellforsch. **52**, 105 (1960).

IURATO, S.: Submicroscopic structure of the membranous labyrinth. II. The epithelium of Corti's ·organ. Z. Zellforsch. **53**, 259 (1961).

IURATO, S.: Submicroscopic structure of the membranous labyrinth. III. The supporting structure of Corti's organ, basilar membrane, limbus spiralis and spiral ligament. Z. Zellforsch. **56**, 40 (1962a).

IURATO, S.: Efferent fibers to the sensory cells of Corti's organ. Exp. Cell Res. **27**, 162 (1962b).

IURATO, S.: Functional implications of the nature and submicroscopic structure of the tectorial and basilar membranes. J. acoust. Soc. Amer. **34**, 1386 (1962c).

IURATO, S.: Fibre efferenti dirette e crociate alle cellule acustiche dell' organo de Corti. Monit. Zool. Ital., Suppl. **72**, 62 (1964).

IURATO, S. (Ed.): Submicroscopic Structure of the Inner Ear. Oxford: Pergamon Press 1967.

IURATO, S., LUCIANO, L., PANNESE, E., REALE, E.: Histochemical localization of acetylcholinesterase (ACHE) activity in the inner ear. Acta oto-laryng. (Stockh.), Suppl. 279 (1971).

IURATO, S., SMITH, C. A., ELDREDGE, D., HENDERSEN, D.: Electron microscopic observations and cochlear potentials after section of the crossed olivo-cochlear tract in the chinchilla. In: Fourth European Region Conf. on Electron Microscopy, Rome 1968.

IVANOV, A. V.: Proiskhozhdenie mnogokletochnykh zhivotnykh, filogeneticheskie ocherki (Origin of Multicellular Animals, Phylogenetic Outlines). Leningrad: Izd. Nauka 1968.

IVANOV, V. P.: Ultrastructural organization of chemoreceptor sensilla in the antennae of the beetle *Acilius sulcatus*. Zh. evolyuts. biokhim. fiziol. **2**, 462 (1968).

IVANOV, V. P.: Electron microscopic study of Johnston's organ of the beetle *Acilius sulcatus*. In the collection of works (Sbornik): Fiziologiya i biokhimiya bespozvonochnykh (Physiology and Biochemistry of Invertebrates), p. 140. Leningrad: Izd. Nauka 1968.

IVANOV, V. P.: Electron microscopic study of insect sensilla, Author's abstract of dissertation, Leningrad 1969a.

IVANOV, V. P.: Ultrastructural organization of chemoreceptors in insects. Trudy Vsesoyuzn. entom. obshch. **53**, 301 (1969b).

IVANOV, V. P., MAMKAEV, YU. V., PEVZNER, R. A.: Electron microscopic study on the statocyst in the acoelic turbellarian *Convoluta convoluta*. Zh. evoluyuts. biokhim. fisiol. **8**, 189 (1972).

IWAYAMA, T., NADA, O.: Histochemically demonstrable ATPase activity in the taste buds of the rat. Exp. Cell Res. **46**, 607 (1967).

JACKSON, R.: The olfactory pigment. J. cell. comp. Physiol. **55**, 143 (1960).

JACKSON, S., FELL, H.: Epidermal fine structure in embryonic chicken skin during atypical differentiation induced by vitamin A in culture. Developm. Biol. **7**, 394 (1963).

JAHN, L.: A possible mechanism for the amplifier effect in the retina. Vision Res. **3**, 25 (1963).

JANDER, R., WATERMAN, T. H.: Sensory discrimination between polarized light and light intensity patterns by Arthropods. J. cell. comp. Physiol. **56**, 137 (1960).

JOHNSTON, C.: Auditory apparatus of the *Culex mosquito*. Quart. J. micr. Sci. (Old series) **3**, 97 (1885).

JOHNSTON, J. W., SANDOVAL, A.: The stereochemical theory of olfaction. 4. The validity of muskiness as a primary odour. Proc. Sci. Sect., Toilet Goods Ass. Special Suppl. **37**, 34 (1962).

KABACHNIK, M. I., BRESTKIN, A. P., MIKHELSON, M. YA.: On the mechanism of the physiological action of organic phosphorus compounds. 9th Mendeleev Congress of General and Applied Chemistry. Moscow: Izd. Nauka 1965.

KAHLENBERG, L.: The relation of the taste of acid salts to their degree of dissociation. J. phys. Chem. **4**, 33 (1900).

KAISSLING, K. E., RENNER, M.: Antennale Rezeptoren für Queensubstanz und Sterzelduft bei der Honigbiene. Z. vergl. Physiol. **59**, 357 (1968).

KANEKO, Y., DALY, J. F.: Activity of acetylcholinesterase on the endolymphatic surface of outer hair cells. Acta oto-laryng. (Stockh.) **67**, 602 (1969).

KARAMYAN, A. I.: On the evolution of the integrative activity of the central nervous system of vertebrates. In: Refleksy golovnogo mozga (Reflexes of the Brain). International conference commemorating the centenary of the publication of the book of this title by I. M. Sechenov. Moscow: Izd. Nauka 1965.

KARAMYAN, A. I.: The Functional Evolution of Vertebrate Brain. Leningrad: Izd. Nauka 1970.

KARASIK, V. M.: Pharmacological characteristics of cholinergic and adrenergic structures. Usp. sovrem. biol. **21** (1), 1 (1946).

KARE, M. R., FICKEN, M. S.: Comparative studies on the sense of taste. In: Olfaction and Taste, I, p. 285. Oxford: Pergamon Press 1963.

KARPENKO, L. D.: Certain chemical changes in mitochondria of the retina during light stimulation. In the collection of works (Sbornik): Materialy 4-oi nauchnoi konferentsii aspirantov Rostovsk. Univ. (Reports of the 4th Scientific Conference of Fellows of Rostov University), p. 217 (1962).

KAVANAU, J. L.: Structure and Function of Biological Membranes. San Francisco: Lioden Day 1965.

KAVANAU, J. L.: Membrane structure and function. Feder. Proc. Symp. Rep. **25**, 1096 (1966).

KAWAMOTO, K., KAKIZAKI, I.: A study on respiratory enzymes in the stria vascularis of the cochlea. J. oto-rhino-Laryng. Soc. Japan **65**, 179.

KAWAMOTO, K., KANEKO, Y.: A study of acetylcholinesterase in the cochlea. J. oto-rhino-laryng. Soc. Jap. **62**, 238 (1959).

KAWATA, S., TAKEDA, H., HAYATA, T.: On the distribution of potassium in the cochlear tissues of normal guinea-pigs. Otol. Fukuoka **9**, 162 (1963).

KEDROVSKII, B. V.: Tsitologiya belkovykh sintezov v zhivotnoi kletke (Cytology of Protein Syntheses in the Animal Cell). Moscow: Izd. Akad. Nauk SSSR 1959.

KENNEDY, E. P.: Recent progress in the biochemistry of membranes. In: Seventh Internat. Congr. of Biochem. Plenary Lecture, p. 6. Tokyo: Science Council 1967.

KERPEL-FRONIUS, S., HAJÓS, F.: A method for the electron microscopic demonstration of cytochrome oxidase in fresh and formalin-prefixed tissues. Histochemie 10, 216 (1967).

KERPEL-FRONIUS, S., HAJÓS, F.: The use of ferricyanide for the light and electron microscopic demonstration of succinic dehydrogenase activity. Histochemie 15, 343 (1968).

KHAN VAN KIEN, L.: Contribution à l'étude de l'histophysiologie de la rétine, en particulier de divers types de cônes à la grenouille et de leurs réponses après action de lumières colorées et monochromatiques. C. R. Ass. Anat. 86, 673 (1955).

KHLOPIN, N. G.: Obshchebiologicheskie i eksperimentalnye osnovy gistologii (General Biological and Experimental Bases of Histology). Moscow: Izd. Akad. Nauk SSSR 1946.

KIBYAKOV, A. V., PLUZHNIKOV, M. S., YANTAREVA, L. I.: The effect of cutting the vestibulocochlear nerve on the acetylcholine content of the inner ear. Fiziol. Zh. SSSR 59, 69 (1973).

KIMURA, K.: Factors affecting the response of taste receptors of rat. Kumamoto med. J. 14, 95 (1961).

KIMURA, K., BEIDLER, L. M.: Microelectrode study of taste bud of the rat. Amer. J. Physiol. 187, 610 (1956).

KIMURA, K., BEIDLER, L. M.: Microelectrode study of taste receptors of rat and hamster. J. cell. comp. Physiol. 58, 131 (1961).

KIMURA, R.: Hairs of the cochlear sensory cells and their attachment to the tectorial membrane. Acta oto-laryng. (Stockh.) 61, 55 (1966).

KIMURA, R., WERSÄLL, J.: Termination of the olivocochlear bundle in relation to the outer hair cells of the organ of Corti in guinea pig. Acta oto-laryng. (Stockh.) 55, 11 (1962).

KINOSITA, H., MURAKAMI, A.: Control of ciliary motion. Physiol. Rev. 47, 53 (1967).

KINZING, H.: Untersuchungen über den Bau der Statocysten einiger dekapoder Crustaceen. Verhandl. Naturhist.-med. Ver. Heidelberg (N. F.) 14, 1 (1919).

KIONKA, H., STRÄTZ, E.: Setzt der Geschmack eines Salzes sich zusammen aus dem Geschmack der einzelnen Ionen oder schmeckt man jedes Salz als Gesamtmolekül? Arch. exp. Path. Pharmacol. 95, 241 (1922).

KISLYAKOV, V. A., ORLOV, I. V.: Physiology of the vestibular system (Present status of the problem). In the collected works (Sbornik): Voprosy fiziologii sensornykh sistem (obzory) (Problems concerning the Physiology of Sensory Systems. Review), p. 4. Moscow—Leningrad: Izd. Nauka 1966.

KISTIAKOWSKY, G.: On the theory of odors. Science 112, 154 (1950).

KLEY, E.: Zur Herkunft der Perilymphe. Z. Laryng. Rhinol. 30, 486 (1951).

KLEMENKOV, V. A., ORLOV, I. V.: Physiology of the vestibular system (Present status of the problem). In the collected works (Sbornik): Voprosy fiziologii sensornykh sistem (obzory) (Problems concerning the Physiology of Sensory Systems. Review), p. 3. Moscow—Leningrad: Izd. Nauka 1966.

KNECHT, S.: Über den Gehörsinn und die Musikalität der Vögel. Z. vergl. Physiol. 27, 169 (1939).

KNECHT, S.: Gesang, Gehör und Musikalität der Vögel. Anat. Anz. 140, 376 (1940).

KOBURG, E.: Autoradiographische Untersuchungen zum Nucleinsäurestoffwechsel der Gewebe der Cochlea. Arch. Ohr.-, Nas.-, Kehlk.-Heilk. 178, 150 (1961).

KOCH, R. B.: Fractionation of olfactory tissue homogenates. Isolation of a concentrated plasma membrane fraction. J. Neurochem. 16, 145 (1969).

KOEHLER, O.: Über die Geotaxis von Paramecium. Arch. Protistenk. 45, 37 (1922).

KOELLE, G. B.: The roles of acetylcholine and acetylcholinesterase in junctional transmission. In: Pharmacology of Cholinergic and Adrenergic Transmission. Proc. Second Internat. Pharmacol. Meeting, p. 29. Oxford: Pergamon Press 1965.

KOELLE, G. B., STEINER, E. L.: The cerebral distributions and intraventricular injection. J. Pharmacol. exp. Ther. 118, 420 (1956).

KOELLE, G. B., WOLFAND, L., FRIEDENWALD, J., ALLEN, R.: Localization of specific cholinesterase in ocular tissues of the cat. Amer. J. Ophthal. 35, 1580 (1952).

KOELLE, J. B.: Electron microscopic localization of cholinesterase in the nervous system. In the collection of works (Sbornik): Biokhimiya i funktsiya nervnoi systemy (Biochemistry and Function of the Nervous System), Reports of International Symposium held on 24—28 Sept. 1965, p. 185. Moscow—Leningrad: Izd. Nauka 1967.

KOELLE, W. A., KOELLE, G. B.: The localization of external functional acetylcholinesterase at the synapses of autonomic ganglia. J. Pharmacol. exp. Ther. **126**, 9 (1959).

KOHLRAUSCH, W.: Über das Schwellgewebe an den Muscheln der Nasenschleimhaut. Arch. Anat., Physiol. Wiss. Med. **149** (1853).

KOICHEV, K. A.: Electron microscopic study of the organ of Corti under conditions of relative rest and following exposure to sound. Arkh. Anat. Gistol. Embriol. **56**, 45 (1969a).

KOICHEV, K. A.: Electron microscopic study of sodium distribution in the organ of Corti of animals in a state of relative rest and exposed to the effect of sound. Tsitologiya **11**, 537 (1969b).

KOICHEV, K. A.: Electron microscopic and cytochemical study of the organ of Corti. Author's abstract of dissertation, Sofia 1969c.

KOIDE, Y., HANDO, R., YOSHIKAWA, Y.: Distribution of some oxidising enzymes in the cochlea. Acta oto-laryng. (Stockh.) **58**, 344 (1964).

KÖLLIKER, A.: Mikroskopische Anatomie, Gewebelehre des Menschen, 2. Aufl., Leipzig 1865.

KOLMER, W.: Gehörorgan. In: Von Möllendorffs Handbuch der mikroskopischen Anatomie des Menschen, Bd. **3**, S. 250. Berlin: Springer 1927.

KOMAI, T.: Studies on Two Aberrant Ctenophores, *Coeloplana* and *Gastrodes*. Kyoto 1922.

KOMNICK, H.: Electronenmikroskopische Lokalisation von $Na^+$ und $Cl^-$ in Zellen und Geweben. Protoplasma (Wien) **55**, 414 (1962).

KONISHI, T., KELSEY, E., SINGLETON, G. T.: Effect of chemical alteration in the endolymph on the cochlear potentials. Acta oto-laryng. (Stockh.) **62**, 393 (1966).

KONISHI, Y., ZOTTERMAN, Y.: Taste functions in fish. In: Olfaction and Taste, **I**, p. 215. Oxford: Pergamon Press 1963.

KONZHUKOVA, E. D.: Morphological changes in lateral-line organs of *Triton taeniatus*, association with environmental conditions. Izv. Akad. Nauk SSSR, Part 1, Ser. biol. **7**, 1505 (1933).

KORN, E. D.: Structure of biological membranes. The unit membrane theory is reevaluted in light of data now available. Science **153**, 1491 (1966).

KOSHTOYANTS, KH. S., KATALIN-ROZHA: On the enzymological foundation of gustatory sensitivity. Biofizika **3**, 689 (1958).

KONSTANYAN, E. G.: The electron microscopic investigation of the olfactory organ in *Triturus vulgaris*. Zh. evoluts. biokhim. fisiol. **7**, 96 (1971).

KOYAMA, N., KURIHARA, K.: Do unique proteins exist in taste buds? J. gen. Physiol. **57**, 3, 297 (1971).

KOZAKOVA, G. V.: On the possible genetic functions of mitochondria. Tsitologiya **7**, 141 (1965).

KREIDL, A.: Weitere Beiträge zur Physiologie des Ohrlabyrinthes (II. Mitth.). Versuche an Krebsen. Sitzber. Akad. Wiss. Wien, Math.-naturw. Kl. Abt. **III**, 102, 149 (1893).

KREPS, E. M.: Comparative biochemistry of muscles and evolutionary theory. Priroda **8—9**, 65 (1933).

KREPS, E. M.: Phospholipids of cellular membranes of the nervous system in the development of the animal world. Report given at the 22nd annual Bakh lecture of 17 March 1966. Leningrad: Izd. Nauka 1967.

KREPS, E. M., VERZHBINSKAYA, N. A.: Brain metabolism in the evolution of vertebrates. Izv. Akad. Nauk SSSR, Ser. biol. **6**, 855 (1959).

KRINSKY, N. J.: The lipoprotein nature of rhodopsin. Arch. Ophthal. **60**, 688 (1958).

KRISTENSEN, H. K.: Examinations after interruption of membranous labyrinth. Acta oto-laryng. (Stockh.) **51**, 382 (1960).

KROHN, A.: Nachträgliche Beobachtungen über den Bau des Auges der Cephalopoden. Verhandl. K. Leopold Karl Acad. Naturforsch. (Nova Acta Corios) **19**, 41 (1839—1842).

KRÜKENBERG, C. F. W.: Über die Stäbchenfarbe der Cephalopoden. Untersuch. Physiol. Inst. Univ. Heidelberg **2**, 58 (1882).

KRUMINS, R.: Die Bortentwicklung bei der Wachsmotte *Galleria mellonella L.* Biol. Zbl. **71**, 183 (1952).

KUBOTA, T., KUBO, J.: Bitterness and chemical structure. Nature **223**, 97—99 (1969).

KUHN, A.: Über Farbenwechsel und Farbensinn von Cephalopoden. Z. vergl. Physiol. **32**, 572 (1950).

KÜHNE, W.: On the Photochemistry of the Retina and Visual Purple. London: Macmillan 1878a.

KÜHNE, W.: Fortgesetzte Untersuchungen über die Retina und die Pigmente des Auges. Untersuch. Physiol. Inst. Univ. Heidelberg **2**, 80 (1878b).

VON KUPFFER, C.: Die Entwicklung der Kopfnerven der Vertebraten. Verhandl. Anat. Gesellsch. **5**, 22 (1891).

KURATA, A.: The morphological studies on the otolith membrane of the guinea-pig maculi utriculi. J. Oto-Rhino-Laryng. Soc. Japan **66**, 453 (1963).

KURIHARA, K.: Isolation of chromoproteins from bovine olfactory tissues. Biochim. biophys. Acta (Amst.) **148**, 328 (1967).

KÜRSCHNER, H. D.: Über die Lactat- und Malatdehydrogenase in den vier Windungen der Cochlea des Meerschweinchens. Diss. Düsseldorf 1968.

KURTIEVA, R. K.: Development of the peripheral end of the human gustatory analyzer. Author's abstract of dissertation, Ashkhabad 1953.

KUSANO, K.: Analysis of the single unit activity of gustatory receptors in the frog tongue. Japan. J. Physiol. **10**, 620 (1960).

KUWABARA, M., NAKA, K.: Response of a signal retinula cell to polarized light. Nature **184**, 455 (1959).

LADMAN, A. J.: The fine structure of rod bipolar synapse in the retina of the albino rat. J. biophys. biochem. Cytol. **4**, 459 (1958).

LANDGREN, S., LILJESTRAND, G., ZOTTERMAN, Y.: Chemical transmission in taste fibre endings. Acta physiol. scand. **30**, 105 (1954).

LANGER, H.: Die Wirkung von Licht auf den chemischen Grundaufbau des Auges von *Calliphora erythrocephalata* Meig. J. Insect. Physiol. **4**, 283 (1960).

LANGER, H.: Nachweis dichroitischer Absorption des Sehfarbstoffes in den Rhabdomeren des Insektenauges. Z. vergl. Physiol. **51**, 258 (1965).

LANGER, H., THORELL, B.: Microspectrophotometry of single rhabdomeres in the insect eye. Exp. Cell Res. **41**, 677 (1966).

LANGLEY, J. N.: On nerve endings and on special excitable substances in cells. Croonian lecture. Proc. roy. Soc. B **78**, 170 (1906).

LANSING, A. T., LAMY, F.: Fine structure of cilia of rotifers. J. biophys. biochem. Cytol. **9**, 799 (1961).

LARRAMENDI, L. M. H., VICTOR, T.: Synapses on the Purkinje cell spines in the mouse: an electron microscopic study. Brain Res. **5**, 15 (1967).

LARSELL, O., McCRADY, E., LARSELL, J. F.: Development of the organ of Corti in relation to the inception of hearing. Arch. Otoloryng. **40**, 233 (1944).

LARSEN, J. R.: Fine structure of the interpseudotracheal papillae of the blowfly. Science **139**, 347 (1944).

LASANSKY, A., DE ROBERTIS, E.: Electron microscopy of retinal photoreceptors. J. biophys. biochem. Cytol. **7**, 493 (1960).

LASHKOV, V. F.: On the peripheral action of the ninth cranial nerve. Izv. Akad. Nauk SSSR, Otd. biol. nauk **3**, 25 (1945).

LAVDOVSKII, M. D.: Histology of the terminal apparatus of the cochlear nerve. Part 1, Dissertation, St. Petersburg 1874a.

LAVDOVSKII, M. D.: Histology of the terminal apparatus of the cochlear nerve. Part 2. Physiological section, conclusions and method of investigation, St. Petersburg 1874b.

LAVERTI, R., MICHAELSON, J. A., SHARMAN, D. F., WHITTAKER, V. P.: The subcellular localization of dopamine and acetylcholine in the dog caudate nucleus. Brit. J. Pharmacol. **21**, 482 (1963).

LAWRENCE, M.: Some physiological factors in inner ear deafness. Ann. Otol. (St. Louis) **69**, 480 (1960).

LAWRENCE, P., KRAUSE, F. B.: Annelid's ciliary photoreceptors. Science **148**, 965 (1965).

LAZAREV, P. P.: Issledovaniya po ionnoi teorii vozbuzhdeniya (Research on the Ionic Stimulation Theory). Moscow 1916.

LAZAREV, P. P.: The theory of gustatory adaptation and its experimental study. Izv. fiziol. inst. **1**, 39 (1920).

LAZAREV, P. P.: Ionnaya teoriya vozbuzhdeniya (Ionic Stimulation Theory). Moscow—Leningrad 1923.

LEBEDINSKII, A. V.: Dynamics of the coordination act in the sensory sphere. Fiziol. Zh. SSSR **19**, 945 (1935).

LEBOUCQ, G.: Contribution à l'étude de l'histogenèse de la rétine chez les mammifères. Arch. Anat. micr. Morph. exp. **16**, 556 (1909).

LEDOUX, A.: Réponses électriques de l'ampoule du canal semi-circulaire à la stimulation calorique. Acta oto-laryngol. (Stockh.) **46**, 290 (1956).

LEHRER, C. M., ORNSTEIN, L.: A diazo coupling method for the electron microscopic localization of cholinesterase. J. biophys. biochem. Cytol. **6**, 399 (1959).

LEIBSON, L. G., VINNIKOV, YA. A., ZHELUDKOVA, Z. P.: Glycogen of the organ of Corti under conditions of relative rest and the effect of sound. Biokhimiya **26**, 70 (1961).

LENINGER, A.: Mitokhondriya (Mitochondria). Moscow: Izd. Mir 1966.

LENTZ, T. L., BARRNETT, R. J.: Fine structure of the nervous system of *Hydra*. Amer. Zool. **5**, 341 (1965).

LEPLAT, G., GEREBTZOFF, M. A.: Localization de l'acétylcholinesterase et des médiateurs diphénoliques dans la rétine. Ann. Oculist. (Paris) **182**, 121 (1956).

LETTVIN, J. Y., GESTELAND, R. G.: Speculation on smell. Cold Spr. Harb. Symp. quant. Biol. **30**, 217 (1965).

LETTVIN, J. Y., PLATT, T. R., WALD, G., BROWN, K. T.: General discussion: Early receptor potential Cold Spr. Harb. Symp. quant. Biol. **30**, 501 (1965).

LEVETEAU, J., MACLEOD, P.: Olfactory discrimination in the rabbit olfactory glomerulus. Science **153**, 175 (1966).

LEVI, R., MAYNERT, E. W.: The subcellular localization of brain-stem norepinephrine and 5-hydroxy-tryptamine in stressed rats. Biochem. Pharmacol. **13**, 615 (1964).

LEWIS, R. P., SHUTE, C. D., SILVER, A.: Confirmation from choline acetylase analyses of a massive cholinergic innervation to the rat hippocampus. J. Physiol. (Lond.) **191**, 215 (1967).

LEYDIG, F.: Über die Haut einiger Süsswasserfische. Z. wissensch. Zool. **3**, 1 (1851).

LIBERMAN, R.: Retinal cholinesterases and glycolysis in rats raised in darkness. Science **135**, 372 (1962).

LINNANE, A. W.: The protein synthesizing system of *Saccharamyces cerevisiae*. Mitochondria and aspects of its genetic control. In: Seventh Internat. Congr. of Biochem., p. 219. Tokyo: Science Council 1967.

LOBANOVA, N. V., RAUTIN, G. N., SPERANSKAYA, N. I.: Spectral characteristics of color vision. Biofizika **8**, 502 (1963).

LOMONOSOV, M. V.: Kurs istinnoi fizicheskoi khimii (Course of Pure Physic Chemistry, 1752—1757). In: Izbr. filosof. soch., Moscow: SOVEKTIZ, 1940.

LOMONOSOV, M. V.: A word on the origin of light, which represent a new theory of colours St. Petersburg 1756.

DE LORENZO, A. J.: The fine structure of synapses in the ciliary ganglion of the chick. J. biophys. biochem. Cytol. **7**, 31 (1960).

DE LORENZO, A. J.: Studies on the ultrastructure and histophysiology of cell membrane, nerve fibres and synaptic junctions in chemoreceptors. In: Olfaction and Taste, I, p. 5. Oxford: Pergamon Press 1963.

LOWENSTEIN, O.: Peripheral mechanisms of equilibrium. Brit. med. Bull. **12**, 114 (1956).

LOWENSTEIN, O., OSBORNE, M. R., THORNHILL, R.: The anatomy and ultrastructure of the labyrinth of the lamprey *(Lampetra fluviatilis L.)*. Proc. roy. Soc. B **170**, 113 (1968).

LOWENSTEIN, O., OSBORNE, M. P., WERSÄLL, J.: Structure and innervation of the sensory epithelia of the labyrinth in the thornback ray *(Raja clavata)*. Proc. roy. Soc. B **178**, 1 (1964).

LOWENSTEIN, O., ROBERTS, T. D. M.: Oscillographic analysis of the gravity and vibration responses from the labyrinth of the thornback ray *(Raja clavata)*. Nature **162**, 852 (1948).

LOWENSTEIN, O., ROBERTS, T. D. M.: The equilibrium function of the otolith organs of the thornback ray *(Raja clavata)*. J. Physiol. (Lond.) **110**, 392 (1949).

LOWENSTEIN, O., ROBERTS, T. D. M.: The localization and analysis of the responses to vibration from the isolated elasmobranch labyrinth. A contribution to the problem of the evolution of hearing in vertebrates. J. Physiol. (Lond.) **114**, 471 (1951).

LOWENSTEIN, O., SAND, A.: The individual and integrated activity of the semicircular canals of the elasmobranch labyrinth. J. Physiol. (Lond.) **99**, 89 (1940).

LOWENSTEIN, O., WERSÄLL, J.: Functional interpretation of the electron microscopic structure of the sensory hairs in the crista of the elasmobranch *Raja clavata* in terms of directional sensitivity. Nature **184**, 1807 (1959).

LOWNDES, A. G.: The swimming of *Monas stigmatica* (Pringsheim) and *Peranema trichophorum* (Ehrbg.) Stein and *Volvox* sp. Additional experiments on the working of a flagellum. Proc. zool. Soc. (Lond.) **114**, 325 (1945).

LUCK, D.: The biogenesis of mitochondria in *Neurospora*. In: Seventh Internat. Congr. of Biochem., Abstr. 11, p. 217. Tokyo: Science Council 1967.

LUCY, J. A.: Globular lipid micelles and cell membranes. J. theor. Biol. 7, 360 (1964).

LUKASHEVICH, T. P.: Change in the activity of oxidizing enzymes in photoreceptors of vertebrates under different illumination conditions. Dokl. Akad. Nauk SSSR 145, 669 (1962).

LUKASHEVICH (TSIRULIS), T. P.: Localization and activity of dehydrases in mitochondria of photoreceptor ellipsoids of vertebrates. Dokl. Akad. Nauk SSSR 156, 1436 (1964).

LUKASHEVICH (TSIRULIS), T. P.: Electron microscopic study of mitochondria of photoreceptor ellipsoids in light and darkness. Tsitologiya 8, 90 (1966).

MACNICHOL, E. E., jr.: Visual receptors as biological transducers. In: Molecular Structure and Functional Activity of Nerve Cells, p. 34. Washington: Amer. Biol. Soc. 1956.

MADDY, A. H.: The chemical organization of the plasma membrane of animal cells. Int. Rev. Cytol. 20, 1 (1966).

MAGNUS, R.: Körperstellung. Experimentelle physiologische Untersuchungen über die einzelnen, bei der Körperstellung in Tätigkeit tretenden Reflexe, über ihr Zusammenwirken und ihre Störungen. Berlin: Springer 1924.

MAGNUS, R.: Ustanovka tela. Eksperimental'no-fiziologicheskoe issledovanie otdelnykh opredelyayushchikh ustanovku tela refleksov, ikh vzaimnykh vliyanii i ikh rastroistv (Positioning of the Body. Experimental Physiological Study of Individual Reflexes Determining the Position of the Body and of their Mutual Interactions). Moscow—Leningrad: Izd. Akad. Nauk SSSR 1962.

MAKAROV, P. O.: Problemy mikrofiziologii nervnoi sistemy (Problems of the Microphysiology of the Nervous System). Moscow: Medgiz 1947.

MALYUKINA, G. A.: On the analyzer of the lateral line of fishes. Vopr. ikhtiol. 5, 3 (1955).

MANDELKERN, L.: Some fundamental molecular mechanisms of contractility in fibrous macromolecules. J. gen. Physicol. 50, 29 (1967).

MANGABEIRA-ALBERNAZ, P. L.: Histochemistry of the connective tissue of the cochlea. Laryngoscope (St. Louis) 71, 1 (1961).

MANN, J.: The Development of the Human Eye. Cambridge Univ. Press 1928.

MANTON, J.: Observations on the fine structure of the zoospore and young germling of *Stigeoclonium*. J. exp. Bot. 15, 399 (1964).

MANUKHIN, B. N.: Fiziologiya adrenoretseptorov (Physiology of Adrenoreceptors). Moscow: Izd. Nauka 1968.

MARTIN, A. R., PILAR, G.: Dual mode of synaptic transmission in the avian ciliary ganglion. J. Physiol. (Lond.) 168, 443 (1963a).

MARTIN, A. R., PILAR, G.: Transmission through the ciliary ganglion of the chick. J. Physiol. (Lond.) 168, 464 (1963b).

MARTINI, V.: Presenza di colinesterasi nelle perilimfa dell orecchio interno del piccione. Boll. Soc. ital. Biol. sper. 16, 70 (1941).

MARX, W. B., DOBELLE, W. H., MACNICHOL, E. F.: Visual pigments of single primate cones. Science 143, 1181 (1964).

MASHANSKII, V. F., MIRKIN, A. S.: On the nonuniform distribution of ATPase on the plasma membrane of mechanoreceptors in connection with the formation of stimulation. Dokl. Akad. Nauk SSSR 184, 1423 (1969).

MATSUSAKA, T.: Etude histochemique de la rétine: L'effet de l'acide iodactique sur la glycogène et l'acide nucléinique du segment interne des cellules visuelles de la rétine. Ann. Oculist. (Paris) 188, 1071 (1956).

MATSUSAKA, T.: ATPase activity in the ciliary rootlet of human retinal rods. J. Cell Biol. 33, 203 (1967).

MATTHEWS, R. G., HUBBARD, R., BROWN, P. K., WALD, G.: Tautomeric forms of metarhodopsin. J. gen. Physiol. 57, 215 (1963).

MATURANA, H., SPERLING, S.: Unidirectional response to angular acceleration recorded from the middle cristal nerve in the statocyst of *Octopus vulgaris*. Nature 197, 815 (1963).

MAYBEE (1939), quoted by MONCRIEFF, R. W. (1946).

MAZO, L. I.: The microphone effect of the cochlea as a method for studying the elaboration of the function of the auditory peripheral apparatus. Probl. fiziol. akustiki 3, 95 (1955).

MAZO, L. I.: Materials dealing with the study of the elaboration and mechanism of the auditory function of the inner ear (bioelectric investigations). Author's abstract of dissertation, Moscow 1958.

MAZOKHIN-PORSHNYAKOV, G. A.: Zrenie nasekomykh (Insect Vision). Moscow: Izd. Nauka 1965.

MAZOKHIN-PORSHNYAKOV, G. A., VISHNEVSKAYA, T. M., GOLUBTSOV, K. V., BOCHAROVA, O. I.: Vision of the large trans-Caspian termite *Anacanthotermes ahngerianus* Jacob (Insecta Isoptera), based on data from electrophysiological tests. Zool. Zh. **46**, 1668 (1967).

McCONNEL, D. G., SCARPELLI, D.: Rhodopsin: an enzyme. Science **139**, 848 (1963).

McCONNEL, D. G., TZAGOLOFF, A., McLENNAN, D. H., GREEN, D. E.: Studies on the electron transfer system. Formation of membranes by purified cytochrome oxidase. J. biol. Chem. **241**, 2373 (1966).

McCRADY, E., jr.: The embryology of the opossum. Amer. anat. mem. **16**, 1 (1938).

McCRADY, E., jr., WEVER, E. G., BRAY, C. W.: The development in the opossum. J. exp. Zool. **75**, 503 (1937).

McINDOO, N. E.: The auditory sense of the honey bee. J. comp. Neurol. **34**, 173 (1922).

McRAE, E. K.: The fine structure of sensory receptor processes in the auricular epithelium of the planarian, *Dugesia tigrina*. Z. Zellforsch. **82**, 479 (1967).

MERKEL, G., VON HARNACK, V. M.: Zur Feinstruktur des „Gehirns" und der Sinnesorgane von *Protodrilis rubropharyngeus* Jaegerstein (Archiannelidae) mit besonderer Berücksichtigung der neurosekretorischen Zellen. Z. Zellforsch. **81**, 222 (1967).

MERKLE, U.: Eine Methode zur morphologischen Erfassung der Ansprechgebiete in der Cochlea des Meerschweinchens. Z. Anat. Entwicklungs-Gesch. **117**, 504 (1953).

MERTON, H.: Versuche zur Geotaxis von *Paramaecium*. Arch. Protistenkunde **85**, 33 (1935).

MEYER ZUM GOTTESBERGE, A.: Autoradiographische Untersuchungen zum Stofftransport in der Cochlea des Meerschweinchens. Arch. Ohr.-, Nas.- u. Kehlk.-Heilk. **178**, 145 (1960).

MICHAELSON, J. A., WHITTAKER, V. P.: The subcellular localization of 5-hydroxytryptamine in guinea-pig brain. Biochem. Pharmacol. **12**, 203 (1963).

MIKHELSON, M. YA.: On the evolution of cholinoreceptors. In: Biokhimiya i funktsiya nervnoi sistemy (Biochemistry and Function of the Nervous System). Transactions of International Symposium, 24—28 September 1965, p. 215. Leningrad: Izd. Nauka 1967.

MIKHELSON, M. YA., ZEIMAL, E. V.: Cholinoreceptors. In: Farmakologiya, khimioterapevticheskie sredstva, toksikologiya, khemoretseptsiya (Pharmacology, Chemotherapeutic Preparations, Toxicology, Chemoreception), p. 7. Moscow: Izd. Itogi nauki, ser. biol. 1967.

MIKHELSON, M. YA., ZEIMAL, E. V.: Atsetilkholin. O molekulyarnom mekhanisme deistviya (Acetylcholine: Molecular Mechanism of Action). Leningrad: Izd. Nauka 1970.

MIKHELSON, M. YA., KHROMOV-BORISOV, N. V.: Chemical mechanism of the physiological action of acetylcholine as a basis for the search for new drugs. Zh. Vsesoyuzn. khim. obshch. im. D. I. Mendeleeva **9**, 418 (1964).

MILLER, D., GRANE, R. K.: The digestive function of the epithelium of the small intestine. I. An intracellular locus of disaccharide and sugar phosphate ester hydrolysis. Biochim. biophys. Acta (Amst.) **52**, 281 (1961).

MILLER, W. H.: Derivatives of cilia in the distal sense cells of the retina of *Pecten*. J. biophys. biochem. Cytol. **4**, 227 (1958).

MILLINGER, A. M.: The fine structure of ampullary electric receptors in *Ameiurus*. Proc. roy. Soc. B **160**, 345 (1964).

MIRKIN, A. S.: Certain characteristics of the structure of isolated mechanoreceptors (Pacini bodies). Dokl. Akad. Nauk SSSR **168**, 484 (1966a).

MIRKIN, A. S.: Resonance phenomena in isolated mechanoreceptors (Pacini bodies) during acoustic stimulation. Biofizika **11**, 638 (1966b).

MIRKIN, A. S.: Reaction of isolated mechanoreceptors (Pacini bodies) to the effect of acoustic pressure. Dokl. Akad. Nauk SSSR **170**, 227 (1966c).

MIRKIN, A. S., TUCHKOV, B. S., MASHANSKII, V. F.: Some characteristic features of the ultrastructure of Pacini bodies. Tsitologiya **9**, 563 (1967).

MITROFANOV, P. I.: Study of the development of vertebrate animals. Proiskhozhdenie nervov i zakladka bokovykh organov (Origin of Nerves and Establishment of Lateral-Line Organs). Warsaw 1892.

MITTELSTAEDT, H.: Physiologie des Gleichgewichtssinnes bei fliegenden Libellen. Z. vergl. Physiol. **32**, 422 (1950).

MIZUKOSHI, O., KONISHI, T., NAKAMURA, F.: Physicochemical process in the hair cells of the organ of Corti. Ann. Otol. (St. Louis) **66**, 106 (1957).

MONCRIEFF, R. W.: The Chemical Senses. New York 1946.

MONCRIEFF, R. W.: The Chemical Senses (2nd ed.). London 1951.

MONCRIEFF, R. W.: An instrument for measuring and classifying odours. J. appl. Physiol. **16**, 742 (1961).

MOODY, M. E., PARRISS, J. R.: The discrimination of polarized light by *Octopus*: a behavioural and morphological study. Z. vergl. Physiol. **44**, 268 (1961).

MOODY, M. F., ROBERTSON, J. D.: The fine structure of some retinal photoreceptors. J. biophys. biochem. Cytol. **7**, 87 (1960).

MORITA, H., YAMASHITA, S.: Generator potential in insect chemoreceptor. Science **130**, 922 (1959).

MORTON, R. A., PITT, G. A. J.: Studies on rhodopsin: pH and the hydrolysis of indicator yellow. Biochem. J. **59**, 128 (1955).

MOULTON, D. G., BEIDLER, L. M.: Structure and function in the peripheral olfactory system. Physiol. Rev. **47**, 1 (1967).

MOUNTFORD, S.: Filamentous organelles in receptor-bipolar synapses of the retina. J. Ultrastruct. Res. **10**, 207 (1964).

MOZELL, M. M.: Olfactory discriminations: electrophysiological spatiotemporal basis. Science **143**, 1336 (1964a).

MOZELL, M. M.: Evidence for sorption as a mechanisms of the olfactory analysis of vapours. Nature **203**, 1181 (1964b).

MÜHLETHALER, K.: Plant cell walls. In: The Cell, **II** (Eds. J. Brachet, A. E. Mirsky), p. 86. New York: Academic Press 1961.

MÜHLETHALER, K.: The ultrastructure of the plastid lamellae. In: Biochemistry of Chloroplasts, **I** (Ed. T. W. Goodwin), p. 49. New York: Acad. Press 1966.

MÜHLETHALER, K., FREY-WYSSLING, A.: Entwicklung und Struktur der Proplastiden. J. biophys. biochem. Cytol. **6**, 507 (1959).

MÜLLER, J.: Zur vergleichenden Physiologie des Gesichtsinnes des Menschen und der Tiere nebst einem Versuch über die Bewegung der Augen und über den menschlichen Blick. Leipzig: C. Cnobloch 1826.

MÜLLER, H.: Anatomisch-physiologische Untersuchung über die Retina bei Menschen und Wirbeltieren. Z. Wissensch. Zool. **8**, 1 (1886).

MULVANEY, B., HEITST, H.: Mapping of the rabbit olfactory sensory apparatus. Anat. Rec. **157**, 377 (1967).

MURRAY, R. G.: Cell types in rabbit taste buds. In: Olfaction and Taste, **III**. New York: Rockefeller Univ. Press 1969.

MURRAY, R. G., MURRAY, A.: The fine structure of·the taste bud of rhesus. Anat. Rec. **138**, 211 (1960).

MURRAY, R. G., MURRAY, A.: Fine structure of rabbit taste buds. In: VI. Internat. Congr. for Electron Micros., p. 485. Kyoto 1966.

MURRAY, R. G., MURRAY, A.: Fine structure· of taste buds of rabbit foliate papillae. J. Ultrastruct. Res. **19**, 327 (1967).

MURRAY, R. G., MURRAY, A., FUJIMOTO, S.: Fine structure of gustatory cells in rabbit taste buds. J. Ultrastruct. Res. **27**, 444 (1969).

MUSEBECK, K., SCHÄTZLE, W.: Histochemischer Nachweis proteingebundener Sulfhydryle in der Meerschweinchenschnecke. Arch. Ohr.-, Nas.- u. Kehlk.-Heilk. **180**, 579 (1962).

NACHIN, K. E.: Wave propagation along flagella. J. exp. Biol. **35**, 796 (1958).

NACHMANSON, D.: Chemical control in nervous activity. In: Acetylcholine in Hormones, Vol. **2** (Eds. Pincus, C., Thimann, K. V.). New York: Academic Press 1950.

NACHMANSON, D.: Chemical and molecular basis of nerve activity. New York: Acad. Press 1959.

NACHMANSON, D.: Chemical and molecular forces regulating the movement of ions. In the collection of works (Sbornik): Problemy evolyutsii funktsii i enzimokhimii protsessov vozbuzhdeniya (Problems of the Evolution of the Function and Enzyme Chemistry of Excitation Processes), p. 215. Moscow: Izd. Akad. Nauk SSSR 1961.

NACHMANSON, D.: Chemical regulation of excitable membranes during the course of electric activity. In the collection of works (Sbornik): Biokhimiya i funktsiya nervnoi sistemy (Biochemistry and Function of the Nervous System). Transactions of International Symposium, 24—28 September 1965, p. 168. Leningrad: Izd. Nauka 1967.

NADAKAVUKAREN, M. J.: Fine structure of negatively stained plant mitochondria. J. Cell Biol. **23**, 193 (1964).

NAFTALIN, L.: Some new proposals regarding acoustic transmission and transduction. In: Cold Spr. Harb. Symp. quant. Biol. **30**, 196 (1965).

NAKA, L., KUWABARA, M.: Two components from the compound eye of the crayfish. J. exp. Biol. **35**, 51 (1959).

NAKAI, Y., HILDING, O.: Adenosinetriphosphatase distribution in the organ of Corti. Histochemical study by light and electron microscopy. Acta oto-laryng. (Stockh.) **64**, 477 (1967).

NAKAI, Y., HILDING, O.: Cochlear development. Some electron microscopic observations of maturation of hair cells, spiral ganglion and Reissner's membrane. Acta oto-laryng. (Stockh.) **66**, 369 (1968).

NASONOV, D. N., RAVDONIK, K. S.: Reaction of isolated cross-striated frog muscles to audible sounds. Fiziol. Zh. SSSR **33**, 569 (1947).

NASONOV, D. N., RAVDONIK, K. S.: Direct effect of audible sounds on nerve cells of isolated spinal ganglions of the rabbit. Dokl. Akad. Nauk SSSR **71**, 985 (1950).

NASONOV, D. N., ROZENTAL, D. L.: Direct effect of audible sounds on the epithelium of renal ducts of the frog, Dokl. Akad. Nauk SSSR **41**, 1163 (1950).

NASS, S., NASS, M. N. K.: Intramitochondrial fibers with DNA characteristics. II. Enzymatic and other hydrolytic treatments. J. Cell Biol. **19**, 613 (1963).

NASU, H., APPONI, G., VIALE, G.: Histochemische Untersuchungen über oxydative Enzyme in der menschlichen Netzhaut. Z. Zellforsch. **56**, 188 (1962).

NATOCHIN, YU. V.: Effect of alcohols on water transport by the skin and bladder of the frog. Dokl. Akad. Nauk SSSR **182**, 1237 (1968).

NEIFAKH, A. A.: Utilization of inhibitors of nucleic metabolism in studying periods of morphogenetic functions of nuclei in the course of their development. In the collection of works (Sbornik): Kletochnaya differentsirovka i induktsionnye mekhanismy (Cellular Differentiation and Induction Mechanisms), p. 38. Moscow: Izd. Nauka 1965.

NEJAD, M. S.: Factors involved in the mechanism of stimulation of gustatory receptors and bare nerve endings on the tongue of the rat. Doct. thesis. Tallahassee 1961.

NELSON, L.: ATP—an energy source for sperm mobility. Biol. Bull. **115**, 326 (1958).

NEMETSCHEK-GANSLER, H., FERNER, H.: Über die Ultrastruktur der Geschmacksknospen. Z. Zellforsch. **63**, 155 (1964).

NEUBERT, K., WÜSTENFELD, E.: Ansprechgebiete im Innenohr. Naturwissenschaften **42**, 350 (1955).

NICKERSON, M.: Adrenergic receptor mechanisms. In: Pharmacology of Cholinergic and Adrenergic transmission, p. 303. Oxford: Pergamon Press 1965.

NIEMI, M., MERENMIES, K.: Cytochemical localization of the oxidative enzyme systems in the retina. I. Diaphorases and dehydrogenases. J. Neurochem. **6**, 200 (1961a).

NIEMI, M., MERENMIES, K.: Cytochemical localization of the oxidative enzyme systems in the retina. II. Cytochrome oxidase. J. Neurochem. **6**, 206 (1961b).

NILSSON, S. E. G.: An electron microscopic classification of the retinal receptors of the leopard frog *(Rana pipiens)*. J. Ultrastruct. Res. **10**, 390 (1964a).

NILSSON, S. E. G.: Receptor cell outer segment development and ultrastructure of the disk membranes in the retina of the tadpole *(Rana pipiens)*. J. Ultrastruct. Res. **11**, 581 (1964b).

NISHIOKA, R. S., HAGADORN, T. R., BERN, H. A.: Ultrastructure of the epistellar body of the octopus. Z. Zellforsch. **57**, 406 (1962).

NOFRE, C., SABADIE, J.: A propos de la protéine linguale dite "sensible aux sucres". C. R. Acad. Sci. **274**, 2913 (1972).

NOMURA, H., SAKADA, S.: On the "water response" of frog's tongue. Japan J. Physiol. **15**, 433 (1965).

O'BRIEN, J. S.: Cell membranes—composition, structure, function. J. theor. Biol. **15**, 307 (1967).

OCHI, J.: Elektronenmikroskopische Untersuchung des Bulbus olfactorius der Ratte während der Entwicklung. Z. Zellforsch. **76**, 839 (1967).

OERTLY, E., MYERS, R. G.: A new theory relating constitution to taste (preliminary paper). Simple relations between the constitution of aliphatic compounds and their sweet taste. J. Amer. chem. Soc. **41**, 855 (1919).

OKANO, M., SUGAWA, J.: Ultrastructure of the respiratory mucous epithelium of the canine nasal cavity. Arch. Histol. Jap. **26**, 1 (1965).

OKANO, M., WEBER, F., FROMMES, S. P.: Electron microscopic studies on the distal border of the canine olfactory epithelium. J. Ultrastruct. Res. **17**, 497 (1967).

ORBELI, L. A.: Physiology and psychology. Fiziol. Zh. SSSR **32** (1946).

ORBELI, L. A.: Basic tasks and methods of evolutionary physiology. In the collection of works (Sbornik): Evolyutsiya funktsii nervnoi sistemy (Evolution of the Function of the Nervous System), p. 7. Leningrad: Izd. Akad. Nauk SSSR 1958.

ORLOV, O. YU.: Color vision systems of vertebrates. Byull. MOIP, otd. biol. **68** (5), 133 (1963).

ORLOV, O. YU., BYZOV, A. L.: Calorimetric studies of the vision of cephalopod mollusks. Dokl. Akad. Nauk SSSR **139**, 723 (1961).

ORLOV, O. YU., MAKSIMOVA, E. M.: On the role of light filters located inside cones (mechanism of the color vision of the lizard and turtle). Dokl. Akad. Nauk SSSR **154**, 463 (1964).

ORMEROD, F. C.: The metabolism of the cochlear and vestibular end-organs. J. Laryng. **75**, 562 (1961).

OSTROVSKII, M. A.: Succinic dehydrogenase activity in the frog retina and variations of this activity under the influence of light. Zh. obshch. biol. **6**, 471 (1961a).

OSTROVSKII, M. A.: Localization of acetylcholinesterase in the frog retina. Zh. obshch. biol. **22**, 474 (1961b).

OSTROVSKII, M. A.: The problem of efferent influences on the retina of the frog eye. Biofizika **7**, 55 (1962).

OSTROVSKII, M. A.: Study of the electroparamagnetic resonance of frozen rhodopsin and retinene solutions. In: Svobodnoradikalnye protsessy v biologicheskikh sistemakh (Free-Radical Processes in Biological Systems), p. 37. Moscow: Abstracts of symposium reports 1964.

OSTROVSKII, M. A.: Study of certain links in the photoenzymatic chain of processes in photoreceptors. Biofizika **10**, 470 (1965).

OSTROVSKII, M. A., FEDOROVICH, I. B.: Enzymatic (ATPase) activity of digitonin extracts of rhodopsin (visual purple) and changes in this activity under the effect of external light. Dokl. Akad. Nauk SSSR **162**, 1992 (1965).

OSTROVSKII, M. A., FEDOROVICH, I. B., GOLUBEV, I. N.: Some aspects of the biophysics of photoreception. Biofizika **12**, 877 (1967).

OSTROVSKII, M. A., FEDOROVICH, I. B., DZHANSKAYA, M. G.: Investigation of primary processes of the photoreceptor act. In: Pervichnye protsessy v retseptornykh elementakh organov chuvstv (Primary Processes in Receptor Elements of Sense Organs), p. 21. Moscow—Leningrad: Izd. Nauka 1966.

OTTOSON, D.: Analysis of the electrical activity of the olfactory epithelium. Acta physiol. scand. **35**, Suppl. 122, 1 (1956).

OTTOSON, D.: Generation and transmission of signals in the olfactory system. In: Olfaction and Taste, I (Ed. Zottermann), p. 35. Oxford: Pergamon Press 1963.

PAK, W. L.: Some properties of the early electrical response in the vertebrate retina. Cold Spr. Harb. Symp. quant. Biol. **30**, 493 (1965).

PAK, W. L., CONE, R. A.: Isolation and identification of the initial peak of the early receptor potential. Nature **204**, 836 (1964).

PAK, W. L., EBREY, T. G.: Visual receptor potential observed at subzero temperatures. Nature **205**, 484 (1965).

PALADE, G. E.: An appraisal of current views on the structure of biological membranes. In: Seventh Internat. Congress of Biochem., p. 1077. Tokyo: Science Council 1967.

PALADE, G. E., PALAY, S. L.: Electron microscope observations of interneuronal and neuromuscular synapses. Anat. Rec. **118**, 335 (1954).

PALAY, S. L.: Synapses in the central nervous system. J. biophys. biochem. Cytol. **2** (Suppl.), 193 (1956).

PALAY, S. L.: The morphology of synapses in the central nervous system. Exp. Cell. Res., Suppl. **5**, 278 (1958).

PALAY, S. L., KARLIN, L. J.: An electron microscopic study of the intestinal villus. The fasting animal. J. biophys. biochem. Cytol. **5**, 363 (1958).

PAPPAS, G. D.: Morphological aspects of synaptic function. In: Fourth European Regional Conference on Electron Microscopy, Rome 1968, p. 531.

PAPPAS, G. D., BENNETT, M. V. L.: Specialized sites involved in electrical transmission between neurons. Ann. N. Y. Acad. Sci. **137**, 495 (1966a).

PAPPAS, G. D., BENNETT, M. V. L.: The fine structure of vesicles associated with excitatory and inhibitory junctions. Biol. Bull. **131**, 381 (1966b).

PARK, R. B.: Subunits of chloroplast structure and quantum conversion in photosynthesis. Int. Rev. Cytol. **20**, 67 (1966).

PARK, R. B., BIGGINS, J.: Quantasome: size and composition. Science **144**, 1009 (1964).

PARKER, G. H.: The movements of the swimming plates in ctenophores, with reference to the theories of ciliary metachronism. J. exp. Zool. **2**, 407 (1905).

PARKER, G. H., STABLER, E. M.: On certain distinctions between taste and smell. Amer. J. Physiol. **32**, 230 (1913).

PARKER, L., SIEGENTHALER, P. A.: Control of chloroplast structure by light. Int. Rev. Cytol. **20**, 97 (1966).

PAVLOV, I. P.: Twenty years of experience in the objective study of the higher nervous activity (behavior) of animals. Conditioned reflexes. Sbornik statei, dokladov, lektsii i rechi (Collection of reports, lectures, and speeches). Moscow—Leningrad: Gosizdat 1928.

PEARSE, A. G.: Intracellular localization of dehydrogenase systems using monotetrazolium salts and metal chelation of their formazans. J. Histochem. Cytochem. **5**, 515 (1957).

PEARSE, A. G.: Localization of oxidative enzymes in rat and chick retina in various physiological conditions. In: The Structure of the Eye, p. 53. New York: Academic Press 1961.

PEARSE, A. G.: Cytochemical localization of ubiquinones in the retina. Nature **205**, 708 (1965).

PEARSON, A. A.: The development of olfactory nerve in man. J. comp. Neurol. **75**, 199 (1941).

PEASE, D. C.: Demonstration of highly ordered pattern upon a mitochondrial surface. J. Cell Biol. **15**, 385 (1962).

PEASE, D. C.: The ultrastructure of flagellar fibrils. J. Cell Biol. **18**, 313 (1963).

PÉNARD, E.: Les Protozoaires considérés sous le rapport de leur perfection organique. Genève 1922.

PENN, R. D., HAGINS, W. A.: Signal transmission along retinal rods and the origin of the electroretinographic a-wave. Nature **223**, 201 (1969).

PESKIN, J. C., LOVE, B. B.: The reaction of L-cysteine with all-*trans*-retinene. Biochim. biophys. Acta (Amst.) **78**, 751 (1965).

VON PETERS, W.: Die Sinnesorgane an den Labellen von *Calliphora erythrocephala* Meig (Diptera). Z. Morphol. Ökol. Tiere **55**, 259 (1963).

PEVZNER, R. A.: Cytohistochemical studies of the taste buds of bony fish (Teleosts) *(Cyprinus carpio* and *Carassius carassius)*. Dokl. Akad. Nauk SSSR **147**, 1187 (1962).

PEVZNER, R. A.: Distribution of succinate-NST-reductase activity in the taste buds of vertebrates. Dokl. Akad. Nauk SSSR **155**, 191 (1964a).

PEVZNER, R. A.: Distribution of acetylcholinesterase activity in the taste buds of vertebrates. Dokl. Akad. Nauk SSSR **155**, 930 (1964b).

PEVZNER, R. A.: Comparative histochemical study of taste buds in vertebrates. Author's abstract of dissertation, Leningrad 1964c.

PEVZNER, R. A.: Cytochemical organization of taste buds in vertebrates. In the collection of works (Sbornik): Pervichnye protsessy v retseptornykh elementakh organov chuvstv (Primary Processes in Receptor Elements of Sense Organs), p. 144. Moscow—Leningrad: Izd. Nauka 1966.

PEVZNER, R. A.: Structural and cytochemical bases of the mechanism of the function of taste buds. Usp. sovrem. Biol. **67**, 53 (1969).

PEVZNER, R. A.: Electron microscopic study of receptor and sustentacular cells in the taste bud of the frog *Rana temporaria*. Tsitologiya **12**, 971 (1970).

PFAFFMANN, C.: Gustatory afferent impulses. J. cell. comp. Physiol. **17**, 243 (1941).

PFAFFMANN, C.: Gustatory nerve impulses in rat, cat and rabbit. J. Neurophysiol. **18**, 429 (1955).

PHILIPPOT, E., GEREBTZOFF, M. A.: Nouvelles recherches sur les lipides de la muqueuse olfactive. J. Physiol. (Paris) **48**, 683 (1956).

PHILIPPOT, E., GEREBTZOFF, M. A.: First results of the analysis of the olfactive pigment. J. Physiol. (Paris) **50**, 451 (1958).

PHILLIPS, D.: Three-dimensional structure of an enzyme molecule. In: Molekuly i kletki (Molecules and Cells), Vol. 3, p. 9. Moscow: Izd. Mir 1968.

PICK, H. L., KARE, M. R.: The effect of extraneous cues on the measurement of taste preference in the chicken. J. comp. physiol. Psychol. **55**, 342 (1962).

PLOTZ, E., PERLMAN, H. B.: A histochemical study of the cochlea. Laryngoscope (St. Louis) **65**, 291 (1955).

PLUZHNIKOV, M. S., YANTAREVA, L. J.: Changes of acetylcholin content in the inner ear lymph following sound stimulation. Fiziolog. Zh. SSSR **57**, 988 (1971).

POINCELOT, R. P., MILLER, P. G., KIMBEL, R. L., jr., ABRAHAMSON, E. W.: Lipid to protein chromophore transfer in the photolysis of visual pigments. Nature **221**, 256 (1969).

POLIKAR, A., BO, SH. A.: Submikroskopicheskie struktury kletok i tkanei v norme i patologii, ikh fiziologicheskoe i patogeneticheskoe znachenie (Submicroscopic Structures of Cells and Tissues under Normal and Pathological Conditions, and their Physiological and Pathogenetic Significance). Leningrad: Medgiz 1962.

POLYAK, S. L.: The Retina. Chicago: University of Chicago Press 1941.

DE PONT, I. I. H. H. M., DAEMEN, F. I. H., BONTING, S. K.: Biochemical aspects of visual process. II. Schiff base formation in phosphatidylethanolamine monolayers upon penetration by retinaldehyde. Biochim. biophys. Acta (Amst.) **3**, 204 (1968).

POPOV, A. V.: Electrophysiological study of the properties of peripheral neurons in the auditory system of the locust. Zh. evolyuts. biokhim. fiziol. **1**, 239 (1965).

POPOV, A. V.: Comparative study of communication sound signals and of certain principles in the organization of the auditory system of cicadas and orthopterans, Tr. Vsesoyuzn. entom. obshch. In: Sovremennye problemy struktury i funktsii nervnoi sistemy nasekomykh (Contemporary Problems of the Structure and Function of the Nervous System of Insects), p. 182. Leningrad: Izd. Nauka 1969.

PORSONS, D.: Negative staining of thinly spread cells and associated virus. J. Cell Biol. **16**, 620 (1963).

PORTER, K. R.: The ground substance: observations from electron microscopy. In: The Cell, Vol. **2** (Eds. J. Brachet, A. Mirsky), p. 621. New York—London: Academic Press 1961.

PORTER, K. R., YAMADA, E.: Studies on the endoplasmic reticulum. V. Its form and differentiation in pigment epithelial cells of the frog retina. J. biophys. biochem. Cytol. **8**, 181 (1960).

PORTUGALOV, V. V.: Ocherki gistofiziologii nervnykh okonchanii (Outlines of the Histophysiology of Nerve Endings). Moscow: Medgiz 1955.

POST, C. T., GOLDSMITH, T. H.: Pigment migration and light adaptation in the eye of the moth, *Galleria mellonella*. Biol. Bull. **128**, 473 (1965).

PRATT, D. C., LIVINGSTON, R., GRELLMAN, K. H.: Flash photolysis of rod particle suspensions. Photochemistry Photobiology **3**, 121 (1964).

PRINGLE, J. W. S.: Physiology of song in cicadas. Nature **172**, 248 (1953).

PRINGLE, J. W. S.: The proprioceptive background to mechanisms of orientation. Erg. Biol. **26**, 1 (1963).

PROSSER, A. P., BROWN, F.: Sravnitel'naya fiziologiya zhivotnykh (Comparative Animals Physiology). Moscow: Izd. Mir 1967.

QUATTRINI, D.: Osservazioni preliminari sulla ultrastruttura delle statocisti dei molluschi gastropodi pulmonati. Boll. Soc. ital. Biol. sper. **43**, 785 (1967a).

QUATTRINI, D.: Alcuni dati morfologici e ultrastrutturali sulla statocisti di *Helix aspersa* Müller (Mollusca Gastropoda Pulmonata). Boll. di Zoologia **34**, 160 (1967b).

RABINOVITCH, M., MOTA, J., YONEDA, S.: Note on histochemical localisation of glycogen and pentose polynucleotides in the visual cells of chick *(Gallus gallus)*. Quart. J. micr. Sci. **95**, 5 (1954).

RAMON Y CAJAL, S.: La rétine des vertébrés. La cellule **9**, 119 (1893).

RASMUSSEN, G. L.: An efferent cochlear bundle. Anat. Rec. **82**, 441 (1946).

RASMUSSEN, G. L.: Further observations of the efferent cochlear bundle. J. comp. Neurol. **99**, 61 (1953).

RASMUSSEN, G. L.: Efferent fibers of the cochlear nerve and cochlear nucleus. In: Neural Mechanisms Auditory and Vestibular Systems (Eds. G. L. Rasmussen, W. F. Windle), p. 105. Springfield/Ill.: Ch. C. Thomas 1960.

RASMUSSEN, G. L., GAČEK, R.: Concerning the question of an efferent fiber component of the vestibular nerve of the cat (Abstract). Anat. Rec. **130**, 361 (1958).

RAUCH, S.: Die Rolle der Elektrolyte zum Hörvorgang. Arch. Ohr.-, Nas.- u. Kehlk.-Heilk. **178**, 126 (1961).

RAUCH, S.: Biochemie des Hörorganes. Stuttgart: Thieme 1964.

RAVIOLA, E., RAVIOLA, Y.: Recherches histochimiques sur la rétine du lapin au cours de son développement post-natal. 2, Groupes-SH et activité acétylcholinesterasique. In: I. Congr. Int. Histochimie et Cytochimie. Paris: Nouvelle Faculté de Medicine, Sect. **21**, 59 (1960).

RAZIN, S., ROTTANA, S., RODWELL, A.: Disaggregation and reassembly of mycoplasma membranes. In: Seventh. Internat. Congr. of Biochem., Abstract II, 327. Tokyo: Science Council 1967.

REESE, T. S.: Olfactory cilia in the frog. J. Cell Biol. **25**, 209 (1965).

RENQUIST, I.: Über den Geschmack. Skand. Arch. Physiol. **38**, 97 (1919).

RETZIUS, G.: Das Gehörorgan der Wirbeltiere. I. Das Gehörorgan der Fische und Amphibien. Stockholm 1881.

RETZIUS, G.: Das Gehörorgan der Wirbeltiere. II. Das Gehörorgan der Vögel und der Säugetiere. Stockholm 1884.

RHODIN, J.: Correlation of ultrastructure and function in normal and experimental changed proximal tubule cells of the mouse kidney. Stockholm: Karolinska Institute 1954.

RHODIN, J.: Anatomy of kidney tubules. Int. Rev. Cytol. **7**, 485 (1958).

RIDDIFORD, L. M.: Antennal proteins of Saturniid moth—their possible role in olfaction. J. Insect Physiol. **16**, 653 (1970).

DE ROBERTIS, E.: Morphogenesis of the retinal rods. An electron microscopic study. J. biophys. biochem. Cytol. **2**, Suppl., 209 (1956).

DE ROBERTIS, E.: Submicroscopic morphology and function of synapse. Exp. Cell. Res. Suppl. **5**, 347 (1958).

DE ROBERTIS, E.: Histophysiology of synapses and neurosecretion. London: Pergamon Press 1964.

DE ROBERTIS, E.: Ultrastructure and cytochemistry of the synaptic region. Science **156**, 907 (1967).

DE ROBERTIS, E.: Isolation and biochemical nature of receptors in the CNS. In: Second International Meeting of the Society for Neurochemistry. Eds. R. Paoletti, R. Fumagalli, and C. Galli, p. 32. Milano: Tamburinied 1969.

DE ROBERTIS, E.: Ultrastructure and cytochemistry of central synapses. Ninth International Congress of Anatomists, Leningrad 1970, p. 42.

DE ROBERTIS, E.: Ultrastructure and cytochemistry of the central synapses. Arkh. Anat. Gistol. Embriol. **60**, 14 (1971).

DE ROBERTIS, E., BENNETT, U. S.: Some features of submicroscopic morphology of synapses in frog and earthworm. J. biophys. biochem. Cytol. **1**, 47 (1955).

DE ROBERTIS, E., FRANCHI, C. N.: Electron microscopic observations on synaptic vesicles in synapses of the retinal rods and cones. J. biophys. biochem. Cytol. **2**, 307 (1956).

DE ROBERTIS, E., DE IRALDI, A. P.: Plurivesicular secretory processes and nerve endings in the pineal gland of the rat. J. biophys. biochem. Cytol. **10**, 361 (1961).

DE ROBERTIS, E., DE IRALDI, A. P., DE LORES, R. A., SALGANNICOFF, L.: Electron microscope observations on nerve endings isolated from rat brain. Anat. Rec. **139**, 220 (1961).

DE ROBERTIS, E., DE IRALDI, A. P., DE LORES, G. R., SALGANICOFF, L.: Cholinergic and noncholinergic nerve ending in brain. J. Neurochem. **9**, 23 (1962).

DE ROBERTIS, E., DE IRALDI, A. P., RODRIGEZ, C., GOMEZ, G. I.: On the isolation of nerve endings and synaptic vesicles. J. biophys. biochem. Cytol. **9**, 229 (1960).

DE ROBERTIS, E., LASANSKY, A.: Submicroscopic organization of retinal cones of the rabbit. J. biophys. biochem. Cytol. **4**, 743 (1958).

ROBERTS, E. (Ed.): Inhibition in the nervous system and gammaaminobutiric acid. New York: Pergamon Press 1960.

ROBERTS, E.: Synaptic neurochemistry: some assumptions. In: Biokhimiya i funktsiya nervnoi sistemy (Biochemistry and Function of the Nervous System). Proceedings of International Symposium, 24—28 September 1965, p. 60. Leningrad: Izd. Nauka 1967.

ROBERTSON, J. D.: The ultrastructure of cell membranes and their derivatives. Biochem. Soc. Symposia **16**, 3 (1959).

ROBERTSON, J. D.: The molecular structure and contact relationships of cell membranes. In: Progress in Biophysics **10**. Oxford: Pergamon Press 1960a.

ROBERTSON, J. D.: Electron microscopy of the motor endplate and the neuromuscular spindle. Amer. J. phys. Med. **39**, 1 (1960b).

ROBERTSON, J. D.: Unit membranes: A review with recent new studies of experimental alterations and a new subunit structure in synaptic membranes. In: Cellular Membranes in Development (Ed. M. Lock), Vol. I. New York: Academic Press 1964.

ROBERTSON, J. D.: Design principles of the unit membranes. In: Principles of Biomolecular Organisation. Ciba Foundation Symposium (Eds. G. E. W. Walsenholme, M. O'Connor), p. 357. Boston: Little Brown 1966.

ROBERTSON, J. D.: Origin of the unit membrane concept. Protoplasma (Wien) **63**, 218 (1967).

RODRIGUEZ-ECHANDIA, E. L.: An electron microscopic study on the cochlear innervation. I. The receptoneural junctions of the outer hair cells. Z. Zellforsch. **78**, 30 (1967).

RODRIGUEZ-ECHANDIA, E. L.: An electron microscopic study on the cochlear innervation. II. The intraepithelial nerve fibers, the neuro-neural synapses and the recepto-neural junctions at the inner hair cell. Z. Zellforsch. **85**, 183 (1968).

ROGGEN, D. R., RASKI, D. J., JONES, N. O.: Cilia in nematode sensory organs. Science **152**, 515 (1966).

RÖHLICH, P.: Fine structural changes induced in photoreceptors by light and prolonged darkness. In: Symposium on Neurobiology of Invertebrates, p. 95. Budapest: Acad. Kiado 1967.

RÖHLICH, P., TAR, E.: The effect of prolonged light deprivation on the fine structure of planarian photoreceptors. Z. Zellforsch. **90**, 507 (1968).

RÖHLICH, P., TÖRÖK, L. I.: Die Feinstrukturen des Auges der Weinbergschnecke *(Helix pomatia* L.). Z. Zellforsch. **60**, 348 (1963).

ROMANOV, S. N.: Reaction of cells in the organism to sounds from an explosion. Fiziol. Zh. SSSR **40**, 1 (1954).

RÖNSCH, G.: Entwicklungsgeschichtliche Untersuchungen zur Zelldifferenzierung am Flügel der Trichoptera, *Limmophilus flavicornis*. Fabr. Z. Morphol. Ökol. Tiere **43**, 1 (1954).

ROSENBAUM, H.: Über den Schwellenwert des sauren Geschmacks. Pflügers Arch. ges. Physiol. **208**, 730 (1925).

ROSENBERG, B., MISRA, T., SWITZER, R.: Mechanism of olfactory transduction. Nature **217**, 423 (1968).

ROSSI, G.: L'acéthylcholinesterase en cours du development de l'oreille interne du cobaye. Acta oto-laryng. (Stockh.) **170**, 1 (1961).

ROSSI, G.: L'innervation efferente des recepteurs vestibulaires. Acta oto-laryng. (Stockh.) **58**, 230 (1964).

ROSSI, G., CORTESINA, G.: Le fibre nervose efferenti cochleari e vestibulari; nuove acquisizioni e conoscenze. Ann. Laring. (Torino) **61**, 296 (1962 a).

ROSSI, G., CORTESINA, G.: The efferent innervation of the inner ear. Panminerva med. **4**, 478 (1962 b).

ROSSI, G., CORTESINA, G.: Research on the efferent innervation of the inner ear. J. Laryng. **77**, 202 (1963).

ROSSI, G., VOENA, G., BUONGIOVANNI, S., CORTESINA, G.: Experimental studies on the local effects of acetylcholine, anticholinergic substances and cholinesterase inhibitors on vestibular function. Acta oto-laryng. (Stockh.) **58**, 159 (1964).

ROTH, L. M.: A study of mosquito behavior. An experimental laboratory study of sexual behavior of *Aedes aegypti* (Linnaeus). Amer. Midl. Nat. **40**, 265 (1948).

ROUILLER, C., FAURÉ-FREMIET, E.: L'ultrastructure des trichocystes fusiformes de *Froutonia atra*. Bull. Micr. appl. **7**, 135 (1957).

RUBIN, M., APOTHEKER, D., LUTMER, R.: The stereochemical theory of olfaction. 3. Structure and odour: 1,4-cyclohexane lactones and related compounds. Proc. Sci. Sect., Toilet Goods Assn. Special Suppl. **37**, 24 (1962).

RUEDI, L., FURRER, W.: Das akustische Trauma. Basel: Karger 1947.

RUPPERT, A., MOUSHEGIAN, G., CALAMBOS, R.: Microelectrode studies of primary vestibular neurons in cat. Exp. Neurol. **5**, 100 (1962).

RUSHTON, W. A. H.: Excitation pools in the frog's retina. J. Physiol. (Lond.) **149**, 327 (1959).

RUSHTON, W. A. H.: The sensitivity of rods under illumination. J. Physiol. (Lond.) **178**, 141 (1965).

SABATINI, D. C., BENSCH, K., BARRNETT, R. J.: Cytochemistry and electron microscopy. The preservation of cellular ultrastructure and enzymatic activity by aldehyde fixation. J. Cell Biol. **17**, 1 (1963).

SAGER, R., PALADE, G. E.: Structure and development of the chlorophast in chlamydomonas. J. Biophys. Biochem. Cytol. **3**, 463 (1957).

SALA, O.: Modifications of the vestibular nerve activity by stimulation of the efferent vestibular system. Experientia (Basel) **19**, 39 (1963).

SAMSONOVA, V. G.: Light and discriminatory sensitivity related to the area, intensity and site of stimulation of the retina. Probl. fiziol. optiki, Izd. Akad. Nauk SSSR **9**, 134 (1950).

SAND, A.: The mechanism of the lateral-line sense organs of fishes. Proc. roy. Soc. B **123**, 472 (1937).

SATIR, P.: On the evolutionary stability of the 9+2 pattern. J. Cell Biol. **12**, 181 (1962).

SATIR, P.: Filament–matrix interaction during ciliary movement: inferences drawn from electron microscopy of the distal end of the ciliary shaft of lamellibranch gill cilia. J. Cell Biol. **23**, 82 (1964).

SATIR, P.: Morphological aspects of ciliary motility. J. gen. Physiol. **50**, 241 (1967).

SATIR, P.: Studies on cilia. III. Further studies on the cilium tip and a "sliding filament" model of ciliary motility. J. Cell Biol. **39**, 77 (1968).

SATO, M., KUSANO, K.: Electrophysiology of gustatory receptors. In: Electr. Activity of Single Cells, p. 77. Tokyo: Igakushoin, Hongo 1960.

SAXEN, L.: The glycogen inclusions of the visual cells and its hypothetical role in the photomechanical responses. Acta anat. (Basel) **25**, 319 (1955).

SCALZI, H. A.: The cytoarchitecture and cytochemistry of gustatory receptors in the rabbit foliate papillae (Abst.). Anat. Rec. **154**, 486 (1966).

SCALZI, H. A.: The cytoarchitecture of gustatory receptors from the rabbit foliate papillae. Z. Zellforsch. **80**, 413 (1967).

SCARPELLI, D. C., CRAIG, E. L.: The fine localization of nucleoside triphosphatase activity in the retina of the frog. J. Cell Biol. **17**, 279 (1963).

SCHATZ, G., HASLBRUNNER, E., TUPPY, H.: Deoxyribonucleic acid associated with yeast mitochondria. Biochem. biophys. Res. Commun. **15**, 127 (1964).

SCHERAGA, H. A.: Contractility and conformation. J. gen. Physicol. **50**, 5 (1967).

SCHIMPER, A. F. W.: Untersuchungen über die Chlorophyllkörper und die ihnen homologen Gebilde. Jahrb. Wiss. Bot. **16**, 1 (1885).

SCHMIDT, W. J.: Doppelbrechung, Dichroismus und Feinbau der Sehzellen vom Frosch. Z. Zellforsch. **22**, 485 (1935).

SCHMIDT, W. J.: Der Einfluss von Kaliumpermanganat auf die Doppelbrechung der Markscheide der Nervenfasern und der Aussenglieder der Sehzellen. Z. Zellforsch. **23**, 261 (1936a).

SCHMIDT, W. J.: Doppelbrechung und Feinbau der Markscheide der Nervenfasern. Z. Zellforsch. **23**, 657 (1936a).

SCHMIDT, W. J.: Polarisationsoptische Analyse eines Eiweiss-Lipoid-Systems erläutert am Aussenglied der Sehzellen. Kolloidzschr. **84**, 137 (1938).

SCHNEIDER, W.: Über den Erschütterungssinn von Käfern und Fliegen. Z. vergl. Physiol. **32**, 287 (1950).

SCHNEIDER, D.: Elektrophysiologische Untersuchungen von Chemo- und Mechanoreceptoren der Antenne des Seidenspinners *Bombyx mori*. Z. vergl. Physiol. **40**, 8 (1957a).

SCHNEIDER, D.: Electrophysiological investigation of the antennal receptors of the silk moth during chemical and mechanical stimulation. Experientia (Basel) **13**, 89 (1957b).

SCHNEIDER, D.: Microelectrodes record electrical impulses in individual sensory nerve cells of a moth's antenna. Phil. Serv. Sci. Ind. **4**, 92 (1957c).

SCHNEIDER, D.: Electrophysiological investigation on the olfactory specificity of sexual attracting substances in different species of moth. J. Insect Physiol. **8**, 15 (1962).

SCHNEIDER, D., LACHER, V., KAISSLING, K. E.: Die Reaktionsweise und das Reaktionsspektrum von Riechzellen bei *Antheraea pernyi* (Lepidoptera, Saturniidae). Z. vergl. Physiol. **48**, 632 (1964).

SCHNAITMAN, C., GREENWALT, J. W.: Enzymatic properties of the inner and outer membranes of rat liver mitochondria. J. Cell Biol. **38**, 158 (1968).

SCHOEN, L.: Mikroabteilungen einzelner zentraler Vestibularis-Neurone von Knochenfischen bei Statolithenreizen. Z. vergl. Physiol. **39**, 399 (1957).

SCHÖNE, H., STEINBRECHT, R. A.: Fine structure of statocyst receptor of *Astacus fluviatilis*. Nature **220**, 184 (1968).

SCHUKNECHT, H., CHURCHILL, J. A., DORAN, R.: The localization of acetylcholinesterase in the cochlea. Arch. Otolaryng. **69**, 549 (1959).

SCHULTZE, E.: Über die becherförmigen Organe der Fische. Z. wiss. Zool. **12**, 222 (1862).

SCHULTZE, M.: Über die Endigungsweise der Geruchsnerven und das Epithelialgewebe der Nasenschleimhaut. Mschr. Berl. Akad. Wiss. **504** (1856).

SCHULTZE, M.: Über die Endigungsweise des Hörnerven im Labyrinth. Müllers Arch. 343 (1858).

SCHULTZE, M.: Zur Anatomie und Physiologie der Retina. Arch. mikr. Anat. **2**, 175 (1866).

SCHULTZE, M.: Die Stäbchen in der Retina der Cephalopoden. Arch. mikr. Anat. **5**, 1 (1869).

SCHWALBE, G.: Über die Geschmacksorgane der Säugetiere und des Menschen. Arch. mikr. Anat. **4**, 154 (1867).

SCHWALBE, J.: Beiträge zur Morphologie und Histologie der tympanalen Sinnesapparate der Ortho-pteren. Zoologica (Stuttg.) **50**, 1 (1906).

SCHWARTZKOPFF, J.: Morphological and physiological properties of the auditory system in birds. In: Proc. 13th Internat. Ornithological Congress. Amer. Ornithol. Union **2**, 1059 (1963).

SECHENOV, I. M.: Refleksy golovnogo mozga. Popytka svesti sposob proiskhozhdeniya psikhicheskikh yavlenii na fiziologicheskie osnovy (Reflexes of the Brain. An Attempt to Reduce the Method of Origin of Psychic Phenomena to Physiological Bases). St. Petersburg: 1863—1865. Leningrad, Izd. Priboi 1926.

SECHENOV, I. M.: Fiziologiya nervnoi sistemy (Physiology of the Nervous System). St. Petersburg 1866.

SEEFELDER, R.: Beiträge zur Histogenese und Histologie der Netzhaut, des Pigmentepithels und der Sehnerven. Arch. Ophthal. **73**, 419 (1910).

SEKOGATI, Y.: On the ATPase activities in the retina and rod outer segments. J. cell. comp. Physiol. **56**, 129 (1960).

SELIGMAN, A. M., KARNOVSKY, M. J., WASSERKRUG, H. L., HAUKER, J. S.: Nondroplet ultrastructural demonstration of cytochrome oxidase activity with a polymerizing osmiophilic reagent, diamino-benzidine (DAB). J. Cell Biol. **38**, 1 (1968).

SERRA, J. A.: Why flagella and cilia have $1+9$ pairs of fibres. Exp. Cell Res. **20**, 395 (1960).

SEVERTSOV, A. N.: Glavnye napravleniya evolyutsionnogo protsessa. Morfobiologicheskaya teoriya evolyutsii (Main Directions of the Evolutionary Process. Morphobiological Theory of Evolution), 3rd Ed., Moscow: Izd. MGU 1967.

SHALLENBERGER, R. S.: Hydrogen bonding and the varying sweetness of the sugars. J. Food Sci. **28**, 584 (1963).

SHALLENBERGER, R. S.: Why do sugars taste sweet? New Sci. **23**, 569 (1964).

SHALLENBERGER, R. S., ACREE, T. E.: Molecular theory of sweet taste. Nature **216**, 480 (1967).

SHALLENBERGER, R. S., ACREE, T. E., GUILD, W. E.: Configuration, conformation and sweetness of hexose anomers. J. Food Sci. **30**, 560 (1965).

SHANNON, C.: Mathematical theory of linkage. In: Roboty po teorii informatsii i kibernetike (Works on the Theory of Information and Cybernetics) IL, p. 243. Moscow 1963.

SHANTHAVEERAPPA, T. R., BOURNE, G. H.: Monoamine oxidase distribution in the rabbit eye. J. Histochem. Cytochem. **12**, 281 (1964).

SHAPOT, V. S.: Interrelations between oxidation processes, combined phosphorylation and biosyntheses in the cell. Usp. sovrem. Biol. **37**, 255 (1954).

SHAW, S. R.: Polarized light responses from crab retinula cells. Nature **211**, 92 (1966).

SHAW, S. R.: Simultaneous recording from two cells in the locust retina. Z. vergl. Physiol. **55**, 183 (1967).

SHEN, S. C., GREENFIELD, P., BOELL, E. J.: Localization of acetylcholinesterase in chick retina during histogenesis. J. comp. Neurol. **106**, 433 (1956).

SHERRINGTON, C. S.: The central nervous system, Vol. **3**. In: A Text-Book of Physiology, 7th Ed. London: Macmillan 1897.

SHIBUYA, T.: Dissociation of olfactory neural response and mucosal potential. Science **143**, 1338 (1964).

SHIMIZU, N., MAEDA, S.: Histochemical studies on glycogen of the retina. Anat. Rec. **112**, 472 (1952).

SHIRO, N., KYOZO, K.: Fine structures of the organ of Corti in the newborn mouse. Nihon Univ. J. Med. **9**, 401 (1967).

SHMAL'GAUZEN, O. I.: Comparative experimental study of the early development stages of olfactory rudiments in amphibians. Dokl. Akad. Nauk SSSR **74**, 863 (1950).

SHVANVICH, V. N.: Kurs obshchei entomologii (General Entomology Course). Moscow—Leningrad: Izd. Sovetskaya nauka 1949.

SIDMAN, R. L.: The structure and concentration of solids in photoreceptor cells studied by refractometry and interference microscopy. J. biophys. biochem. Cytol. **3**, 15 (1957).

SIDMAN, R. L., WISLOCKI, C. B.: Histochemical observations on rods and cones in retinas of vertebrates. J. Histochem. Cytochem. **2**, 413 (1954).

SIEKEVITZ, P.: Biogenesis of membranes. In: Seventh Internat. Congr. of Biochem. Abstract **11**, 225 (1967).

SILLMAN, A. J., ITO, H., TOMITA, T.: Studies on the mass receptor potential of the isolated frog retina. I. General properties of the response. Vision Res. **9**, 1435 (1969a).

Sillman, A. J., Ito, H., Tomita, T.: Studies on the mass receptor potential of the isolated frog retina. II. On the bases of the ionic mechanism. Vision Res. **9**, 1443 (1969b).

Silvester, N. B., Holwill, M. E.: Molecular hypothesis of flagellar activity. Nature **205**, 665 (1965).

Simidzu, M.: Cellular physiology of taste. I. Cytochemical study of enzymes in the gustatory elements of the tongue epithelium. J. Physiol. Soc. Japan **19**, 254 (abstract) (1957).

Sirlin, G., Jacob, J., Kato, K.: The relation of messenger to nucleolar RNA. Exp. Cell Res. **24**, 355 (1962).

Sjöstrand, F. S.: The ultrastructure of the outer segments of rods and cones of the eye as revealed by the electron microscope. J. cell. comp. Physiol. **42**, 15 (1953a).

Sjöstrand, F. S.: The ultrastructure of the inner segments of the guinea-pig eye as revealed by electron microscope. J. cell. comp. Physiol. **42**, 45 (1953b).

Sjöstrand, F. S.: Ultrastructure of retinal rod synapses of the guinea pig eye as revealed by the three-dimensional reconstruction from serial sections. J. Ultrastruct. Res. **2**, 122 (1958).

Sjöstrand, F. S.: The ultrastructure of retinal photoreceptors of the vertebrate eye. Ergebn. Biol. **21**, 128 (1959a).

Sjöstrand, F. S.: Fine structure of cytoplasm: the organization of membranous layers. Rev. Mod. Physics **31**, 301 (1959b).

Sjöstrand, F. S.: Electron microscopy of the retina. In: The structure of the Eye, p. 1. New York: Acad. Press 1961.

Sjöstrand, F. S.: A new repeat structural element of mitochondrial and certain cytoplasmic membranes. Nature **199**, 1262 (1963).

Sjöstrand, F. S.: The structure of cellular membranes. Protoplasma (Wien) **63**, 248 (1967).

Sjöstrand, F. S., Barajas, L.: Effect of modifications in conformation of protein molecules on structure of mitochondrial membranes. J. Ultrastruct. Res. **25**, 121 (1968).

Sjöstrand, F. S., Elfvin, L. G.: The granular structure, demonstrated in frozen-dried tissue. J. Ultrastruct. Res. **10**, 263 (1964).

Skouby, A. P., Zilstorff-Pedersen, K.: The influence of acetylcholine, menthol and strychnine on taste receptors in man. Acta physiol. scand. **34**, 250 (1955).

von Skramlik, E.: The fundamental substrates of taste. In: Olfaction and taste, I, p. 125. Oxford: Pergamon Press 1963.

Slautterback, D. B.: Nematocyst development. In: The biology of *Hydra* and of some other Coelenterata (Eds. H. M. Lenhoff, W. F. Loomis), p. 77. Miami: Florida Univ. Press 1961.

Slautterback, D. B.: Cytoplasmic microtubules. I. *Hydra.* J. Cell Biol. **18**, 367 (1963).

Slautterback, D. B.: The cnidoblast-musculoepithelial cell complex in the tentacles of *Hydra.* Z. Zellforsch. **79**, 296 (1967).

Slautterback, D. B., Fawcett, D. W.: The development of the cnidoblasts of *Hydra.* J. biophys. biochem. Cytol. **5**, 441 (1959).

Slifer, E. H.: The fine structure of insect sense organs. Int. Rev. Cytol. **2**, 125 (1961).

Slifer, E. H., Prestage, J. H., Beams, H. W.: The chemoreceptors and other sense organs on the antennal flagellum of the grasshopper (Orthoptera, Acrididae). J. Morph. **105**, 154 (1959).

Slifer, E. H., Sekhon, S. S.: Fine structure of the sense organs on the antennal flagellum of the honey bee, *Apis mellifera* Linnaeus. J. Morph. **109**, 351 (1961).

Smirnov, G. D.: The ultrastructure of synapses and the problem of synaptic transmission. Usp. sovrem. Biol. **63**, 249 (1967).

Smith, C. A.: Capillary areas of the membranous labyrinth. Ann. Otol. (St. Louis) **63**, 435 (1954).

Smith, C. A.: Structure of the stria vascularis and the spiral prominence. Ann. Otol. (St. Louis) **66**, 521 (1957).

Smith, C. A.: Innervation pattern in the cochlea: the inner hair cell. Ann. Otol. (St. Louis) **70**, 504 (1961).

Smith, C. A.: Innervation of the cochlea. Rev. Panamer. Otorhinolaryng. Bronchosc. **1**, 77 (1967).

Smith, C. A.: Electron microscopy of the inner ear. Ann. Otol. (St. Louis) **77**, 629 (1968a).

Smith, C. A.: Structure and functions of inhibitory neuronal mechanisms. Oxford: Pergamon Press 1968b.

Smith, C. A., Rasmussen, G. L.: Recent observations on the olivocochlear bundle. Ann. Otol. (St. Louis) **72**, 489 (1963).

SMITH, C. A., RASMUSSEN, G. L.: Nerve endings in the maculae and cristae of the chinchilla vestibuli, with a special reference to the efferents. In: Third Symp. on the Role of the Vestibular Organs in Space Exploration, p. 183. Pensacola/U.S.A. 1967.

SMITH, C. A., SJÖSTRAND, F. S.: Structure of the nerve endings on the external hair cells of the guinea pig cochlea as studied by serial section. J. Ultrastruct. Res. **5**, 523 (1961).

SNODGRASS, R. E.: The morphology of insect sense organs and the sensory nervous system. Smiths. Misc. Coll. **77**, 1 (1926).

SNODGRASS, R. E.: Principles of Insect Morphology. New York: McGraw-Hill 1935.

DE SNOO, K.: Das trinkende Kind im Uterus. Z. Geburtsh. Gynäk. **105**, 88 (1937).

SNYAKIN, P. G.: Funktsional'naya mobil'nost' setchatki (Functional Mobility of the Retina). Moscow: Medgiz 1948.

SOTTOCASA, C. L., KUYLENSTIERNA, B., ERNSTER, L., BERGSTRAND, A.: An electron-transport system associated with outer membrane of liver mitochondria. J. Cell Biol. **32**, 415 (1967).

SPIRIN, A. S.: A model of a functioning ribosome—the joining and breaking of ribosome subparticles. Izv. Akad. Nauk SSSR **2**, 169 (1970).

SPOENDLIN, H.: Elektronenmikroskopische Untersuchungen am cortischen Organ des Meerschweinchens. Pract. Oto-rhino-laryng. (Basel) **19**, 192 (1957).

SPOENDLIN, H.: Submikroskopische Veränderung am cortischen Organ des Meerschweinchens nach akustischer Belastung. (Vorläuf. Mitt.). Pract. Oto-rhino-laryng. (Basel) **20**, 197 (1958).

SPOENDLIN, H.: Submikroskopische Organisation der Sinneselemente im cortischen Organ des Meerschweinchens. Pract. Oto-rhino-laryng. (Basel) **21**, 34 (1959).

SPOENDLIN, H.: Ultrastructural features of the organ of Corti in normal and acoustically stimulated animals. Ann. Otol. (St. Louis) **71**, 657 (1962).

SPOENDLIN, H.: Ultrastructural studies of the labyrinth in squirrel monkeys. In: Symposium on the Role of the Vestibular Organs in Space Exploration, p. 7. Washington: NASA 1965.

SPOENDLIN, H.: Ultrastructure of the vestibular sense organ. In: The Vestibular System and Its Diseases (Ed. R. J. Wolfson), p. 39. Philadelphia: University of Pennsylvania Press 1966.

SPOENDLIN, H., BALOGH, K., jr.: Histochemische Darstellung von Dehydrogenasen in der Schnecke lebender Tiere. Arch. Ohr.-, Nas.- u. Kehlk.-Heilk. **182**, 579 (1963a).

SPOENDLIN, H., BALOGH, K., jr.: Histochemical localization of dehydrogenase in the cochlea of living animals. Laryngoscope (St. Louis) **73**, 1061 (1963b).

SPOENDLIN, H., GAČEK, R.: Electron microscopic study of the efferent and afferent innervation of the organ of Corti in the cat. Ann. Otol. (St. Louis) **72**, 660 (1963).

STAEHELIN, L. A.: The interpretation of freeze-etched artificial and biological membranes. J. Ultrastruct. Res. **22**, 326 (1968).

STENSIÖ, E. A.: The Downtonian and Devonian Vertebrates of Spitzbergen. I. Family Cephalaspodoae. Oslo: Skrift of Svalbard 1927.

STEURER, O.: Beiträge zur pathologischen Anatomie und Pathogenese der Taubstummheit. Z. Hals-, Nas.- u. Ohrenheilk. **3**, 172 (1922).

STEVENS, B. J., SWIFT, H.: RNA-transport from nucleus to cytoplasm in *Chironomus* salivary glands. J. Cell Biol. **31**, 55 (1966).

STILES, W. S.: Colour vision: the approach through increment-threshold sensitivity. Proc. nat. Acad. Sci. (Wash.) **45**, 100 (1959).

STILES, W. S.: Foveal threshold sensitivity of fields of different colors. Science **145**, 1016 (1964).

STOCKHAMMER, K.: Zur Wahrnehmung der Schwingungsrichtung linear polarisierten Lichtes bei Insekten. Z. vergl. Physiol. **38**, 30 (1956).

STONE, L.: The development of lateral-line sense organs in Amphibians observed in living and vital stained preparations. J. comp. Neurol. **57**, 507 (1933).

STOSSBERG, M.: Die Zellvorgänge bei der Entwicklung der Flügelschuppen von *Ephestia kühniella*. Z. Morph. Ökol. Tiere **34**, 173 (1938).

VAN DER STRICHT, O.: The genesis and structure of the membrana tectoria and the crista spiralis of the cochlea. Publication 21. Contrib. Embryol. Carneg. Inst. **7**, 55 (1918).

VAN DER STRICHT, O.: Les membranes tectorielles des crîtes et des taches acoustiques. Arch. Biol. (Liege) **31**, 299 (1921).

SVANIDZE, I. K.: Cytophotometry of the retina under different eye illumination conditions. Tr. Inst. fiziologii AN Gruz. SSR **13**, 169 (1963).

SVIDERSKAYA, G. E.: Effect of sound on the locomotor activity of chick embryos. Byull. éksp. Biol. Med. **66**, 7 (1967).

SVIDERSKAYA, G. E., GRIGOR'EVA, G. I.: Change in the vital staining of embryonic tissues during the action of sound. Tsitologiya **11**, 1179 (1969).

SZENTÁGOTHAI, J.: The structure of the autonomic interneuronal synapse. Acta neuroveg. (Wien) 253 (1963).

SZENTÁGOTHAI, J. (with the participation of A. Gemeri, R. Shaba, I. Shasha, D. Sekel, Z. Oltvani): Rol' otdel'nykh labirintnykh retseptorov pri orientatsii glaz i golovy v prostranstve (Role of Individual Labyrinth Receptors During the Orientation of the Eyes and Head in Space). Leningrad: Izd. Nauka 1967.

TAKAGI, K., AKAO, M., TAKAHASHI, A.: Tritium-labelled acetylcholine receptor in the smooth muscle of the small intestine of the dog. Life Sci. **4**, 2165 (1865).

TAKAGI, M.: Studies on the ultraviolet-spectral displacements of cattle rhodopsin. Biochim. biophys. Acta (Amst.) **66**, 328 (1963).

TAKAGI, S. F., OMURA, K.: Microelectrode study on the electrical activity of the olfactory epithelium. J. Physiol. Soc. Japan **22**, 768 (1960).

TAKAGI, S. F., OMURA, K.: Responses of the olfactory receptor cells to odours. Proc. Jap. Acad. **39**, 253 (1963).

TAKAGI, S. F., SHIBUYA, T.: Electrical activity of lower olfactory nervous system of toad. In: Electrical Activity of Singe Cells, p. 1. Tokyo 1960a.

TAKAGI, S. F., SHIBUYA, T.: The "on" and "off" responses observed in the lower olfactory pathway. Japan. J. Physiol. **10**, 99 (1960b).

TAKAGI, S. F., WYSE, G., KITAMURA, H., ITO, K.: The roles of sodium and potassium ions in the generation of the electroolfactogramm. J. gen. Physiol. **51**, 552 (1968).

TAKAGI, S. F., YAJIMA, T.: Electrical activity and histological change in the degenerating olfactory epithelium. J. gen. Physiol. **48**, 559 (1965).

TAKAHASHI, K.: Study on the distribution of several chemical substances in membranous labyrinth of normal guinea pig. J. oto-rhino-laryng. Soc. Japan **64**, 266 (1961).

TAKASAKA, T., SMITH, C. A.: The structure and innervation of the pigeon's basilar papilla. J. Ultrastruct. Res. **35**, 20 (1971).

TASAKI, I.: Impulses in individual auditory nerve fibers of guinea pig. J. Neurophysiol. **16**, 97 (1957a).

TASAKI, I.: Hearing. Ann. Rev. Physiol. **19**, 417 (1957b).

TASAKI, I.: Afferent impulses in auditory nerve fibers and the mechanism of impulse initiation in the cochlea. In: Neural Mechanisms of Auditory and Vestibular Systems (Eds. G. L. Rasmussen, W. F. Windle), p. 40. Springfield/Ill.: Ch. C. Thomas 1960.

TASAKI, I., DAVIS, H., ELDREDGE, D. H.: Exploration of cochlear potentials in guinea pig with a microelectrode. J. acoust. Soc. Amer. **26**, 765 (1954).

TASAKI, I., FERNANDEZ, C.: Modification of cochlear microphonics and action potentials by KCl solution and by direct current. J. Neurophysiol. **15**, 497 (1952).

TASAKI, K., KARITA, K.: Intraretinal discrimination of horizontal and vertical planes of polarized light by Octopus. Nature **209**, 934 (1966).

TASAKI, K., NORTON, A. S., FUKUDA, Y.: Regional and directional differences in the lateral spread of retinal potentials in the octopus. Nature **198**, 1206 (1963).

TASAKI, K., OIKAWA, T., NORTON, A. S.: The dual nature of the octopus electroretinogramm. Vision Res. **3**, 61 (1963).

TASAKI, I., SPYROPOPOULOS, C. S.: Stria vascularis as source of endocochlear potential. J. Neurophysiol. **22**, 149 (1959).

TATEDA, H., BEIDLER, L. M.: The receptor potential of the taste cell of the rat. J. gen. Physiol. **47**, 479 (1964).

TAXI, J.: Etude au microscope électronique de synapses ganglionnaires chez quelques Vertébrés. In: Proc. IV. Internat. Congr. Neuropathol. (Ed. H. Jacob), Vol. **2**, p. 197. Stuttgart: Thieme 1962.

TERAYAMA, J., HOLZ, E., BECK, C.: Adrenergic innervation of the cochlea. Ann. Otol. (St. Louis) **75**, 69 (1966).

DE THE, G.: Ultrastructural cytochemistry of the cellular membranes. In: The Membranes, p. 121. New York: Academic Press 1968.

THOMPSON, H. W.: Some comments on theories of smell. In: Molecular Structure and Organoleptic Quality, p. 103. London 1957.

THURM, U.: On insect mechanoreceptor. I. Fine structure and adequate stimulus. Cold Spr. Harb. Symp. quant. Biol. **30**, 75 (1965a).

THURM, U.: On insect mechanoreceptor. II. Receptor potentials. Cold Spr. Harb. Symp. quant. Biol. **30**, 83 (1965b).

THUNEBERG, L., ROSTGAARD, J.: Motility of microvilli. A film demonstration. J. Ultrastruct. Res. **29**, 578 (1969).

TITOVA, L. K.: Razvitie retseptornykh struktur vnutrennego ukha pozvonochnykh (Development of Receptor Structures in the Inner Ear of Vertebrates). Leningrad: Izd. Nauka 1968.

TITOVA, L. K., ARONOVA, M. Z.: Cholinesterase in the lateral-line organs of bony fish (teleosts). Dokl. Akad. Nauk SSSR **155**, 974 (1964).

TITOVA, L. K., VINNIKOV, YA. A.: Comparative histochemical study of cholinesterases in receptor structures of the labyrinth of vertebrates. In the collection of works (Sbornik): Evolyutsiya funktsii (Evolution of Function), p. 249. Moscow—Leningrad: Izd. Nauka 1964.

TITOVA, L. K., GRIBAKIN, F. G.: Electron microscopic studies of the development of Corti's organ of the domestic hen. Arkh. Anat., Gistol. Embriol. **53**, 40 (1967).

TODD, R. B., BOWMAN, W.: The Physiological Anatomy and Physiology of Man, Vol. **2**, p. 1. London 1847.

TOKUJASU, K., YAMADA, E.: The fine structure of the retina studied with electron microscope. IV. Morphogenesis of outer segments of retinal rods. J. biophys. biochem. Cytol. **6**, 225 (1959).

TOMITA, T.: Electrophysiological study of the mechanisms subserving color coding in the fish retina. Cold Spr. Harb. Symp. quant. Biol. **30**, 559 (1965).

TOMITA, T., KANEKA, A., MURAKAMI, M., PAULTER, E. D.: Spectral response curves of single cones in the carp. Vision Res. **7**, 519 (1967).

TONNDORF, J., DUVALL, A. J., RENEAU, J. R.: Permeability of intracochlear membranes to various vital stains. Ann. Otol. (St. Louis) **71**, 801 (1962).

TORREY, T. W.: The relation of taste buds to their nerve fibres. Proc. nat. Acad. Sci. (Wash.) **17**, 591 (1931).

TORREY, T. W.: The relation of taste buds to their nerve fibres. J. comp. Neurol. **59**, 203 (1934).

TOYODA, J., NOSAKI, H., TOMITA, T.: Light-induced resistance changes in single photoreceptors of *Necturus* and *Gekko*. Vision Res. **9**, 455 (1969).

TRET'YAKOV, D. K.: Organy chuvstv rechnoi minogi (Sense Organs of the River Lamprey). Odessa 1916.

TRUJILLO-CENOZ, O.: Some aspects of the structural organization of the arthropod eye. Cold Spr. Harb. Symp. quant. Biol. **30**, 371 (1965).

TRUMEN, D. E. S., KORNER, A.: Incorporation of amino acids into the protein of isolated mitochondria. A search for optimum conditions and a relationship to oxidative phosphorylations. Biochem. J. **83**, 588 (1962).

TSCHACHOTIN, S.: Die Statocyste der Heteropoden. Z. wiss. Zool. **90**, 343 (1908).

TURPAEV, T. M.: Mediatornaya funktsiya atsetilkholina i priroda kholinoretseptora (The Mediator Function of Acetylcholine and the Nature of the Cholinoreceptor). Moscow: Izd. Akad. Nauk SSSR 1962.

TURPAEV, T. M.: Regulation of the mediator process by means of a biochemical feedback mechanism. In: Biokhimiya i funktsiya nervnoi sistemy (Biochemistry and Function of the Nervous System). Proceedings of International Symposium, 24—28 September 1965, p. 234. Leningrad: Izd. Nauka 1967.

UCHIZONO, K.: Characteristics of excitatory and inhibitory synapses in the central nervous system of the cat. Nature **207**, 642 (1965).

UCHIZONO, K.: Inhibitory synapses on the stretch receptor neuron of the crayfish. Nature **214**, 833 (1967).

UCHIZONO, K.: Inhibitory and excitatory synapses in vertebrate animals. In: Structure and Function of Inhibitory Neural Mechanisms (Ed. C. von Euler *et al.*), p. 33. Oxford: Pergamon Press 1968.

UENO, K.: Morphogenesis of the retinal cone studied with electron microscope. Jap. J. Ophthal. **5**, 114 (1961).

VON UEXKÜLL, J.: Die Schwimmbewegungen der *Rhizostoma pulmo*. Mitt. Zool. Sta. Neapel **14**, 620 (1901).

UGOLEV, A. M.: Fiziologiya i patologiya pristenochnogo (kontaktnogo) pishchevareniya (Physiology and Pathology of Parietal [Contact] Digestion). Leningrad: Izd. Nauka 1967.

ULEHLA, V.: Ultramikroskopische Studien über Geisselbewegung. Biol. Zbl. **31**, 654 (1911).

UNGAR, G.: Molecular organisation of neural information processing. In: Structure and Function of nervous tissue. IV. Acad. Press. **215** (1972).

UTINA, I. A., BYZOV, A. L.: Study of the functional properties of photoreceptors in the retina in the dark and under illumination with constant and blinking light. Biofizika **5**, 749 (1965).

VANDENHEUVEL, F. A.: Structural studies of biological membranes: the structure of myelin. Ann. N. Y. Acad. Sci. **122**, 57 (1965).

VAVILOV, S. I.: Mikrostruktura sveta (The Microstructure of Light). Moscow 1950.

VERNE, J.: La cytochemie des phosphatases alcalines chez les vertébrés. Ann. biol. **29**, 517 (1956).

VERWORN, M.: Psycho-physiologische Protisten-Studien. Experimentelle Untersuchungen. Jena: Fischer 1889.

VERWORN, M.: Studien zur Physiologie der Flimmerbewegung. Pflügers Arch. ges. Physiol. **48**, 149 (1891).

VERZHBINSKAYA, N. A.: Changes in the enzymic systems of the energic brain metabolism in vertebrate phylogenese. In: Biokhimia nervnoi sistemi, p. 193. Izd. Kiev 1954.

VETOKHIN, I. A.: The work of the ciliated epithelium of the gastrovascular system in the jellyfish *Aurelia aurita*. Works of the Murmansk Biological Station **2**, 107 (1926a).

VETOKHIN, I. A.: Processes of stimulation in the bell of the jellyfish *Aurelia aurita* and regulation of the movement of this animal in seawater. Russ. fiziol. Zh. **9**, 517 (1926b).

VILLEGAS, G. M.: Electron microscopic study of the vertebrate retina. J. gen. Physiol. **43**, Suppl. **2**, 15 (1960).

VILLEGAS, G. M.: Ultrastructure of the human retina. J. Anat. (Lond.) **98**, 501 (1964).

VILSTRUP, TH., JENSEN, C. E.: Three reports on the chemical composition of the fluids of the labyrinth. Ann. Otol. (St. Louis) **63**, 151 (1954).

VILSTRUP, TH., JENSEN, C. E.: On the displacement potential in acid mucopolysaccharides. Acta oto-laryng. (Stockh.) Suppl. **163**, 42 (1961).

DE VINCENTIS, M.: Sulla distribuzione e metabolismo degli acidi nucleinici nella retina, Congr. Soc. Oftal. Ital. Rom **38**, 11 (1949).

DE VINCENTIS, M.: Ulteriore contributo istochemico al metabolismo degli RNA della retine in condizioni di luce et di oscurita. Bull. Soc. ital. Biol. sper. **29**, 1 (1953).

VINNICHENKO, L. N.: Electron microscopic studies of the lamprey kidney. In the collection of works (Sbornik): Elektronnaya mikroskopiya kletok (Electron Microscopy of Animal Cells), p. 5. Moscow—Leningrad: Izd. Nauka 1967.

VINNIKOV, YA. A.: Experimental phylo-ontogenetic classification of receptors (sense organs) in vertebrates. Zh. obshch. biol. **7**, 345 (1946).

VINNIKOV, YA. A.: Setchatka glaza pozvonochnykh (The Retina of the Eye of Vertebrates). Moscow: Medgiz 1947.

VINNIKOV, YA. A.: On the structure of the olfactory organ. Arkh. Anat. Gistol. Embriol. **33**, 49 (1956a).

VINNIKOV, YA. A.: The olfactomotor reaction of receptor cells of the olfactory organ. Usp. sovrem. biol. **41**, 353 (1956b).

VINNIKOV, YA. A.: The problem of evolutionary cytochemistry and histochemistry. Tsitologiya **1**, 141 (1959a).

VINNIKOV, YA. A.: Problems of evolutionary morphology of analyzers. Arkh. Anat. Gistol. Embriol. **37**, 3 (1959b).

VINNIKOV, YA. A.: Mechanochemical and structural bases of the function of the receptors in sense organs. In the collection of works (Sbornik): Molekulyarnaya biologiya, problemy i perspektivy (Molecular Biology, Problems and Prospects), p. 304. Moscow: Izd. Nauka 1964.

VINNIKOV, YA. A.: Structural and cytochemical organization of receptor cells of sense organs in the light of the evolution of their functions. Zh. evolyuts. biokhim. fiziol. **1**, 67 (1965a).

VINNIKOV, YA. A.: Characteristic features of the cellular and subcellular organization of sense organs in the light of problems concerned with bionics. In the collection of works (Sbornik): Bionika (Bionics), p. 91. Moscow: Izd. Nauka 1965b.

VINNIKOV, YA. A.: Structural and cytochemical bases of the mechanism of the function of sense organ receptors. In the collection of works (Sbornik): Nervnaya kletka (Nerve Cell), p. 7. Leningrad: Izd. LGU 1966a.

VINNIKOV, YA. A.: On some general structural and cytochemical mechanisms of the function of sense organ receptors. In the collection of works (Sbornik): Pervichnye protsessy v retseptornykh elementakh organov chuvstv (Primary processes in the receptor elements of sense organs), p. 189. Moscow—Leningrad: Izd. Nauka 1966b.

VINNIKOV, YA. A.: Principles of structural, chemical and functional organization of sensory receptors. Cold Spr. Harb. Symp. quant. Biol. **30**, 293 (1966c).

VINNIKOV, YA. A.: The development and growth of cell membranes. Zh. evolyuts. biokhim. fiziol. **2**, 175 (1966d).

VINNIKOV, YA. A.: Some structural and cytochemical characteristics of synaptic transmission associated with the function of mitochondria. In the collection of works (Sbornik): Biokhimiya i funktsiya nervnoi sistemy (Biochemistry and Function of the Nervous System). Proceedings of International Symposium 1965, p. 8. Leningrad: Izd. Nauka 1967a.

VINNIKOV, YA. A.: The problem of the modelling of a universal sensory pickup unit. In the collection of works (Sbornik): Voprosy bioniki (Problems of Bionics), p. 19. Moscow: Izd. Nauka 1967b.

VINNIKOV, YA. A.: De certaines particularités structurales et cytochimiques de la transmission synaptique en rapport à la fonction des mitochondries. Ann. Histochim. **12**, 97 (1967c).

VINNIKOV, YA. A.: Some regularities in cellular and subcellular evolution of structure, chemistry and function of sense organs. Progr. Brain Res. **22**, 518 (1968).

VINNIKOV, YA. A.: The ultrastructural and cytochemical bases of the mechanism of function of the sense organ receptors. In: The Structure and Function of Nervous Tissue (G. H. Bourne, Ed.), p. 265. New York: Academic Press 1969.

VINNIKOV, YA. A.: Cellular and molecular bases of the evolution of the sense organs. J. Evolut. Biochem. Physiol. **6**, 483 (1970a).

VINNIKOV, YA. A.: The evolution of the structural, cytochemical and functional organization in the sense organs. Arck. Anat. Gistol. Embriol. **58**, 21 (1970b).

VINNIKOV, YA. A., GAZENKO, O. G., BRONSHTEIN, A. A., TSIRULIS, T. P., IVANOV, V. P., PYATKINA, G. A.: Structural, cytochemical and functional organization of statocysts of Cephalopoda. In: Symposium on Neurobiology of Invertebrates, p. 29. Budapest: Akad. Kiado 1967.

VINNIKOV, YA. A., GAZENKO, O. G., BRONSHTEIN, A. A., TSIRULIS, T. P., IVANOV, V. P., PYATKINA, G. A.: Cytochemical and electron microscopic study of the statocysts of cephalopod molluscs. Zh. evoluts. biokhim. fiziol. **4**, 10 (1968).

VINNIKOV, YA. A., GAZENKO, O. G., TITOVA, L. K., BRONSHTEIN, A. A.: Morphological and histochemical study of the labyrinth of animals under altered gravitational field conditions. I. The utricle. Izv. Akad. Nauk SSSR, ser. biol. **2**, 222 (1963a).

VINNIKOV, YA. A., GAZENKO, O. G., TITOVA, L. K., OSIPOVA, I. V., BRONSHTEIN, A. A.: Histochemical and ultrastructural changes of the receptor cells on the utricle under altered gravitational field conditions. Dokl. Akad. Nauk SSSR **153**, 450 (1963b).

VINNIKOV, YA. A., GAZENKO, O. G., TITOVA, L. K., BRONSHTEIN, A. A., OSIPOVA, I. V., GOVARDOVSKII, V. I., ARONOVA, M. Z., ZHINKIN, I. L.: Electron microscopic and histochemical studies of the utricle of some vertebrates under relative rest conditions and after the action of accelerations. In the collection of works (Sbornik): Funktsionalnaya evolyutsiya nervnoi sistemy (Functional Evolution of the Nervous System), p. 170. Moscow—Leningrad: Izd. Nauka 1965.

VINNIKOV, YA. A., GAZENKO, O. G., TITOVA, L. K., BRONSHTEIN, A. A., PEVZNER, R. A., ARONOVA, M. Z., VASILYEV, P. V.: Electron microscopic study of mitochondria in the synapse region of the utricle of the inner ear of vertebrates. Dokl. Akad. Nauk SSSR **166**, 1447 (1966).

VINNIKOV, YA. A., GAZENKO, O. G., TITOVA, L. K., BRONSHTEIN, A. A., TSIRULIS, T. P., PEVZNER, R. A., GOVARDOVSKII, V. I., GRIBAKIN, F. G., IVANOV, V. P., ARONOVA, M. Z., CHEKHONADSKII, N. A.: Retseptor gravitatsii. Evolyutsiya strukturnoi, tsitokhimicheskoi i funktsionalnoi organizatsii. V serii "Problemy Kosmicheskoi Biologii" t. 12. (Receptor of Gravity. Cytochemical and Functional Organization. In: The Problems of Cosmic Biology, vol. 12). Leningrad: Izd. Nauka 1971.

VINNIKOV, YA. A., GOVARDOVSKII, V. I., OSIPOVA, I. V.: The structural organization of the gravitation organ (utricle) in the pigeon. Biofizika **10**, 641 (1965a).

VINNIKOV, YA. A., GOVARDOVSKII, V. I., OSIPOVA, I. V.: Electron microscopic study of the gravitation organ (utricle) in the pike *(Esox lucius)*. Biofizika **10**, 1003 (1965b).

VINNIKOV, YA. A., GOVYRIN, V. A., LEONTEVA, G. P., ANICHIN, V. F.: The adrenergic innervation of the organ of Corti. Dokl. Akad. Nauk SSSR **171**, 484 (1966).

VINNIKOV, YA. A., KOICHEV, K.: Sodium localization in the spiral organ during relative quiet and after exposure to sound. Nature **233**, 641 (1969).

VINNIKOV, YA. A., OSIPOVA, I. V., TITOVA, L. K., GOVARDOVSKII, V. I.: Electron microscopic study of the organ of Corti of birds. Zh. obshch. biol. **26**, 138 (1965).

VINNIKOV, YA. A., SOKOLOVA, M. M.: Sorption of a vital dye by hair cells of the organ of Corti of the guinea pig under relative rest conditions and after exposure to sound. Dokl. Akad. Nauk SSSR **116**, 892 (1961).

VINNIKOV, YA. A., TITOVA, L. K.: Histophysiological characteristics of the olfactory receptor. Dokl. Akad. Nauk SSSR **65**, 903 (1949).

VINNIKOV, YA. A., TITOVA, L. K.: Morfologiya organa obonyaniya (Morphology of the Olfactory Organ). Moscow: Medgiz 1957a.

VINNIKOV, YA. A., TITOVA, L. K.: Presence and distribution of glycogen in the organ of Corti during relative rest and sound exposure. Dokl. Akad. Nauk SSSR **116**, 892 (1957b).

VINNIKOV, YA. A., TITOVA, L. K.: Presence and distribution of acid phosphatase in the organ of Corti of animals under relative rest conditions and after exposure to sound. Byull. éksp. Biol. Med. **10**, 60 (1957c).

VINNIKOV, YA. A., TITOVA, L. K.: Presence and distribution of alkaline phosphatase in the organ of Corti of animals under relative rest conditions and after exposure to sound. Byull. éksp. Biol. Med. **3**, 101 (1958a).

VINNIKOV, YA. A., TITOVA, L. K.: Presence and distribution of a specific acetylcholinesterase in the organ of Corti of animals under relative rest conditions and after exposure to sound. Dokl. Akad. Nauk SSSR **149**, 164 (1958b).

VINNIKOV, YA. A., TITOVA, L. K.: Distribution of nucleic acids in hair cells of the organ of Corti of animals under relative rest conditions and after exposure to sound. Byull. éksp. Biol. Med. **4**, 73 (1958c).

VINNIKOV, YA. A., TITOVA, L. K.: Presence and distribution of succindehydrase and cytochromoxidase in the organ of Corti of animals under relative rest conditions and after exposure to sound. Dokl. Akad. Nauk SSSR **122**, 921 (1958d).

VINNIKOV, YA. A., TITOVA, L. K.: Method of intra-vital isolation of the membranous labyrinth (of the cochlea and vestibule), preparation and description of plane preparations of the organ of Corti. Arkh. Anat., Gistol. Embriol. **36**, 82 (1959).

VINNIKOV, YA. A., TITOVA, L. K.: Kortiev organ. Gistophisiologya i gistokhimiya (The Organ of Corti. Histophysiology and Histochemistry). Moscow—Leningrad: Izd. Akad. Nauk SSSR 1961.

VINNIKOV, YA. A., TITOVA, L. K.: Activity of dehydrogenases in mitochondria of nerve endings in the synapse region of the inner ear of vertebrates. Dokl. Akad. Nauk SSSR **142**, 484 (1962a).

VINNIKOV, YA. A., TITOVA, L. K.: Cytophysiological and cytochemical studies of the hair cells of the organ of Corti (cytochemical theory of hearing). Usp. sovrem. Biol. **53**, 105 (1962b).

VINNIKOV, YA. A., TITOVA, L. K.: Histochemische Untersuchungen des cortischen Organs. Z. mikr.-anat. Forsch. **69**, 42 (1962c).

VINNIKOV, YA. A., TITOVA, L. K.: Cytophysiology and cytochemistry of the organ of Corti: a cytochemical theory of hearing. Int. Rev. Cytol. **14**, 157 (1963).

VINNIKOV, YA. A., TITOVA, L. K.: The Organ of Corti. Its Histophysiology and Histochemistry. New York: Consultants Bureau 1964.

VINNIKOV, YA. A., TITOVA, L. K., ARONOVA, M. Z.: Vergleichende histochemische Untersuchung der Cholinesterasen in den rezeptorischen Strukturen des Labyrinths und in den Organen der Seitenlinie bei den Wirbeltieren. Acta histochem. (Jena) **22**, 120 (1965).

VON VINTSCHGAU, M.: Beobachtungen über Veränderungen der Schmeckbecher nach Durchschneidung des Nervus Glosso-pharyngeus. Pflügers Arch. ges. Physiol. **23**, 1 (1880).

VOGEL, R.: Über ein tympanales Sinnesorgan, das mutmassliche Hörorgan der Singzikade. Z. Anat. Entwickl.-Gesch. **67**, 190 (1923).

VOLKENSHTEIN, M. V.: Molekuly i zhizn. Vvedenie v molekulyarnuyn biofiziku (Molecules and Life. Introduction to Molecular Biophysics). Moscow: Izd. Nauka 1965.

VOSTEEN, K. H.: Darstellung der Bernsteinsäuredehydrogenase in der Schnecke des Meerschweinchens. Arch. Ohr.-, Nas.- u. Kehlk.-Heilk. **168**, 295 (1956).

VOSTEEN, K. H.: Die Lokalisation verschiedener Atmungsfermente in der Schnecke. Arch. Ohr.-, Nas.- u. Kehlk.-Heilk. **171**, 369 (1958).

VOSTEEN, K. H.: Elektronenmikroskopische Untersuchungen über die Verteilung von Glycogen im Ductus cochlearis bei Meerschweinchen. Pract. oto-rhino-laryng. (Basel) **26**, 400 (1964).

VOYNO-YASENETSKII, A. V.: Materials from a study of the motor function in ontogenesis. In: Funktsionalnaya evolyutsiya nervnoi sistemy (Functional Evolution of the Nervous System), p. 92. Moscow—Leningrad: Izd. Nauka 1965.

DE VRIES, H., KUIPER, W.: Optics of the insect eye. Ann. N. Y. Acad. Sci. **74**, 195 (1958).

DE VRIES, H., SPOOR, A., JIELOF, R.: Properties of the eye with respect to light. Physica **19**, 419 (1953).

DE VRIES, H., STUIVER, M.: The absolute sensitivity of the human sense of smell. In: Sensory Communication (Ed. W. A. Rosenblitz), p. 159. Cambridge/Mass.: M.I.T. Press 1961.

WADDINGTON, C.: Morfogenez i kletka (Morphogenesis and the Cell). Moscow: Izd. Mir 1964.

WADDINGTON, C. H., PERRY, M. M.: The ultrastructure of the developing eye of Drosophila. Proc. Roy. Soc. B **133**, 155 (1960).

WALD, G.: Vitamin A and vision. Collect. Net. **14**, 1 (1939).

WALD, G.: The distribution and evolution of visual system. In: Comparative Biochemistry (Eds. M. Florkin, H. S. Mason), Vol. **1**, p. 311. New York: Academic Press 1960.

WALD, G.: General discussion of retinal structure in relation to the visual process. In: The structure of the eye, p. 101. New York: Academic Press 1961a.

WALD, G.: The molecular organization of visual systems. In: Light and Life (Eds. W. D. McElroy, B. Glass), p. 724. Baltimore: Johns Hopkins Univ. Press 1961b.

WALD, G.: The receptors of human color vision. Science **145**, 1007 (1964).

WALD, G.: Visual excitation and blood clotting. Science **150**, 1028 (1965).

WALD, G.: A molecular basis of visual excitation. Nature **219**, 800 (1968).

WALD, G., BROWN, P. K.: The molar extinction of rhodopsin. J. gen. Physiol. **37**, 189 (1953).

WALD, G., BROWN, P. K., GIBBONS, J. R.: Visual excitation: a chemoanatomical study. Symp. Soc. exp. Biol. **16**, 32 (1962).

WALD, G., BROWN, P. K., GIBBONS, J. R.: The problem of visual excitation. J. Opt. Soc. Amer. **53**, 20 (1963).

WALD, G., BROWN, P. K., SMITH, P. H.: Iodopsin. J. gen. Physiol. **38**, 623 (1954—1955).

WALD, G., HUBBARD, R.: The reduction of retinene to vitamin $A_1$ in vitro. J. gen. Physiol. **32**, 367 (1949).

WALLACH, D. E. H.: Membrane lipids and the conformations of membrane proteins. J. gen. Physiol. **54**, 3 (1969).

WALTMAN, B.: Electrical properties and fine structure of the ampullary canals of Lorenzini. Acta physiol. scand. **66**, Suppl. 264, 3 (1966).

WASSER, P. G.: Curare and cholinergic receptor in the motor endplate. In: Curare and Curare-like agents (Ed. D. Bovel et al.), p. 219. Amsterdam: Elsevier 1959.

WEALE, R. A.: Photo-sensitive reactions in fovea of normal and cone-monochromatic observers. Optica acta **6**, 158 (1959).

WEBER, E. G.: Die Lehre von Tastsinn und Gemeingefühl. Braunschweig 1851.

WECKER, H., FISCHER, F.: Über den Azetilcholinesterasegehalt der subretinalen Flüssigkeit bei ruprurellen Netzhautablösungen. Ophthalmologica (Basel) **96**, 348 (1939).

WEIBEL, E. R.: Zur Kenntnis der Differenzierungsvorgänge im Epithel des Ductus cochlearis. Acta anat. (Basel) **29**, 53 (1957).

WEIER, T., BISALPUTRA, T., HARRISON, A.: Subunits in chloroplast membranes of Scenedesmus quadricauda. J. Ultrastruct. Res. **15**, 38 (1966).

WEISSBLUTH, M.: The physics of hemoglobin. In: Structura i svyaz (Structure and Communication), p. 11. Moscow: Izd. Mir 1969.

WERSÄLL, J.: Studies on the structure and innervation of the sensory epithelium of the cristae ampullares in the guinea pig. Acta oto-laryng. (Stockh.), Suppl. **126**, 1 (1956).

WERSÄLL, J.: Vestibular receptor cells in fish and mammals. Acta oto-laryng. (Stockh.), Suppl. **163**, 25 (1961).

WERSÄLL, J., FLOCK, A.: Physiological aspects of the structure of vestibular end organs. Internat. vestib. Symp. Uppsala. Acta oto-laryng. (Stockh.), Suppl. **192**, 85 (1963).

WERSÄLL, J., FLOCK, A., LUNDQUIST, P. G.: Structural basis for directional sensitivity in cochlear and vestibular sensory receptors. Cold Spr. Harb. Symp. quant. Biol. **30**, 115 (1965).

WERSÄLL, J., HILDING, K., LUNDQUIST, P. G.: Ultrastruktur und Innervation der cochlearen Haarzellen. Arch. Ohr.-, Nas.- u. Kehlk.-Heilk. **178**, 106 (1961).

WEVER, E. G., VERNON, J. A.: The auditory sensitivity of Orthoptera. Proc. nat. Acad. Sci. (Wash.) **45**, 413 (1959).

WHALEY, W. G., KERHART, J. E., MOLLENHAUER, H. H.: The dynamics of cytoplasmic membranes during development. In: Cellular Membranes in Development (Ed. M. Locke), p. 135. New York: Academic Press 1964.

WHITTAKER, V. P.: The application of subcellular fractionation techniques to the study of brain function. Progr. Biophys. Molec. Biol. **15**, 39 (1965).

WHITTAKER, V. P.: Isolation of nerve endings and synaptic vesicles from the central nervous system. In: Biokhimiya i funktsiya nervnoi sistemy (Biochemistry and Function of the Nervous System). Proceedings of International Symposium, 24—28 September 1965. Leningrad: Izd. Nauka 1967.

WHITTAKER, V. P., GRAY, F. G.: The synapse: biology and morphology. Brit. med. Bull. **18**, 223 (1962).

WIEBERG, K. B.: Physical Organic Chemistry. New York: John Wiley 1964.

WILLIAMS, J., PORSONS, D.: Density-gradient centrifugation of sonical mitochondria fragments. In: VI. Internat. Congr. Biochem. Abstr. **8**, 670 (1964).

WINDLE, W. F.: Physiology of the Fetus. Origin and Extent of Function in Prenatal Life, p. 188. Philadelphia and London: Saunders 1940.

WINTER, M., GAUTSCHI, F.: Odour and constitution. XX. Synthesis of cis- and trans-3-Hexenal. Helv. chim. acta **45** (7), 2567 (1962).

WISLOCKI, G. B., LADMAN, A. J.: Selective staining of the otholitic membranes, cupulae and tectorial membrane of the inner ear. Anat. Rec. **118**, 416 (1954).

WISLOCKI, G. B., SIDMAN, R.: The chemical morphology of the retina. J. comp. Neurol. **101**, 53 (1954).

WITTMAACK, K.: Über Bau und Funktion der Membrana tectoria. Acta oto-laryng. (Stockh.) **24**, 397 (1936).

WOLBARSHT, M. L.: Receptor sites in insect chemoreceptors. Cold Spr. Harb. Symp. quant. Biol. **30**, 281 (1965).

WOLBARSHT, M. L., DETHIER, V. G.: Electrical activity in the chemoreceptors of the blowfly. I. Responses to chemical and mechanical stimulation. J. gen. Physiol. **42**, 393 (1958).

WOLFF, H. G.: Einige Ergebnisse zur Ultrastruktur der Statocysten von Limax maximus, Limax flavus und Arion empiricorum (Pulmonata). Z. Zellforsch. **100**, 251 (1969).

WOLFF, H. G.: Efferente Aktivität in den Statonerven einiger Landpulmonaten (Gastropoda). Z. vergl. Physiol. **70**, 401 (1970).

WOLFF, H. G.: Statocysten-Funktion bei einigen Landpulmonaten (Gastropoda). Z. vergl. Physiol. **69**, 326 (1970b).

WOLKEN, J. J.: A molecular morphology of Euglena gracilis var. bicillaris. J. Protozool. **3**, 211 (1956).

WOLKEN, J. J.: Retinal structure. Mollusc Cephalopods: Octopus, Sepia. J. biophys. biochem. Cytol. **4**, 835 (1958).

WOLKEN, J. J.: A structural model for a retinal rod. In: The Structure of the Eye, p. 173. New York: Academic Press 1961.

WOLKEN, J. J.: An eye pigment of the cockroach. Exp. Eye Res. **2**, 182 (1962).

WOLKEN, J. J.: Structure and molecular organization of retinal photoreceptors. J. Opt. Soc. Amer. **53**, 1 (1964).

WOLKEN, J. J.: Lipids and the molecular structure of photoreceptors. J. Amer. Oil Chemistry **43**, 271 (1966).

WOLKEN, J. J., BOWNESS, J. M., SCHEER, J. J.: The visual complex of the insect: retinene in the housefly. Biochim. biophys. Acta (Amst.) **43**, 531 (1960).

WOLKEN, J. J., CAPENOS, J., TURANO, A.: Photoreceptor structures. 3. Drosophila melanogaster. J. biophys. biochem. Cytol. **3**, 441 (1957).

WOLKEN, J. J., GUPTA, P. D.: Photoreceptor structures. The retinal cells of the cockroach eye. J. biophys. biochem. Cytol. **9**, 720 (1961).

WOLKEN, J. J., MELLON, A. D., CONTIS, G.: Photoreceptor structures. J. Exp. Zool. **134**, 383 (1957).

WOLKEN, J. J., SCHEER, J. H.: An eye pigment of the cockroach. Exp. Eye Res. **2**, 182 (1963).

WRIGHT, M. R.: Maintenance of denervated taste organ in adult Triturus viridescens. Proc. Soc. exp. Biol. **76**, 463 (1951).

WRIGHT, M. R.: Persistence of taste organs in tongue grafted to liver. Proc. Soc. exp. Biol. (N. Y.) **97**, 367 (1958).

WRIGHT, M. R.: Taste organs in tongue-to-liver grafts in the newt Triturus viridescens. J. exp. Zool. **156**, 377 (1964).

WRIGHT, R. H.: The Science of Smell. London: Allen & Unwin 1964.

WRIGHT, R. H.: Nauka o zapakhakh (The Science of Smell). Moscow: Izd. Mir 1966.

WRIGHT, R. H., HUGHES, I. R., HENDRIX, D. E.: Olfactory Coding. Nature 216, 404 (1967).

WÜSTENFELD, E., SPRENGER, E. H.: Variationstatistische Untersuchungen an den Sinneszellkernen des cortischen Organs von Meerschweinchen. Z. Zellforsch. 48, 728 (1958).

YAKOVLEV, V. A., TITOVA, L. K., BRONSHTEIN, A. A., VINNIKOV, YA. A.: Localization and cytochemical characteristics of proteins in hair cells of Corti's organ in a state of relative rest and under the effect of sound. Dokl. Akad. Nauk SSSR 136, 459 (1961).

YAMADA, E.: The fine structure of the paraboloid of the retina as revealed by electron microscopy. Anat. Rec. 136, 352 (1960).

YAMADA, E., ISHIKAVA, T.: Fine structure of the horizontal cells in some vertebrate retinae. Cold Spr. Harb. Symp. quant. Biol. 30, 383 (1965).

YAMADA, K.: Gustatory and thermal responses in the glossopharyngeal nerve of the rabbit and cat. J. Japan. Physiol. 17, 94 (1967).

YAMAMOTO, T., TASAKI, K., SUGAWARA, Y., TONOSAKI, A.: Fine structure of the octopus retina. J. Cell Biol. 25, 345 (1965).

YASUSUMI, G., DEGUCHI, N.: Submicroscopic structure of the compound eye as revealed by electron microscopy. J. Ultrastruct. Res. 1, 259 (1958).

YOSHIZAWA, T., WALD, G.: Pre-lumirhodopsin and the bleaching of visual pigments. Nature 197, 1279 (1963).

YOUNG, J. Z.: The statocysts of Octopus vulgaris. Proc. roy. Soc. B 152, 3 (1960).

YOUNG, J. Z.: A Model of the Brain. Oxford: Clarendon Press 1964.

YOUNG, R. W.: Passage of newly formed protein through the connecting cilium of retinal rods in the frog. J. Ultrastruct. Res. 23, 462 (1968).

YOUNG, R. W.: An hypothesis to account for a basic distinction between rods and cones. Vision Res. 11, 1 (1971).

YOUNG, R. W., DROZ, B.: The renewal of protein in retinal rods and cones. J. Cell Biol. 39, 169 (1968).

YOUNG, TH.: The Bakerian lecture. On the theory of light and colors. Phil. Trans. roy. Soc. 92, 12 (1802).

YUR'EVA, G. YU.: On the role of reactive groups of protein complexes in the stimulation of a gustatory receptor. Biofizika 11, 665 (1957).

YUR'EVA, G. YU.: Concerning the problem of the enzymochemical basis of gustatory sensitivity. Author's abstract of dissertation, Moscow 1960a.

YUR'EVA, G. YU.: Concerning the problem of the role of reactive protein groups in gustatory reception. Fiziol. Zh. SSSR 46, 1071 (1960b).

ZAGORUL'KO, T. M.: On consecutive images in the visual system. Usp. sovrem. Biol. 25, 231 (1948).

ZALEWSKI, A. A.: Changes in phosphatase enzymes following denervation of the vallate papilla of the rat. Exp. Neurol. 22, 40 (1968).

ZALEWSKI, A. A.: Role of nerve and epithelium in the regulation of alkaline phosphatase activity in gustatory papillae. Exp. Neurol. 23, 18 (1969).

ZAVARZIN, A. A.: Histologische Studien über Insekten. III. Über das sensible Nervensystem der Larven von Meldortha vulgaris. Z. wiss. Zool. 100, 447 (1912).

ZAVARZIN, A. A.: Gistologicheshkoe issledovanie chuvstvitel'noi sistemy opticheskikh gangliev naseko-mykh (Histological Study of the Sensory System of Optical Ganglions of Insects). St. Petersburg 1913.

ZAVARZIN, A. A.: Ocherki po evolyutsionnoi gistologii nervnoi sistemy (Outlines on the Evolutionary Histology of the Nervous System). Moscow—Leningrad: Medgiz 1941.

ZBARSKII, I. B.: Structure and function of the nuclear membrane, Usp. sovrem. Biol. 67, 323 (1969).

ZONANA, H. V.: Fine structure of the squid retina. Bull. Johns Hopk. Hosp. 109, 185 (1961).

ZORZOLI, G., BORIANI, A.: Recherches histochimiques sur les cellules ciliées de l'organe de Corti soumises à des stimulations acoustiques. Rev. Laryng. (Bordeaux) 79, 213 (1958).

ZOTTERMAN, Y.: The neural mechanism of taste. In: Progress Brain Res. 23, 139 (1967).

ŽUPANČIČ, A. O.: The mode of action of acetylcholine. A theory extended to a hypothesis on the mode of action of other biologically active substances. Acta physiol. scand. 29, 63 (1953).

# Addendum

BROWN, P. K.: Rhodopsin rotates in the visual receptor membrane. Nature New Biol. **236**, 35 (1972).

BUDELMANN, B.-U., BARBER, V. G., WEST, S.: Scaning electron-microscopical studies of the arrangements and numbers of hair cells in the statocysts of Octopus vulgaris, Sepia officinalis and Loligo vulgaris. Brain Res. **56**, 25 (1973).

BUDELMANN, B.-U., WOLF, H. G.: Gravity response from angular acceleration receptors in Octopus vulgaris. J. comp. Physiol. **85**, 283 (1973).

CONE, R. A.: Rotational diffusion of rhodopsin in the visual pigment membrane. Natur New Biol. **236**, 39 (1972).

DAEMEN, F. J. M., DE GRIP, W. J., JANSEN, P. A. A.: Biochemical aspects of the visual process, XX. The molecular weight of rhodopsin. Biochim. biophys. Acta **271**, 419 (1972).

DRATZ, E. A., GAW, J. A., SCHWARTZ, S., CHING, WEI-MEI: Molecular organization of photoreceptor membranes of rod outer segments. Nature New Biol. **237**, 99 (1972).

FLOCK, A., LAM, D. M. K.: Neurotransmitter synthesis in inner ear and lateral line sense organs. Nature **299**, 142 (1974).

GERNANDT, B. E.: Vestibular mechanisms. In: Handbook of Physiology sec. I. Neurophysiology, vol. I (Eds. J. Field, H. Magoun, V. E. Hall). American Physiological Society, Washington 1959).

GOVARDOVSKII, V. I.: Some properties and the dinamic of endolymph fluid of the statocysts in Cephalopods. Zh. evoluts. biokh. fisiol. **7**, 410 (1971 b).

GRIBAKIN, F. G.: Perception of polarized lite in insects by filter mechanisme. Nature **246**, 357 (1973).

GRIBAKIN, F. G.: Functional morphology of the compound eye of the honey bee. In: The Compound Eye and Vision of Insect. (Ed. Horridge, G. A.) Clarendon Press, Oxford (1974).

LOWENSTEIN, O.: Physiology of the vestibular receptors. In: Progress in Brain Research (Eds. A. Brodal, O. Pompeiano), p. 19. Elsevier Publishing Company. Amsterdam (1972).

RAWELINS, F. A.: A time sequence autoradiographic study of the in vitro incorporation of ($I,2-H^3$) cholesterol into peripheral nerves myelin. Cell Biology. **58**, 42 (1973).

ROSENTAL, J. M., NORRIS, D. M.: Chemosensory mechanism in american Cockroach olfaction and gustation. Nature **224**, 370 (1973).

TITOVA, L. K., ARONOVA, M. Z., TSIRULIS, T. P., KHARKEEVICH, T. A.: Electronmicroscopic and cytochemical study of the gravity receptor of invertebrates. In the collection of works: Mekhanizmy raboty retseptornykh elementov organov chuvstv. (Mechanisms of action of the receptor elements of sensory organs). p. 162. Leningrad: Izd. Nauka (1973).

VINNIKOV, YA. A.: Evolution of the gravity receptor. Minerva otorinolaringologica **24**, 1 (1974).

# Subject Index